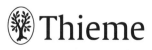

Burgerstein's Handbook of Nutrition

Micronutrients in the
Prevention and Therapy
of Disease

Michael Zimmermann, M.D.
Senior Scientist
Director of Postgraduate Studies
The Laboratory for Human Nutrition
Swiss Federal Institute of Technology
Zürich, Switzerland

88 illustrations
164 tables

Thieme
Stuttgart · New York

Library of Congress Cataloging-in-Publication Data is available from the publisher

9th German edition published 2000 by Karl F. Haug Verlag, Hüthig Medizin-Verlage GmbH & Co. KG, Heidelberg.

Titel of the German edition: Burgerstein's Handbuch Nährstoffe: Vorbeugen und heilen durch ausgewogene Ernährung

Important Note: Medicine is an everchanging science undergoing continual development. Research and clinical experience are continually expanding our knowledge, in particular our knowledge of proper treatment and drug therapy. Insofar as this book mentions any dosage or application, readers may rest assured that the authors, editors, and publishers have made every effort to ensure that such references are in accordance with the state of knowledge at the time of production of the book.
Nevertheless, this does not involve, imply, or express any guarantee or responsibility on the part of the publishers in respect to any dosage instructions and forms of application stated in the book. Every user is requested to examine carefully the manufacturer's leaflets accompanying each drug and to check, if necessary in consultation with a physician or specialist, whether the dosage schedules mentioned therein or the contraindications stated by the manufacturers differ from the statements made in the present book. Such examination is particularly important with drugs that are either rarely used or have been newly released on the market. Every dosage schedule or every form of application used is entirely at the user's own risk and responsibility. The authors and publishers request every user to report to the publishers any discrepancies or inaccuracies noticed.

© 2001 Georg Thieme Verlag.
Rüdigerstrasse 14,
D-70469 Stuttgart, Germany
Thieme New York, 333 Seventh Avenue.
New York, NY 10001, USA

Typesetting and printing by Gulde Druck, Tübingen

Printed in Germany.

ISBN 3-13-127951-6 (GTV)
ISBN 1-58890-062-2 (TNY)   1 2 3 4 5

Preface

As a medical doctor focusing on metabolism and nutrition, colleagues ask me where they can find reliable information on vitamins and minerals and their application in medicine. Although an abundance of material is available, most is of two types: on the one side, skeptical and stubbornly conservative; on the other, biased and unsubstantiated. This book aims for the middle. In writing it, I have tried to be objective and evidence-based, but also open-minded. I have drawn from the scientific literature, as well as my own clinical experience.

No longer "alternative" therapy, micronutrients are taking their rightful place in mainstream medicine. We now have convincing evidence of their efficacy in preventive medicine and therapeutics. This book is generously referenced to direct the reader towards in-depth reviews and original articles in this rapidly expanding field. It is intended as a resource for doctors and other health professions allied to medicine. Although micronutrients are generally available over the counter, interested members of the public should consult with their doctor or pharmacist. Nutrition and metabolism are complex and individual. Prudent use of micronutrients as therapy should always be medically supervised.

With some modification, this book is essentially the first English translation of *Burgerstein's Handbuch Nährstoffe* (Karl F. Haug Verlag, Heidelberg). This classic Swiss text, written by Dr. Lothar Burgenstein, first appeared in 1982. Dr. Burgerstein died in 1987 at age 92, but his book has been carefully updated through nine German editions and continues to be a leader in the field. The latest editions have been bestsellers. I would like to acknowledge the contributions of several people to this book. The spirit of Lothar Burgenstein certainly motivated its writing. Hugo Schurgast made substantial contributions to the text and appendices. Uli Burgerstein provided constant support and encouragement, and much insightful criticism.

Michael Zimmermann
Zürich, May 2001

Contents

4 Micronutrition through the Life Cycle

5 Micronutrients as Prevention and Therapy

Appendix

1 The Basic Principles of Micronutrition

The Role of Micronutrients in Prevention and Therapy

A remarkable shift in nutritional research has occurred in the past 50 years. In the first half of the 20th century, nutritional science focused on the discovery of vitamins and description of classic vitamin and mineral deficiency diseases, such as scurvy (vitamin C deficiency) and rickets (vitamin D deficiency). Widespread efforts were then made to fortify the food supply to prevent vitamin and mineral deficiencies. Grains were enriched with B vitamins and iron, salt was iodized, water was fluoridated, and milk and margarine were fortified with vitamins A and D. These measures have essentially eliminated many previously common disorders, including pellagra, beri beri, and rickets. However, vitamin and mineral deficiencies remain widespread. For example, there is a high prevalence of inadequate intakes of iron and folic acid among women[1,2], and deficiencies of vitamin D, vitamin B12, and calcium are common among older adults.[3,4] Preventive nutrition must continue to emphasize the importance of a healthy and varied diet.

Today nutrition is moving into exciting new areas of prevention and medical therapy, particularly with regard to *micronutrients*. The term "micronutrients" refers to the vitamins, minerals, trace elements, amino acids, and essential fatty acids found in our diets, normally in only very small amounts (milligram or microgram levels). Modern medicine is discovering that with optimum "micronutrition" illnesses can be treated, and in many cases prevented, without relying on more costly (and potentially more dangerous) drugs and surgery. This new paradigm began with the work of pioneering biochemists in the 1960s, led by Dr. Linus Pauling, twice winner of the Nobel Prize. Pauling realized that many micronutrients have significant and far-reaching health effects beyond simple prevention of the classic deficiency diseases. He realized that many chronic illnesses occur when micronutrient deficiencies or imbalances cripple the body's biochemistry and metabolism.[5] Although initially Pauling's ideas met with skepticism within the scientific community, time and the progress of scientific research have shown the value of his basic principles. Correcting deficiencies and imbalances by providing the missing nutrients–often at levels greater than those normally found in the diet–has proved to be a powerful new therapeutic approach.[6–8] Pauling termed this new medicine "orthomolecular medicine," which he defined as

"...the preservation of good health and the treatment of disease by varying the concentrations in the human body of substances that are normally present in the body and are required for health.[5]"

Approximately 45 essential micronutrients are necessary for life and must be supplied by the diet because they cannot be synthesized in the human body. Why are these substances so critical for health? Micronutrients are basic components of every cell in the body. They serve as chemical messengers, building blocks, and enzymes. For tissues to function efficiently all of them need to be present in the right amount, in the right place, and at the right time. Micronutrients are constantly being metabolized, broken down, and excreted and need to be quickly replaced. Because most are not stored in the body in large amounts, regular daily intake is important to maintain tissue levels. An erratic supply weakens cells and forces them to "limp along", thus increasing vulnerability to disease.

Mechanism of Action

How can micronutrients help prevent and treat disease? The first way is the elimination of a chronic deficiency. If the diet is low in an essential nutrient, body reserves become depleted. If the deficiency is severe, clear symptoms develop quickly over a period of weeks. For example, if vitamin C intake falls sharply, scurvy develops after several weeks. Gums begin to bleed, the skin becomes hyperkeratotic, rough, and dry, and capillary hemorrhages appear in the skin.[9] In contrast, marginal nutrient deficiencies only gradually impair cell metabolism, and the ill effects may be subtle, becoming evident only after years or decades. Long-term, marginal intakes of vitamin C[9] or selenium[10] during adulthood, although not producing clear symptoms from day to day, may increase the risk of certain forms of cancer. This point was dramatically made in a recent multicenter trial by the Nutritional Prevention of Cancer Study Group, in which boosting selenium intake by supplementation in 1300 middle-aged men reduced their risk of cancer by 50% (see Table).[10] The level of micronutrition adequate for day-to-day survival is often not sufficient for lifelong, optimum health.

Specific and localized tissue deficiencies of vitamins may occur despite adequate levels in the blood and in many other tissues. For example, localized deficiencies of folate,[11] vitamin E,[12] and vitamin A[13] in the bronchopulmonary tree of smokers may increase the risk of cancer. Similarly, folate deficiency in

Reduced risk of cancer developing in adult men receiving a daily 200 µg selenium supplement compared with placebo

Cancer sites	Reduced risk
Lung	46%
Prostate	63%
Colorectal	58%
Total cancer	37%

(Adapted from Clark LC, et al. JAMA. 1996;276:1957–63)

the uterine cervix of women taking oral contraceptives and in the colon in ulcerative colitis may increase the risk of dysplasia in these tissues.[11]

The second way a micronutrient can treat illness or help prevent disease is by enhancing healthy pathways of cell metabolism. Supplementing dietary calcium intake during adolescence and adulthood reduces turnover of bone and promotes mineral deposition into the skeleton[14,15]. This can help maintain bone mineral density and greatly reduce the risk of osteoporosis and bone fractures in later life. Many trace elements are essential cofactors in enzyme systems, and boosting intake stimulates activity of the enzymes. Selenium is an essential component of glutathione peroxidase, an important antioxidant enzyme. Increasing selenium intake increases enzyme activity and reduces vulnerability to oxidative stress.[16,17]

Certain micronutrients–at levels of intake far greater than those in usual diets–develop beneficial new actions that are not apparent at lower doses. A good example is niacin. In low doses, niacin, as a component of nicotinamide adenine dinucleotide (NAD^+), plays an important role in energy production in cells. At doses 10 to 100 times higher, niacin begins to influence lipid metabolism in the liver, lowering low-density lipoprotein (LDL) cholesterol and triglycerides in the blood, and increasing high-density lipoprotein (HDL) cholesterol. High-dose niacin is recommended as first-line therapy for certain forms of hyperlipidemia.[18] While normal dietary intake of folic acid supports growth of red blood cells and helps prevent anemia, higher doses (two to four times normal dietary levels) during early pregnancy provide powerful protection against birth defects. For women planning a pregnancy, taking a multivitamin containing adequate folic acid can reduce the risk of having a baby with a birth defect by 25–50%. The reduction in risk is particularly strong for neural tube defects (defects of the spine) and cleft lip and palate.[19,22] High-dose supplements of vitamin B6 and zinc can enhance T cell activity and may increase resistance to infection.[21]

Vitamin E is another micronutrient that develops new, beneficial actions at higher doses (Fig 1.1). Clear signs of deficiency are prevented at doses of approximately 8–10 mg/day in healthy adults. Increasing intake to 150–200 mg/day reduces the risk of coronary heart disease by 40% in adult men and women.[22] An intake of 200–400 mg/day can help protect the lungs from the oxidative stress of air pollution. Boosting intake to even higher levels–around 800 mg–may enhance the immune response and increase the body's ability to fight infection.[23]

Biochemical function of micronutrients: examples of classical vs. newer roles

Micronutrient	Classical roles	Newer roles
Niacin	Coenzyme in energy metabolism	Reduction of blood LDL cholesterol[18]
Folic acid	Hematopoiesis	Prevention of birth defects[19]
Vitamin E	Growth, reproduction	Antioxidant, immune function[20]
Vitamin B6	Coenzyme in protein metabolism	Immune function[21]
Iron	Hematopoiesis	Mental function, immune system

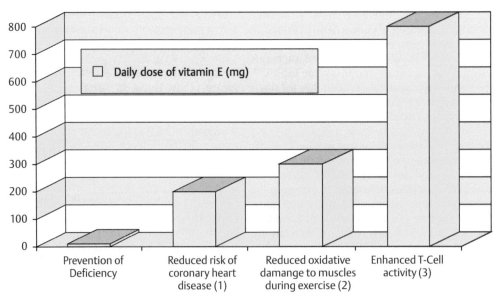

Fig. 1.1: Biochemical roles of vitamin E at increasing doses. (Sources: Stampfer MJ, et al. N Eng J Med. 1923;328:1444; Rokitzki L, et al. Int J Sports Nutr. 1994;4:253; Meydani SN, et al. Am J Clin Nutr. 1990;52:557.)

Variability in Micronutrient Requirements among Individuals

Professor RJ Williams, a chemist who played a key role in the discoveries of pantothenic acid and folic acid, emphasized the broad variability in micronutrient needs within the population. He developed the concept of "biochemical individuality," a fundamental principle of micronutrient prevention and therapy, describing it as follows:

"Each individual has a distinctive nutrient environment of his or her own, because while the list of nutrients needed by all of us may be the same, the respective amounts needed are necessarily not the same for all individuals.[24]"

Put simply, each person has unique nutritional requirements. Depending on one's individual genetic makeup, striking variability can exist in the body's biochemistry. A nutrient intake sufficient for one person may be inadequate for another. For example, 2 mg/day of vitamin B6 is adequate for good health in most people, yet some individuals with inherited defects in vitamin B6 metabolism need up to 30 to 100 times this amount.[25] The absorption and daily requirement for calcium can vary four- to fivefold among healthy middle-aged women.[26] Normal plasma concentrations for 1,25 $(OH)_2$ vitamin D (the activated form of the vitamin) vary between 15 and 45 pg/ml in healthy adults. [9] In the 10% of the population who are heterozygous for the hemochromatosis gene (see pp. 68), dietary iron intakes that normally maintain health may be toxic in the long-term.[27]

Biochemical individuality also helps explain why different people react differently to dietary factors. For example, a high intake of salt will increase blood pressure in the one-third of the adult population who are "salt-sensitive,"[28] while others simply excrete the excess without ill effects. A high amount of dietary cholesterol may produce hypercholesterolemia in some people, but not all.[29]

Moreover, besides these genetic differences, nutritional requirements can be profoundly influenced by many factors, including age, environment, and lifestyle choices. A smoker's requirement for vitamin C is two to three times that of a nonsmoker.[30] Pregnancy doubles a woman's need for iron. Strenuous athletic training sharply increases requirements for the vitamin B complex and magnesium.[31] Therefore, across the population, there a broad range of optimum intakes for the essential nutrients. Factors which cause nutritional needs to vary from person to person are shown in the table below and are considered in detail in later sections.

Factors that cause nutritional needs to vary from person to person

Genetic differences (biochemical individuality)	Growth during childhood and adolescence, aging
Pregnancy and breastfeeding	Gender
Illness, infection, or surgery	Regular alcohol or caffeine intake
Smoking	Dietary factors, levels of intake for fat, carbohydrates, fiber, and protein
Drug-nutrient interactions	Exposure to environmental pollutants
Psychological and emotional stress	Activity and exercise level

Safety

Vitamins, minerals and trace elements, like all substances, can be toxic if taken in sufficiently high amounts. Toxicity has been reported for vitamins A, D, K, B6, niacin, and many of the minerals and trace elements.[32] However, micronutrients generally provide safer therapy than traditional drugs. Many of the vitamins have large therapeutic indices and are free from adverse side effects even at doses of 10 to 20 times the normal dietary intake.[32,33] In contrast, the therapeutic index is narrow for many drugs and adverse side effects are common. Despite thorough testing, many drugs are found to have side effects that become apparent only after years of use. An example is the discovery that short-acting calcium channel blockers, used widely to treat high blood pressure, may actually increase the risk of sudden cardiac death.[34] Hospitals regularly admit people with aspirin-induced gastrointestinal bleeding, digitalis toxicity, or diuretic-induced mineral depletion. In the US, caring for patients suffering from adverse drug side effects accounts for approximately 20% of all hospital costs. The annual cost of such care is estimated to be in excess of US$ 2 billion.[35]

In many instances drugs are life-saving, and no one would want to be without them. However, for many of the common chronic diseases, including cardiovascular disease and arthritis, drugs provide only symptomatic relief. New research is showing that micronutrients can be beneficial in these difficult-to-treat diseases.[6,8,36] No longer alternative therapy, micronutrients are taking their rightful place in mainstream medicine and becoming cornerstones of both prevention and treatment.

References

1. Schott TO, Johnson WG. Folic acid: influence on the outcome of pregnancy. Am J Clin Nutr. 2000;71:1295S.
2. Looker AC, et al. Prevalence of iron deficiency in the United States. JAMA. 1997;277:973.
3. Thomas MK, et al. Hypovitaminosis D in medical inpatients. N Engl J Med. 1998;338:777.
4. Lindenbaum J, et al. Prevalence of cobalamin deficiency in the Framingham elderly population. Am J Clin Nutr. 1994;60:2.
5. Pauling L. How to Live Longer and Feel Better. WH Freeman, New York, 1986
6. Sauberlich HE, Machlin LJ, eds. Beyond Deficiency: New views on the function and health effects of vitamins. Ann NY Acad Sci. 1992;669:1–404.
7. Werbach M. Textbook of Nutritional Medicine. Tarzana, CA: Third Line Press; 1999.
8. Bendich A, Butterworth CE, eds. Micronutrients in Health and Disease Prevention. New York: Marcel Dekker; 1991.
9. Gershoff SN. Vitamin C: New roles, new requirements? Nutr Rev. 1993;51:313.
10. Clark LC, et al. Effects of selenium supplementation for cancer prevention in patients with carcinoma of the skin. JAMA. 1996;276 :1957.
11. Heimburger DC. Localized deficiencies of folic acid in the aerodigestive tissues. Ann NY Acad Sci. 1992;669:87.
12. Pacht ER, et al. Deficiency of vitamin E in the alveolar fluid of smokers. J Clin Invest. 1986;77:789.
13. Biesalski HK, Stofft E. Biochemical, morphological, and functional aspects of systemic and localized vitamin A deficiency in the respiratory tree. Ann NY Acad Sci. 1992;669:325.
14. Heaney RP. Bone mass, nutrition and other lifestyle factors. Nutr Rev. 1996;54:S3.
15. Teegarden D, Weaver CM. Calcium supplementation increases bone density in adolescent girls. Nutr Rev. 1994;52:171.
16. Burk FR. Selenium in Biology and Human Health. New York: Springer Verlag; 1993.
17. Rayman MP. The importance of selenium to human health. Lancet. 2000;356:233.
18. Swain R, Kaplan B. Vitamins as therapy in the 1990s. J Am B Fam Pract. 1995;8:206.
19. Shaw GM, et al. Risks of orofacial clefts in children born to women using multivitamins containing folic acid periconceptionally. Lancet. 1995;345:393.
20. Meydani SN, Beharka AA. Recent developments in vitamin E and immune response. Nutr Rev. 1998;56;S49.
21. Rall LC, Meydani SN. Vitamin B6 and immune competence. Nutr Rev. 1993;51:217.

22. Czeizel AE, et al. Prevention of the first occurrence of neural-tube defects by periconceptional vitamin supplementation. N Engl J Med. 1992;327:1832.
23. Byers T. Vitamin E supplements and coronary heart disease. Nutr Rev. 1993;51:333.
24. Williams RJ. Biochemical Individuality. Austin: University of Texas Press; 1975.
25. Leklem JE. Vitamin B6. In: Shils ME, et al, eds. Modern Nutrition in Health and Disease. Baltimore: Williams & Wilkins; 1999:413.
26. Heaney RP, Recker RR. Distribution of calcium absorption in middle-aged women. Am J Clin Nutr. 1986;43:299.
27. Lynch SR. Iron overload: prevalence and impact on health. Nutr Rev. 1995;53:255.
28. Dustan HP, Kirk KA. The case for or against salt in hypertension. Hypertension. 1989;13:696.
29. McNamara DJ, et al. Heterogeneity of cholesterol homeostasis in man: Response to changes in dietary fat quality and cholesterol quantity. J Clin Invest. 1987;79:1729.
30. Schectman G. Estimating ascorbic acid requirements for cigarette smokers. Ann NY Acad Sci. 1993;686:335.
31. Armstrong LA, Maresh CM: Vitamin and mineral supplements as nutritional aids to exercise performance and health. Nutr Rev. 1996;54:S149.
32. Hathcock JN. Vitamins and minerals: Efficacy and safety. Am J Clin Nutr. 1997;66:427.
33. Bendich A. Safety issues regarding the use of vitamin supplements. Ann NY Acad Sci. 1992;669:300.
34. Furberg CD, et al. Nifedipine: dose related increase in mortality in patients with coronary heart disease. Circulation. 1995;92:1326.
35. Classen DC, et al. Adverse drug events in hospitalized patients: Excess length of stay, extra costs and attributable mortality. JAMA. 1997;277:301.
36. Bendich A, Deckelbaum RJ. Preventive Nutrition. Torowa, NJ: Humana Press; 1997.

2 Micronutrients in Foods

Micronutrients in the Diets of Industrialized Countries

In the USA and Western Europe, agriculture and the food industry produce enough to feed the population and export large quantities of food. Despite this, many people are poorly nourished: they are oversupplied with foods rich in fat, protein, sugar, and salt, and undersupplied with complex carbohydrates, fiber, vitamins, and minerals. Dietary surveys have repeatedly found that micronutrient deficiencies are widespread in the industrialized countries. For example:

● In many large cities in Europe, a quarter of older adults are deficient in vitamin B6, a nutrient vital to the health of the immune system.[1]

● The average selenium intake in adults in the UK, in Germany, and in Sweden is only 25–35% of the recommended level.[2]

● In the USA almost 50% of young women have low iron stores, and more than two-thirds of women develop iron deficiency during pregnancy.[3]

● In the USA, vitamin D deficiency is found in about 25% of infants[4] and 30–60% of older adults.[5,6]

● The intake of folic acid in 75–95% of young women in Europe is below the level currently recommended to prevent birth defects.[7]

Why are vitamin and mineral deficiencies so widespread? Five major factors contribute to the problem:

1. Food refining, processing, and storage causes loss of micronutrients.[8,9] Modern food processing depletes foods of their natural vitamin, mineral, and fiber content and often adds sodium, fat, and food additives. White flour has only about 15% of the vitamin E, 25% of the vitamin B6, and less than 1% of the chromium found in whole-wheat flour.[8,9] Potato chips have almost

Common dietary deficiencies of micronutrients in the USA and Western Europe*

USA	Western Europe
Vitamin B6	Vitamin B6
Folic acid	Folic acid
Vitamin A	Vitamin A
Vitamin C	Vitamin C
Vitamin D	Vitamin D
	Thiamin
	Riboflavin
Calcium	
Magnesium	Calcium
Zinc	Iodine
Iron	Iron

* Mean intakes among broad segments of the population are less than 70% of the RDAs (1989) and/or the European Community PRIs (1992).
(Sources: Life Sciences Research Office, DHHS. 1989; 89:1255; Hurrell RF. Bibl Nutr Dieta. 1989;43:125; Block G, et al. Ann NY Acad Sci. 1993;678:245; de Groot, et al, eds. Eur J Clin Nutr. 1996;50:S1–127; USDA NFS rep. no. 91–2, 1995.)

none of the fiber and vitamin C found in potatoes but are high in sodium and fat. Many frozen vegetables lose nearly half of their vitamin B6 content. Oranges and other fruit, picked green and poorly stored, can lose most or all of their vitamin C content.[8]

2. Modern, intensive agricultural methods deplete the soil of minerals and trace elements. Intensive agriculture, combined with industrial pollution and acid rain, reduces the mineral content of soils. The mineral and trace-element content of many foods varies considerably depending on the soils in which they are grown. Although healthy plants will grow in soils depleted in selenium and zinc, their mineral content will be sharply reduced.

3. People often make the wrong choices in their diets. Typical diets in the industrialized countries emphasize meat, refined grains, whole-milk products, and processed

Loss of micronutrients in food processing and preparation

Food	Method	Micronutrients	Loss (%)
Chicken	Deep frozen	Thiamin, riboflavin, niacin	20–40
Fish	Canned	B vitamins	70
Milk	Pasteurization	Thiamin, vitamin B6, folate	5–10
Milk	Sterilization	Vitamin B6, folate, vitamin B12	35–90
Beef	Roasted	Thiamin, vitamin B6, pantothenic acid	35–60
Pulses (beans, lentils)	Boiling	Copper, iron, zinc, B vitamins	15–50
Strawberries, apricots	Deep frozen	Vitamin C	20–45
Vegetables	Boiling	Thiamin, riboflavin, folate, vitamin C, carotenoids	30–75
Vegetables	Steaming	Thiamin, folate, vitamin C	30–40
Vegetables (spinach, cabbage, leeks)	Boiling	Magnesium, zinc, calcium	25–40
Vegetables	Boiling and canning	Vitamin A	20–30
White rice	Boiling	Thiamin, riboflavin, vitamin B6	50
Whole-wheat pasta	Boiling	Iron, magnesium	25–40
Plant oils (safflower oil, soybean oil)	Heat extraction and refining	Vitamin E	50–70

Sources: Karmas E, Harris RS, eds. Nutritional Evaluation of Food Processing. 3rd ed. New York: AVI; 1988. Biesalski HK, et al, eds. The Vitamins. Stuttgart: Georg Thieme Verlag; 1997.

foods. As a result, intakes of sodium, fat, and cholesterol are many times higher than recommended levels, while intakes of fiber, essential fatty acids, and micronutrients are often low.[10]

4. Polluted urban and industrial environments increase micronutrient requirements. In the major cities of Europe and the USA, millions of people are regularly exposed to air pollution (NO_2 and O_3) above safe levels.[11] Pollution in the air, water, and food supply can sharply increase the body's need for antioxidants. High intake of vitamins E and C helps protect against lung damage caused by air pollution.[12] Selenium-dependent and zinc-dependent enzyme systems reduce toxicity from heavy metals and other xenobiotics,[13] while vitamin C is needed to protect the digestive tract from carcinogens in foods.[14]

5. Alcohol, tobacco, caffeine, and medicinal drugs all interfere with absorption and/or utilization of micronutrients. More than 90% of older adults take medication daily, and many of the most commonly prescribed drugs impair nutritional health.[15,16] Thiazide diuretics deplete stores of potassium and magnesium in the body. The contraceptive pill impairs metabolism of folate and vitamin B6 and increases the requirement for these vitamins.[17] Smoking sharply depletes stores of vitamin C and vitamin B12 in the body, and alcohol consumption causes widespread loss of iron, zinc, magnesium, and many of the B vitamins.[18]

The Difference between the Diet of Our Distant Ancestors and Our Diet Today

In the industrialized countries diets have changed remarkably over the past 100 years. This dietary shift, combined with an increasingly sedentary lifestyle, is a major cause of many common diseases–heart disease, osteoporosis, tooth decay, high blood pressure, and diabetes. These disorders, so prevalent now, were rare before the 20th century. For thousands of years, humans adapted to and thrived on a diet radically different from today's diet.[19,20] Looking at the diet of our ancestors provides an insight into what foods and nutrients humans were genetically "designed" to consume for good health.

● Our distant ancestors ate a diet consisting mainly of fresh plant foods, including nuts, seeds, roots, wild grains and beans, and fruits. Carbohydrates were eaten as whole grains, and were rich in fiber, vitamin E, and minerals. Refined carbohydrates and sucrose, although practically absent from our ancestors' diet, contribute over half of the energy in today's diet.[19,20]

● Our original diet was much lower in total fat. Moreover, the ratio of polyunsaturated fat from plant oils to saturated fat from animal products was 3 to 4 : 1. In contrast, modern diets contain two to three times more saturated fat than polyunsaturated fat.[19,20] Our ancestors ate wild game that was low in total fat (only about 4% fat) but provided rich amounts of beneficial omega-3 fatty acids (see pp. 89). In contrast, today's beef and pork are typically 25–30% fat, but lack omega-3 fatty acids.

● Our ancestors' diet was much richer in vitamins and minerals. It had three to four times as much calcium and magnesium as our present diet, six times the vitamin C content, and much more fiber, vitamin E, and zinc.[19,20]

● Our ancestors' diet contained about 16 times more potassium than sodium. This ratio has been sharply reversed–modern diets contain four times more sodium than potassium.[19,20]

Clearly, our modern diet is dramatically different to the diet our species was "brought up on." Humans were not designed to thrive on a highly refined, micronutrient-depleted diet rich in simple sugars, animal fat, sodium, and food additives.

Comparison of Paleolithic and current diets

	Diet of late Paleolithic man (hunters/gatherers eating 65% plant foods and 35% meat)	Current diet in industrialized Western countries
Total fat intake (% of calories)	21	42
Ratio of saturated : polyunsaturated fat	1 : 3	2 : 1
Fiber (g/day)	45	20
Sodium (mg/day)	690	2300–7000
Calcium (mg/day)	1600	740
Vitamin C (mg/day)	400	90

Adapted from: Eaton SB. N Engl J Med. 1985;312:283.

Food Sources of Micronutrients

Vegetables and Fruits

Vegetables and fruits are the cornerstones of a healthy diet. They are rich sources of vitamins, minerals, complex carbohydrates, and fiber. Some, such as peas and corn, are also good sources of protein. Moreover, vegetables and fruits are generally inexpensive, contain no cholesterol, have little or no fat, and are low in calories. A high intake of vegetables, particularly of the *Brassica* family (broccoli, cabbage, cauliflower, and Brussels sprouts) can sharply reduce the risk of cancer.[10] These vegetables contain compounds that can help the body detoxify and clear potential carcinogens. In addition, fruits and vegetables are rich sources of antioxidant nutrients, such as beta carotene and vitamin C, that may also protect against cancer and heart disease.[21,22]

Until recently, vegetables and fruits tended to be available on a regional and seasonal basis: asparagus in the spring, tomatoes in the summer, and cabbages in the fall. But today, worldwide distribution has made most food available all year round. This greater availability, however, has come at a price. Large-scale mechanized growing and harvesting methods, combined with a need for foodstuffs to withstand the rigors of long-distance transport and storage, have led to an emphasis on hardiness and a long 'shelf-life' as opposed to flavor, freshness, and nutrient content. The nutritional value of much of today's produce is further reduced by modern intensive agriculture that depletes the soil of important minerals (such as zinc and selenium) so that plants grown on these soils are less nutritious. Furthermore, vegetables and fruits can lose most of their vitamins, particularly fragile ones like riboflavin and vitamin C, when carelessly stored.[8] Fresh produce should ideally be stored in a cool dark place; nutrient losses are accelerated when produce is exposed for long periods to light, heat, or air.

Many nutrients are concentrated in or just beneath the skin of produce. For example, nearly all the fiber in an apple is contained in the peel, and much of the vitamin C in potatoes is concentrated just beneath the skin. If apples, pears, potatoes, and other produce are agrichemical-free, they should be washed thoroughly and the skin left on. The rules for maintaining micronutrient content when cooking vegetables are simple: minimal water, a covered pot, and the shortest possible cooking time.

To get the most micronutrients from fruits, eat them in their fresh, raw state. Some vegetables are healthier if thoroughly cooked, whereas others are much healthier if eaten raw. Levels of oxalic acid, a substance present in spinach and other greens that can block absorption of calcium and iron,[23] are reduced by cooking. Also, natural toxins found in cabbages, cauliflower, and mushrooms are heat labile and destroyed by cooking. Mushrooms, beets and beet greens, spinach, cabbage, broccoli, cauliflower, brussel sprouts, peas, beans, and eggplant are all healthier if cooked. On the other hand, most other vegetables, including onions and garlic, are more nutritious when consumed raw.

How nutritious are canned and frozen vegetables and fruits? Most frozen produce is processed without cooking, so most of the micronutrient content is conserved. But canned vegetables and fruits undergo a heating process that destroys much of the vitamin C and B vitamins.[8] Also, minerals leach out of canned food into the water, and unless the liquid in the can is used in food preparation, the minerals will be lost. Large amounts of sodium are added during the processing and canning of vegetables. Canned fruit is often conserved in heavily sugared water. A fresh peach has about 70 calories; a canned peach, with the added sugar, contains about 180 calories. When available, fruit that is conserved in its own juice is preferable.

Meat (Beef, Pork, Lamb, and Poultry)

Meat is exceptionally rich in iron, zinc, and vitamins B6 and B12. Moreover, the micronutrients in meat tend to be highly bioavailable. About 20% of the iron in meat is absorbed, compared to only 2–5% from most plant foods.[23] In the average US diet, meat provides 70–75% of the total dietary zinc requirement and almost all of the vitamin B12 requirement. At the same time, meat is the major source of saturated fat and cholesterol in the diet of the industrialized countries. A high meat intake may increase the risk of heart disease, stroke, and colon cancer. A large study in the USA found that women who eat meat (beef, pork, or lamb) at least once a day are twice as likely to develop colon cancer as those with a lower meat intake.[24] Women who regularly eat chicken or fish rather than red meat cut their risk by about 50%. Moderation when eating meat is the key: eating too much is harmful, but occasional consumption of meat can provide important nutrients without adding too much fat to the diet. For the average adult, a small serving of beef sirloin (80–100 g) will provide the full daily vitamin B12 requirement, half the daily protein and zinc requirements, and one-third of the daily iron, niacin, and riboflavin requirements.

Eggs

Eggs are one of nature's most nutritious foods. The protein in eggs contains a perfect balance of all the essential amino acids: one large egg contains about 8 g of protein, or about one-sixth of the daily protein requirement. Eggs are also rich in the fat-soluble vitamins A, E, and D, and are an excellent source of sulfur and iron. The egg white contains most of the protein; the yolk contains almost all the vitamins and minerals. The yolk is one of the richest natural sources of choline and lecithin but it also contains about 250 mg of cholesterol. People with high blood cholesterol, who need to limit their cholesterol consumption, should eat eggs only rarely. However, for most people with normal blood cholesterol, eating eggs regularly will provide important nutrients and have little or no effect on blood cholesterol.[25] Although it is sometimes claimed that darker yellow yolks contain more nutrients than pale ones, the yolk color depends mainly on the content of xanthophylls (natural yellow pigments in chicken feed).

Milk and Milk Products

A single glass of milk supplies about one-quarter of the daily protein and vitamin D requirements. Milk and milk products are also very important sources of calcium, in a form that is easily absorbed and processed by the body. In the USA and much of Europe, milk products account for 60–85% of total calcium intake. However, three potential health problems are associated with milk:

1. Many people do not produce enough lactase to completely digest the lactose in milk. If lactose is poorly digested, it can cause cramps, gas, and diarrhea. This inherited condition is termed "lactose intolerance" and most often affects Asians, African-Americans, and other populations that traditionally consume few milk products. Although most infants and children can absorb lactose, lactase activity tends to decline with age. Lactose-intolerant people can often eat small amounts of yogurt, buttermilk, and some cheeses because most of the lactose in these foods has been fermented by bacteria.

2. Milk allergy can be a trigger of asthma, eczema, arthritis, and other symptoms.[26] A milk allergy is almost always a reaction to the proteins in cow's milk, whereas lactose intolerance is a reaction to the lactose. Therefore, unlike lactose-intolerant individuals, people with a milk allergy must often avoid all milk products, including yogurt and cheese.

3. Whole milk is rich in fat. Fat accounts for half the calories in milk, almost all of which is saturated fat. Low-fat milk is as nutritious

as whole milk except that most of the vitamins A and D are lost when the fat is removed (in many "fortified" low-fat milks, they are replaced later). Skimmed milk contains nearly all of the protein and minerals contained in whole milk. Some milk products are nearly all fat: about two-thirds of the calories in cream are fat, and butter is 100% milk fat. Adults who wish to reduce their saturated fat intake should drink low-fat milk in place of whole milk and eat butter and cream only rarely.

Pasteurization reduces the levels of several of the B vitamins in milk by about 10–15%. However, milk sterilized by extremely high heat (UHT) loses up to 35% of its thiamin, vitamin B6, and biotin content and 75–95% of its folate and vitamin B12 content.[27]

Cheese is basically concentrated milk with added salt: about a liter of milk is used to make 100 g of most cheeses. Cheese is high in protein and calcium but rich in saturated fat, sodium, and cholesterol. Several of the B vitamins present in milk are lost during the cheese-making process. Many soft cheeses (and cottage cheese) lose much of their calcium content as well.[27]

Fish

Like meat, eggs, and milk, fish is an excellent source of vitamins, minerals, and complete protein. Unlike these other animal foods, however, fish is low in fat, calories, and cholesterol. For example, compared with a serving of beef sirloin a serving of trout contains only half the calories and one-quarter the fat, but provides equal amounts of protein and B vitamins. Not only is most fish low in fat, the fat in fish also has high amounts of omega-3 fats (see pp. 89), which may reduce the risk of coronary heart disease and high blood pressure.[28,29] Farm-raised fish tends to have lower amounts of the omega-3 fats than fish from open waters. Salt-water fish is the richest natural source of iodine, and both fresh-water and salt-water fish are good sources of iron, selenium, and potassium.[27]

A potential problem with eating fish is the hazard of chemical pollution. Water pollutants become concentrated in fish from polluted rivers, lakes, or coastal waters (particularly large carnivorous fish at the top of the food chain). Swordfish, tuna, and bluefish caught from polluted coastal waters typically contain large amounts of mercury and other chemicals. Smaller fish, such as sardines and herrings that feed mainly on tiny marine organisms, as well as larger fish that live farther offshore in cleaner waters, are less likely to be contaminated. Before cooking large fish, the fatty areas and the dark meat just beneath the skin should be trimmed off since this is where most of the chemicals and heavy metals accumulate.

When buying canned fish (such as tuna or salmon), choose those packed in water and not oil. Adding oil doubles the amount of calories and may reduce the omega-3 fat content of the fish by 20–30%. Also, the sodium content of canned fish should be carefully checked. Depending on how much salt is added during processing, the sodium content can be as high as 500 mg per serving (low-salt types or those with no salt added contain only 40–100 mg per serving).

Cereals, Bread, Wheat Bran, and Wheat Germ

Whole grains are the best natural sources of complex carbohydrates and fiber. Populations eating large amounts of whole-grain products (e.g., Africa and Asia) have far fewer intestinal and bowel problems–such as constipation, hemorrhoids, diverticulitis, and colon cancer–compared to Western populations consuming mainly refined carbohydrates.[30]

In industrialized countries most grains are refined to make them quicker to cook, easier to chew, and storable for longer periods. However, refining removes healthful portions of grains and strips away many important nutrients. White flour and rice, through refining, lose more than 80% of the original vitamin and mineral content found in the whole grain.[8,9] Two vital components of wheat are lost during refining–the germ and bran. The wheat germ (the small, dark point on the end of the wheat kernel) contains most of the B vitamins and essential amino acids and is rich in vitamin E, minerals, and trace elements (magnesium, zinc, and selenium). The wheat bran is the hull of the wheat kernel. It contains B vitamins and minerals and is especially rich in fiber. Because whole-grain products retain most of the germ and bran, they are much more nutritious than their refined counterparts (Fig. 2.1).

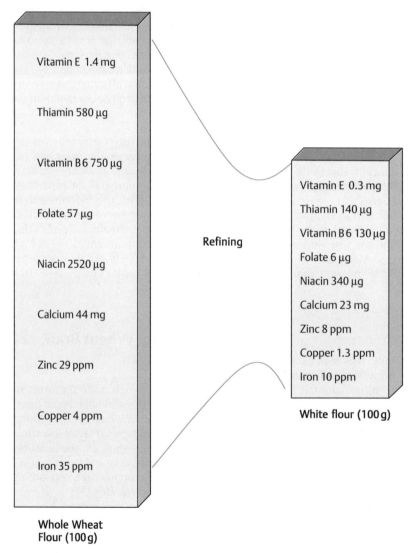

Vitamin E 1.4 mg

Thiamin 580 µg

Vitamin B 6 750 µg

Folate 57 µg

Niacin 2520 µg

Calcium 44 mg

Zinc 29 ppm

Copper 4 ppm

Iron 35 ppm

Whole Wheat Flour (100 g)

Refining

Vitamin E 0.3 mg

Thiamin 140 µg

Vitamin B 6 130 µg

Folate 6 µg

Niacin 340 µg

Calcium 23 mg

Zinc 8 ppm

Copper 1.3 ppm

Iron 10 ppm

White flour (100 g)

Fig. 2.1: Loss of micronutrients in the milling and refining of wheat flour. (Source: Pederson B, et al. World Rev Nutr Diet. 1989;60:1)

Salt

Salt contains the essential mineral sodium. Although the daily sodium requirement is low (about 200–300 mg/day), the average diet in the industrialized countries contains 4–6 g of sodium, about twenty times the daily requirement.[10] In about one-third of adults high intakes of sodium (especially when combined with low intakes of potassium and calcium) increase blood pressure (Fig. 2.2).[31,32] Excess sodium intake also increases urinary calcium excretion and may increase the risk of osteoporosis.[33]

Where does all this extra sodium come from? Less than 10% comes from the natural sodium content of food; about 75% comes from salt that has been added during production and

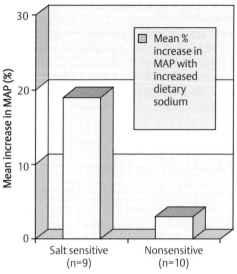

Fig. 2.2: Elevation of blood pressure in salt-sensitive individuals through an increase in dietary salt intake. 15 g of salt was added daily to the diets of 19 adults with essential hypertension. 50% showed no significant increase in mean arterial pressure (MAP) and 50% showed a sharp rise in MAP. Mean increase in MAP in the salt-sensitve group was 19%. (Adapted from Kawalski T, et al. Am J Med. 1978;64:193)

Foods containing the highest levels of sodium

> 400 mg sodium/100 g
Most breads, potato chips, canned soups and vegetables

> 800 mg sodium/100 g
Most cheeses, processed meats and sausages, cornflakes and other breakfast cereals, salted nuts, olives, condiments (soy sauce, ketchup, mustard)

Examples of high sodium : potassium ratios in processed foods

Food	Serving size	Sodium (mg)	Sodium: potassium ratio	Comments
Smoked salmon	100 g	1800	5 : 1	Fresh salmon has only 100 mg sodium/100 g
Sausages	One, large	350–1100	6 : 1	
Cornflakes	50 g	600	10 : 1	Most processed breakfast cereals are high in sodium and low in potassium
Canned vegetable soup	100 g	500	4 : 1	
Canned corn	100 g	400–1100	6 : 1	Fresh corn contains only trace amounts of sodium and has a sodium : potassium ratio of 1 : 140. Most canned vegetables are loaded with salt.
Cheeses	100 g	200–1000	9 : 1	Cottage cheese, parmesan, romano, and gorgonzola are examples of cheeses with a very high sodium content

processing, and only about 15% is added during cooking or at the table. [34] Natural, fresh foods are typically very low in sodium and have a healthy ratio of sodium to potassium. In contrast, cheese, processed meats (such as sausages), salty snacks like crackers, nuts, and chips, canned vegetables, sauces, and soups contain high amounts. For example, a fresh to-mato contains only 10 mg of sodium and 280 mg of potassium, while an average bowl of canned tomato soup contains 1200 mg of sodium and 400 mg of potassium. A typical sausage contains more than 800 mg of sodium but only 150 mg of potassium, and 100 g of parmesan cheese contains more than 1200 mg of sodium.

Vegetarian Diets

For thousands of years humans were hunters and gatherers who consumed mainly fruits, leaves, roots, and seeds, supplemented occasionally with meat when it was available. Plant foods have a low energy density–they contain few calories for their bulk–so to obtain 2500 kcals/day eating only fruits, leaves, and roots, around 7–8 kg of these foods would need to be eaten each day. Therefore, consumption of some meat, which is a concentrated form of energy, minerals, and protein, had obvious advantages.

Vegetarianism is a general term encompassing diets that contain no food of animal origin ("vegan") and plant-based diets that contain dairy products ("lactovegetarian") or dairy products and eggs ("lacto-ovovegetarian"). Although meat is a concentrated source of energy, protein, iron, and zinc, it is not an absolute dietary requirement for humans. Lacto-ovovegetarian diets provide optimum nutrition if foods are carefully chosen. However, strict vegans need to be particularly careful when choosing foods or they may not obtain enough of several important micronutrients. The potential deficiencies in vegetarian diets are as follows.

Vitamins

Vitamins B12 and D are found only in animal products. Although certain vegetarian foods (such as miso, tempeh, seaweeds, and spirulina) have been recommended as potential sources of vitamin B12, they contain only compounds that resemble vitamin B12 but that are not active.[35] Therefore, strict vegan diets need to include a vitamin B12 supplement and/or plant foods, such as soy milk or tofu, that have been enriched with the vitamin.[35] Although vitamin D is found only in animal products, daily requirements are low (5–10 µg/day), and with adequate exposure to the sun the body is able to synthesize adequate vitamin D.[36] Vegans who live in northern climates with long, dark winters may develop vitamin D deficiency.[37]

Minerals

Meat, milk, and eggs are the richest sources of iron, zinc, and calcium. Although some plant foods contain these minerals, they are poorly absorbed compared with those found in meat or milk. For example, although a serving of lentils and a serving of veal may contain similar amounts of iron, the iron in the veal is about five times more bioavailable.[23] Women vegetarians, because of their increased need for calcium and iron, need to choose foods carefully to obtain adequate amounts. (See pp. 59 and 66 for good plant sources for these minerals.) An effective way to increase absorption of iron from food is to eat vitamin C-rich foods, drink a large glass of orange juice or take a vitamin C supplement with each meal. Vitamin C can overcome the inhibitors of iron absorption in plant foods, and double or even triple the amount of iron absorbed.[23]

Protein

Many grains and legumes are very good sources of protein. However, unlike the protein in meat, fish, milk, and eggs, the protein in plants is incomplete–that is, the amounts of one or more of the essential amino acids present are inadequate. It is therefore important to combine proteins that complement one another so that a complete set of amino acids is provided. Examples of complete protein combinations are legumes (such as beans, lentils, peas, or peanuts) together with whole-grain rice, bread, or other cereals. These protein combinations do not necessarily need to be eaten at the same meal; as long as a variety of complementary proteins are eaten regularly (such as within a day or two of each other), the body is provided with adequate complete protein.

Following a strict vegan diet may be problematic during times when nutritional needs are particularly high. During pregnancy and lactation, for example, the amount of iron, zinc, and calcium needed is higher than that which can be obtained from a typical vegan diet.[38,39] Because these minerals are vital for the health of the developing baby, vegan mothers should consider taking a multimineral supplement.[38,39] Also, a vegan diet may not be optimum during early childhood (before 5 years of age). Children fed strict vegan diets often do not grow as well as children fed mixed diets. They tend to be smaller and lighter and are at greater risk for rickets, because of vitamin D deficiency, as well as for iron-deficiency anemia.[40]

In vegetarian diets variety is the key to healthy eating. To get all the essential nutrients it is important to eat a wide range of foods: fruits, vegetables, nuts, seeds, legumes, whole-grain cereals, and soy products. It is important to choose plant foods that are carefully grown and stored to maintain their nutrient content.

What are the health benefits of a vegetarian or semivegetarian diet? Vegetarians are less at risk for heart attack and diabetes.[41] The risk of vegetarians suffering a heart attack is around two-thirds lower than that of meat eaters.[42] High blood pressure, obesity, and high blood cholesterol are also less likely in vegetarians. Vegetarians suffer less from many digestive disorders, including gallbladder disease, constipation, and colon cancer.[41,43] Studies in Germany, England, and the USA have found that vegetarian diets may reduce the risk of cancer–particularly lung, ovarian, and breast cancer–by up to 50%.[43]

References

1. Dirren HM. EURONUT/SENECA: A European study of nutrition and health in the elderly. Nutr Rev. 1994;52:S38.
2. Rayman MP. The importance of selenium to human health. Lancet. 2000;356:233.
3. Yip R. Iron supplementation during pregnancy: Is it effective? Am J Clin Nutr. 1996;63:853.
4. Zeghoud F, et al. Subclinical vitamin D deficiency in neonates: Definition and response to vitamin D supplements. Am J Clin Nutr. 1997;65:771.
5. Thomas MK, et al. Hypovitaminosis D in medical inpatients. N Engl J Med. 1998;338;777.
6. Lindenbaum J, et al. Prevalence of cobalamin deficiency in the Framingham elderly population. Am J Clin Nutr. 1994;60:2.
7. de Bree A, et al. Folate intake in Europe: Recommended, actual, and desired intake. Eur J Clin Nutr. 1997;51:643.
8. Karmas E, Harris RS, eds. Nutritional Evaluation of Food Processing. 3rd ed. New York: Van Nostrand Reinhold; 1988.
9. Williams AW, Erdman JW. Food processing: Nutrition, safety, and quality balance. In: Modern Nutrition in Health and Disease. Shils ME, Olson JA, Shike M, Ross AC, eds. Baltimore: Williams & Wilkins; 1999:1813.
10. Truswell AS. Dietary goals and guidelines: national and international perspectives. In: Modern Nutrition in Health and Disease. Shils ME, Olson JA, Shike M, Ross AC, eds. Baltimore: Williams & Wilkins; 1999:1727.
11. Bree, et al. A more stringent and longer-term standard for atmospheric ozone. Toxicol Appl Pharmacol. 1990;103:377.
12. Menzel, DB. Antioxidant vitamins and prevention of lung disease. Ann NY Acad Sci. 1992;669:141.
13. Flora SJS, et al. Adjuvants for therapeutic chelating drugs in lead intoxication. Trace Element Electrolytes. 1995;12:131.
14. Sauberlich HE. Pharmacology of vitamin C. Annu Rev Nutr. 1994;14:371.
15. Handbook on Drug and Nutrient Interactions. Chicago: American Dietetic Association; 1994.
16. Thomas JA. Drug-nutrient interactions. Nutr Rev. 1995;53:271.
17. Prasad AS, et al. Effect of oral contraceptives on nutrients: vitamin B6, B12 and folic acid. Am J Obstet Gynaecol. 1976;125:1063.

18. Odeleye OE, Watson RR. Alcohol-related nutritional derangements. In: Watson RR, Watzl B, eds. Nutrition and Alcohol. Boca Raton: CRC Press; 1992.

19. Eaton SB. Paleolithic nutrition–a consideration of its nature and current implications. N Engl J Med. 1985;312:283.

20. Eaton SB. Paleolithic nutrition revisited. Eur J Clin Nutr. 1997;51:207.

21. Steinmetz KA, et al. Vegetables, fruit, and cancer prevention: A review. J Am Diet Assoc. 1996;96:1027.

22. Diaz MN, et al. Antioxidants and atherosclerotic heart disease. N Engl J Med. 1997;337:408.

23. Hurrell RF. Bioavailability of iron. Eur J Clin Nutr. 1997;51:S4.

24. Willet WC, et al. Relation of meat, fat and fiber intake to the risk of colon cancer in a prospective study among women. N Engl J Med. 1990;323:1664.

25. McNamara DJ, et al. Heterogeneity of cholesterol homeostasis in man: Response to changes in dietary fat quality and cholesterol quantity. J Clin Invest. 1987;79:1729.

26. Terho EO, Savolainen J: Review: Diagnosis of food hypersensitivity. Eur J Clin Nutr. 1996;50:1.

27. Holland B, et al, eds. McCance and Widdowson's The Composition of Foods. 5th ed. Cambridge, UK: Royal Society of Chemistry; 1991.

28. Schmidt EB, et al. N-3 fatty acids from fish and coronary artery disease: Implications for public health. Publ Health Nutr. 2000;3:1.

29. Nair SSD, et al. Prevention of cardiac arrhythmia by dietary (n-3) PUFAs and their mechanism of action. J Nutr. 1997;127:383.

30. Mount, JL. The Food and Health of Western Man. London, Tonbridge: Charles Knight & Co.; 1975.

31. Midgley JP, et al. Effect of reduced dietary sodium on blood pressure. A meta-analysis of randomized controlled trials. JAMA. 1996;275:1590.

32. Tarek F, et al. Salt–more adverse effects. Lancet. 1996;348:250.

33. Devine A, et al. A longitudinal study of the effects of sodium and calcium intake on regional bone density in postmenopausal women. Am J Clin Nutr. 1995;62:740.

34. James WP, Ralph A, Sanchez-Castillo CP. The dominance of salt in manufactured food in the sodium intake of affluent societies. Lancet. 1987;1:426.

35. Herbert V, et al. Folic acid and vitamin B12. In: Shils ME, Olson JA, Shike M., eds. Modern Nutrition in Health and Disease. 8th ed. Philadelphia: Lea & Febiger; 1994:402.

36. Institute of Medicine, Food and Nutrition Board. Dietary Reference Intakes for Calcium, Phosphorus, Magnesium, Vitamin D, and Fluoride. Washington D.C.: National Academy Press; 1997.

37. Utiger RD. The need for more vitamin D. N Engl J Med. 1998;338:828.

38. Institute of Medicine. Nutrition during Pregnancy. Washington, D.C.: National Academy Press; 1991.

39. Institute of Medicine. Nutrition during Lactation. Washington, D.C.: National Academy Press; 1991.

40. Dagniele PC, et al. Effects of macrobiotic diets on linear growth in infants and children until ten years of age. Eur J Clin Nutr. 1994;48:S103.

41. Johnston PK. Nutritional implications of vegetarian diets. In: Shils ME, Olson JA, Shike M, Ross AC, eds. Modern Nutrition in Health and Disease. Baltimore: Williams & Wilkins; 1999:1755.

42. Rottka H. Vegetarianism-Pro and Con: The Berlin Vegetarian Study. In: Kluthe R, Kasper H, eds. Fleisch in der Ernährung. Stuttgart: Georg Thieme Verlag; 1994.

43. Trock B, et al. Dietary fiber, vegetables and colon cancer: Critical review and meta-analysis of the epidemiologic evidence. J Natl Cancer Inst. 1990;82:650.

3 The Micronutrients

Vitamins

Vitamin A and Carotenoids

Vitamin A in animal foods (meat, milk, and eggs) is mainly in the form of retinol combined with fatty acids (usually with palmitic acid, as retinyl palmitate). In the body retinol can be converted to retinal or retinoic acid, both of which have specific functions. Retinal plays a central role in the function of the retina, while retinoic acid helps regulate gene expression and cell development. All of these compounds–retinol, retinal, and retinoic acid–are referred to collectively as vitamin A. Vitamin A is carried in the blood on a specialized transport protein, retinol-binding protein (RBP),[1] that is synthesized in the liver.

Carotenoids are a family of compounds found in plant foods that can be converted by the body to vitamin A. The most common carotene in foods is beta-carotene. A beta-carotene molecule can be absorbed intact or can be split into two molecules of vitamin A by intestinal cells and absorbed as vitamin A. A large carrot containing about 15 mg of beta-carotene supplies enough vitamin A to satisfy the adult daily requirement. Other carotenoids, such as alpha-carotene and gamma-carotene, are present in small amounts in foods and also can be converted to vitamin A, though less efficiently than beta-carotene.[2]

Functions

Vision. In the eye vitamin A plays a central role in the transformation of light energy into the nerve impulses the brain perceives as vision.[3] The rod and cone cells of the retinal epithelium are rich in retinal. When light enters the eye, a molecule of retinal absorbs the energy and changes shape, triggering a nerve impulse.

Skin and mucus membrane health. Vitamin A promotes proper growth and development of the cells lining the skin and mucous membranes in the respiratory, gastrointestinal, and genitourinary tracts.[4] It plays a central role in maintaining the health and integrity of the skin.

Immune system. Vitamin A increases resistance to infection by maintaining the integrity of the skin and mucous membrane barriers against bacteria, viruses, and parasites. In addition, vitamin A enhances antibody production by white blood cells and increases the number and activity of T cells.[5] During childhood, vitamin A supports growth and development of T cells in the thymus gland. Carotenoids also can increase activity of T cells and natural killer (NK) cells and enhance production of tumor necrosis factor alpha (Fig. 3.1).[6]

Hormone synthesis. Vitamin A is required for steroid hormone synthesis, including production of corticosteroids in the adrenal gland and androgens and estrogens in the testes and ovaries.

Reproduction. Optimum vitamin A status maintains sperm count and motility in males.[5] In females, deficiency is associated with infertility and spontaneous abortion.

Growth and development. Vitamin A controls cell growth and development.[7] Children deficient in vitamin A fail to grow and develop normally.

Red blood cells. Vitamin A plays an important role in mobilizing iron stores to build new red blood cells.[5]

Several different units are used to indicate the amount of vitamin A in foods and supplements

1 retinol equivalent (RE) =	1 µg of retinol
	6 µg of beta-carotene
	12 µg of other carotenoids
	3.33 IU (international units) of vitamin A

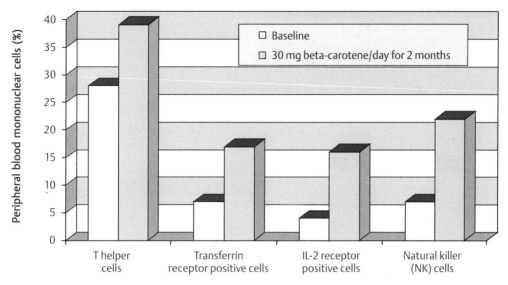

Fig. 3.**1**: **Beta-carotene and immune function.** Supplemental beta-carotene (30/mg/day) for 2 months given to healthy adults significantly increased the number of circulating white blood cells. (Adapted from Watson RR, et al. Am J Clin Nutr. 1991;53:90)

Nervous system. Vitamin A helps maintain the protective sheath (myelin) around nerves, both in peripheral nerves and in the brain.

Skeleton. Vitamin A participates in bone formation, particularly during childhood growth and during fracture healing.

Increased Risk of Deficiency

● Children and adolescents are particularly at risk.[8] If childrens' diets are low in vitamin A, deficiency develops quickly because of small body stores and sharply increased needs for growth.

● Stress, infection, or surgery increases vitamin A requirements.

● Fat malabsorption due to liver or biliary disorders, Crohn's disease, chronic pancreatitis, sprue, or cystic fibrosis causes poor absorption of vitamin A.[7]

● Newborns (and particularly premature infants) have very low stores of vitamin A and do not absorb vitamin A efficiently.

● Many drugs interfere with vitamin A metabolism. For example, cholesterol-lowering drugs and laxatives decrease absorption, whereas barbiturates decrease liver stores (see Appendix I for more details).

● In diabetes and hypothyroidism conversion of carotenes to vitamin A is impaired.

● Heavy alcohol consumption interferes with absorption, storage, and metabolism of vitamin A.

● Cigarette smoking and air pollution increase requirements for vitamin A. Toxic metals, such as cadmium, increase breakdown and loss of vitamin A from the body.

● Repeated and lengthy exposure to bright sunlight, particularly in lighter-skinned people, breaks down beta-carotene in the skin and retinal in the eyes.[5]

Signs and Symptoms of Deficiency

- Dryness, itching, and redness of the conjunctiva
- Inability to adapt to and see in dim light (night blindness)
- Dry, rough, itchy skin with rash
- Dry, brittle hair and nails
- Loss of sense of smell, taste, and appetite
- Fatigue
- Anemia
- Poor growth
- Increased vulnerability to infections[5,6]
- Increased risk of cancer of the throat, lung, bladder, cervix, prostate, esophagus, stomach, and colon[9]
- Impaired reproduction and fertility
- Increased risk of kidney stones

Good Dietary Sources

Vitamin A in foods is found in two forms: as retinol in animal products and as carotenes in plants. Carotenes give many fruits and vegetables their yellow/orange color.

Foods rich in pre-formed vitamin A (retinol)	Serving size	µg
Beef liver	100 g	9100
Cod liver oil	10 g	2550
Egg	1 whole	110
Cheddar cheese	30 g	95
Butter	10 g	59
Whole milk	1 dl	30

Foods rich in beta-carotene (and other carotenoids)	Serving size	µg vit-amin A
Carrot	1, large	810
Sweet potato	1, large	920
Spinach	100 mg	460
Apricots	3	290
Peach	1, large	200

Recommended Daily Intakes

Recommendations for daily intake of beta-carotene for prevention are in the range of 2–6 mg. The usual therapeutic dose range is 15–45 mg/day.[10] Carotene supplements derived from natural sources are preferable. They contain, along with beta-carotene, a mixture of carotenoids, including lutein, alpha-carotene, and lycopene, and may have additional health benefits. For example, lycopene is a potent antioxidant[11] and may decrease the risk of prostate cancer and cataract.

Recommended daily intakes for vitamin A (retinol equivalents)		
	Prevention of deficiency	
	UK RNI (1991)	USA RDA (1989)
Adult men	700	1000
Adult women*	600	800
	Therapeutic dose range	
	Pauling (1986)	Werbach (1990/99)
Adult men	6000–12000	3000–45000
Adult women*	6000–12000	3000–45000

* excluding pregnant or lactating women. Women planning a pregnancy or who are pregnant should not exceed a daily intake of 2500 RE (from both food and supplements). See page 129 for a discussion of vitamin A in pregnancy.

Preferred Form and Dosage Schedule

Vitamin A *Can be toxic*	Retinol ester (e.g. retinol palmitate)	Take with meals
Beta carotene *Not toxic*	Natural source beta-carotene, such as that derived from the sea algae Dunaliella salina, contains both the cis- and trans-isomers of beta carotene. It may have a broader range of activity and is preferrable to synthetic beta carotene (containing only the trans-isomer)	Take with meals

Use in Prevention and Therapy

Infectious diseases. Infections of the skin (fungal infections, acne, impetigo, boils), influenza, conjunctivitis, ear infections (otits externa and media), bronchitis and pneumonia, and infectious diarrheal disease may benefit from vitamin A. Even in children who are not vitamin A deficient, vitamin A can lessen the severity of communicable infectious diseases.[5,12,13] For example, vitamin A supplements taken with measles or infectious diarrhea can reduce complications and mortality by more than 50%.[5,13]

Skin and scalp/hair disorders. Vitamin A helps maintain skin health and may be beneficial in cases of dry skin, dandruff, premature aging of skin,[14] eczema, and psoriasis.

Traumatic injury. Vitamin A plays a major role in the healing of wounds and bony fractures.

Gynecologic disorders. Vitamin A may be beneficial in reducing menstrual symptoms (heavy menstrual bleeding, breast tenderness) and in benign fibrocystic breast disease.

Protection against carcinogens. Vitamin A is one of nature's primary anticancer substances, particularly in the skin and mucous membranes. Ample intakes of vitamin A have been shown to protect against cancers of the lung, bladder, prostate, larynx, esophagus, stomach, and colon. Vitamin A can prevent precancerous lesions, such as oral leukoplakia (white patches on the lips and mouth often found in smokers) and cervical dysplasia, from developing and may produce regression and disappearance of these disorders.[15] As a cancer treatment, large doses of retinoic acid may reduce growth and recurrence of certain forms of skin cancer.[16] As an antioxidant, beta-carotene helps provide protection against damage from many xenobiotics (such as polychlorinated biphenyls [PCBs]). It may also reduce the risk of skin cancer associated with exposure to sunlight[6] and radiation.[2]

Respiratory disorders. Vitamin A may reduce symptoms and severity of chronic obstructive pulmonary disease and asthma, particularly in regular smokers.[17]

Gastric ulcers. Vitamin A helps maintain gastric mucus production and may reduce stress ulceration in traumatized or burned patients.

Cataract. Ample intake of vitamin A and beta-carotene may reduce the risk of developing cataract.

Anemia. The combination of iron plus vitamin A may be more effective than iron alone in treating iron-deficiency anemia.

Toxicity

High doses of vitamin A can produce severe toxicity.[19] However, toxicity is not usually observed in adults at doses lower than 15000 RE, even when taken for long periods (weeks to months). Infants and children are more susceptible than adults to vitamin A toxicity. Vitamin A is a teratogen and high doses (more than 10000 RE) may produce birth defects, even with exposure as short as 1 week in early pregnancy.[20] Pregnant women should avoid excess intake of vitamin A from supplements and from vitamin A-rich foods, such as liver (100 mg contains nearly 10000 μg retinol). Total daily intake of vitamin A should not exceed 2500 RE during pregnancy. Because their conversion to retinol in the body is tightly regulated, carotenes do not produce vitamin A toxicity. People with the skin disorder erythropoetic protoporphyria are routinely given 100–200 mg (170–330000 IU) of beta-carotene per day for long periods without ill effects. Chronic high intakes (amounts equal to

Signs and symptoms of vitamin A toxicity
• Bone pain and joint swelling
• Nausea, vomiting, and diarrhea
• Dry skin and lips
• Hair loss
• Headache and blurred vision
• Enlargement of the liver and spleen
• Reduced thyroid activity
• High blood calcium

approximately 1 kg carrots per day) can cause a benign, reversible yellowing of the skin and nails. There is no evidence that beta-carotene, at any dose level, produces birth defects. Because beta-carotene supplements do not produce vitamin A toxicity, in many cases they may be preferable to taking preformed vitamin A.

References

1. Vieira AV, et al. Retinoids: Transport, metabolism and mechanisms of action. J Endocrinol. 1995;146:201.
2. Canfield LM, et al. Carotenoids and human health. Ann NY Acad Sci. 1994;691:1–300.
3. Sommer A. Vitamin A: Its effect on childhood sight and life. Nutr Rev. 1994;52:60.
4. De Luca LM, et al. Vitamin A in epithelial differentiation and skin carcinogenesis. Nutr Rev. 1994;52:45.
5. Semba RD. The impact of vitamin A on immunity and infection. In: Bendich A, Deckelbaum RJ, eds. Preventive Nutrition. Totawa, NJ: Humana Press; 1997:337.
6. Schmidt K. Interaction of antioxidative micronutrients with host defense mechanisms: A critical review. Int J Nutr Res. 1997;67:307.
7. Olson JA. Vitamin A. In: Ziegler EE, Filer LJ, eds. Present Knowledge in Nutrition. Washington DC: ILSI Press; 1996.
8. Spannus-Martin DJ, et al. The vitamin A statuses of young children of several ethnic groups in a socioeconomically disadvantaged urban population. FASEB J. 1994;8:940.
9. Menkes MS, et al. Serum beta-carotene, vitamins A and E, selenium and the risk of lung cancer. N Engl J Med. 1986;315:1250.
10. Erdman JW, et al. Beta-carotene and the carotenoids: Beyond the intervention trials. Nutr Rev. 1996;54:185.
11. Stahl W, Sies H. Lycopene: A biologically important carotenoid for humans? Arch Biochem Biophys. 1996;336:1.
12. Ross AC, Stephenson CB. Vitamin A and retinoids in antiviral responses. FASEB J. 1996;10:979.
13. Barreto ML, et al. Effect of vitamin A supplementation on diarrhea and acute lower respiratory tract infections in young children in Brazil. Lancet. 1994;344:228.
14. Saurat JH. Retinoids and ageing. Horm Res. 1995;43:89.
15. Garewal HS, Schantz S. Emerging role of beta-carotene and antioxidant nutrients in prevention of oral cancer. Arch Otolaryngol Head Neck Surg. 1995;121:141
16. De Luca LM, et al. Retinoids in differentiation and neoplasia. Sci Am Sci Med. 1995;4:28.
17. Sergio AR, et al. Assessment of vitamin A status in chronic obstructive pulmonary disease patients and healthy smokers. Am J Clin Nutr. 1996;64:928.
18. Suharno D, et al. Supplementation with vitamin A and iron for nutritional anemia in Indonesia. Lancet. 1993;342:1325.
19. Chytil F. Safety aspects of vitamin A administration. Eur J Clin Nutr. 1996;50:S21.
20. Rothman KJ. Teratogenicity of high vitamin A intake. N Engl J Med. 1995;333:1369.

Vitamin D

Vitamin D is the only vitamin whose biologically active form is a hormone. The term "vitamin D" refers to a family of related compounds. Vitamin D3 (also called cholecalciferol) is the form synthesized from cholesterol in sun-exposed skin. For healthy children and adults, exposing the hands, face, and arms on a clear summer day for 10–15 minutes several times each week provides adequate vitamin D. Vitamin D3 is the natural form of the vitamin found in animal products such as eggs, fish, and liver. Another form of vitamin D, vitamin D2 (ergocalciferol), is synthesized by certain fungi and is used in many supplements and as a food fortifier. However, vitamin D3 is the preferred form for humans as its bioavailability is twice that of vitamin D2.[1]

After absorption from foods or production in the skin, vitamin D is stored as 25-OH-vitamin D in the liver. When needed by the body, it is subsequently activated to 1,25 -OH-vitamin D by the kidney.[1] Thus, a healthy liver and kidneys are essential for optimum vitamin D status. (1 μg vitamin D = 40 IU vitamin D.)

Functions

Calcium metabolism. The principal function of vitamin D is to regulate calcium levels in the blood and tissues. A fall in blood calcium will trigger production of active vitamin D, which stimulates calcium absorption from the diet, increases release of calcium from bones, and slows renal excretion.

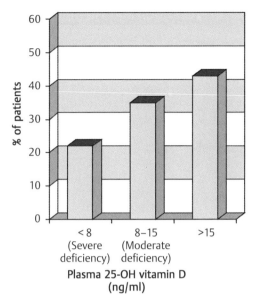

Fig. 3.2: **Vitamin D deficiency is common in hospitalized patients.** In a study of 290 patients on a general ward, 57% were deficient in vitamin D and 22% severely deficient. Adapted from Thomas MK, et al. N Engl J Med. 1998;338:777.

Skeletal health. Vitamin D is essential for normal bone growth during childhood and for maintaining bone density and strength during adulthood. Vitamin D enhances calcium absorption from foods and increases calcium and mineral deposition into the skeleton.[2]

Cell growth and development. Vitamin D is an important regulator of cell development throughout the body, particularly in white blood cells and epithelial cells.

Immune system. Vitamin D enhances the activity and response of white blood cells in infection. *any autoimmune disease, cancer*

Increased Risk of Deficiency

● Because vitamin D is found only in animal foods, strict vegetarian diets sharply increase the risk of deficiency if sunlight exposure is inadequate.

● Many elderly people are at high risk for deficiency because of poor diets and inadequate sunlight exposure.[3] Also, older people are much less efficient at synthesizing vitamin D in the skin and, compared with younger adults, produce less than half the amount of vitamin D from sun exposure.[4] Moreover, the kidneys of elderly people are less efficient at activating stored forms of vitamin D.[5]

● Because of reduced sunlight intensity and duration, people living in northern latitudes, particularly in the winter season, are at risk for deficiency if dietary intake is low.[6] A sunscreen with a sun protection factor (SPF) higher than eight completely prevents skin synthesis of vitamin D.

● People with fat malabsorption as a result of liver or biliary disease, Crohn disease, chronic pancreatitis, sprue, cystic fibrosis, and abetalipoproteinemia absorb vitamin D poorly.

● The ability of people with chronic kidney failure to activate stored forms of vitamin D is impaired.

Signs and Symptoms of Deficiency

Children
- Delayed growth and development (child begins crawling and walking late)
- Irritability and restlessness
- Rickets: softening of bones, spinal deformities, bowed legs and knock knees, enlargement of the rib-sternum joints
- Delayed tooth eruption and poorly formed tooth enamel
- Impaired immune response with increased risk of infection

Adolescents
- Impaired growth of bones and musculature
- Swelling and pain at the end of long bones, especially at the knee
- Impaired immune response with increased risk of infection

Adults
- Loss of bone mineral from the skeleton with increased risk of osteoporosis and fractures
- Hearing loss and ringing in the ears

continued

- Muscle weakness, particularly around the hip and pelvis
- Possible increased risk of colorectal and breast cancer
- Possible increased risk of high blood pressure[7]
- Impaired immune response with increased risk of infection

Good Dietary Sources

Food	Serving size	μg
Salmon	100 g	16
Tuna	100 g	5
Eggs	1, medium	1
Calf liver	100 mg	1
Emmentaler cheese	30 mg	0.33
Butter	10 mg	0.1

Recommended Daily Intakes

Recommended daily intakes for vitamin D (μg)		
	Prevention of deficiency	
	UK RNI (1991)	USA DRI (1997)
Adult men	0–10	5–15
Adult women*	0–10	5–15
	Therapeutic dose range	
	Pauling (1986)	Werbach (1990)
Adult men	20	10–40
Adult women*	20	10–40

* excluding pregnant or lactating women.

Preferred Form and Dosage Schedule

Cholecalciferol (vitamin D3) is generally preferable to ergocalciferol (vitamin D2)	Take with meals

Use in Prevention and Therapy

Bone disorders. Vitamin D is effective at treating rickets in children. Together with calcium, it can slow or prevent bone loss in individuals at risk of osteoporosis and reduce the fracture rate in individuals with osteoporosis.[8,9]

Psoriasis. Vitamin D, due to its ability to regulate epithelial cell growth and development, can reduce the hyperproliferation of skin cells in psoriasis and may reduce the severity of the disease.[10]

Immunity. Vitamin D can stimulate white blood cells and may enhance resistance to infection.[11]

Hearing disorders. In certain individuals vitamin D, together with calcium, can reduce symptoms of tinnitus and improve hearing loss.

Cancer prevention. Ample intake of vitamin D may reduce the risk of colorectal and breast cancer.[12]

Toxicity

There is a wide range of susceptibilty to the toxicity of vitamin D2. Intakes of more than 100 μg per day may cause hypercalcemia and calcium deposition into soft tissues in children. Chronic intakes of more than 1000 μg vitamin D per day in adults can cause renal calcification and calcification of other soft tissues.

References

1. Trang HM, et al. Evidence that vitamin D3 increases serum 25-hydroxyvitamin D more efficiently than does vitamin D2. Am J Clin Nutr. 1998;68:854–8.
2. Fraser DR. Vitamin D. Lancet. 1995;345:104.
3. Villareal DT, Civitelli R, Chines A, et al. Subclinical vitamin D deficiency in postmenopausal women with low vertebral bone mass. J Clin Endocrinol Metab. 1991;72:628.
4. National Research Council. Vitamin D. In: Recom-

mended Dietary Allowances. 10th ed. Washington DC: National Academy Press; 1989:92.

5. Russell RM, Suter PM. Vitamin requirements of elderly people: An update. Am J Clin Nutr. 1993;58:4.
6. Dawson-Hughes B, et al. Plasma calcidiol, season and serum parathyroid hormone concentrations in healthy elderly men and women. Am J Clin Nutr. 1997;65:67.
7. Sowers MR, et al. The association of intakes of vitamin D and calcium with blood pressure among women. Am J Clin Nutr. 1985;42:135.
8. Dawson-Hughes B, et al. Effect of vitamin D supplementation on wintertime and overall bone loss in healthy postmenopausal women. Ann Intern Med. 1991;115:505.
9. Reid IR. Therapy of osteoporosis: calcium, vitamin D, and exercise. Am J Med Sci. 1996;312(6):278.
10. Lowe KE. Vitamin D and psoriasis. Nutr Rev. 1992;50:138.
11. Casteels K, et al. Immunomodulatory effects of 1,25-dihydroxyvitamin D3. Curr Opin Nephrol Hypertens. 1995;4:313.
12. Garland C, et al. Dietary vitamin D and calcium and risk of colorectal cancer: A 19-year prospective study in men. Lancet. 1985;1:307.

Vitamin E

Vitamin E is a general term for a group of compounds, each with varying degrees of vitamin E activity. The most abundant and active form of vitamin E is alpha-tocopherol, but significant amounts of beta-tocopherols, gamma-tocopherols, and delta-tocopherols are also found in the diet. The relative activities of the tocopherols vary considerably and are important in assessing the vitamin E content of foods or supplements. For example, although soybean oil has a higher total tocopherol content than sunflower oil, most of the vitamin E in soy is gamma-tocopherol; in sunflower oil most of the vitamin E is alpha-tocopherol, giving the oil a greater level of vitamin E activity. In addition, the liver metabolizes and excretes gamma-tocopherol more rapidly than alpha-tocopherol. The naturally occurring isomer of vitamin E (d-alpha-tocopherol) has approximately 50% greater bioavailability and potency in the body than synthetic vitamin E (dl-alpha-tocopherol) (Fig. 3.3).[1]

Vitamin E form	Relative biologic activity
Alpha-tocopherol	100
Beta-tocopherol	50
Gamma-tocopherol	10–30
Delta-tocopherol	1

Functions

Antioxidant action. Vitamin E is an important lipid-soluble antioxidant that scavenges free radicals in tissues and protects cellular components.[2] It works together with glutathione peroxidase and vitamin C in limiting free radical damage. Vitamin E also protects cellular proteins from oxidative damage during ischemic events, such as angina pectoris, heart attack, and stroke.

Antithrombotic action. Vitamin E slows down the action of thrombin (a blood clotting protein) and reduces platelet aggregation by inhibiting thromboxane.[3] Although vitamin E is a natural "blood thinner" it does not increase risk of bleeding in healthy people.

Increased Risk of Deficiency

● Many people do not obtain adequate dietary vitamin E. In most foods vitamin E is removed by processing. For example, refined flour and white rice lose nearly all of the vitamin originally present in the whole grain.

● The consumption of polyunsaturated fatty acids (PUFAs) has steadily increased in the USA and Europe over the past several decades. Because vitamin E is required in tissues to protect PUFAs from oxidation, the need for vitamin E increases with increased intake of PUFAs.[4] The greater the intake of PUFAs, the greater the risk of vitamin E deficiency if dietary intake of the vitamin is marginal.

● Vitamin E requirements are sharply increased by urban environments, air and water pollution, certain food pesticides and additives, and radiation.[5]

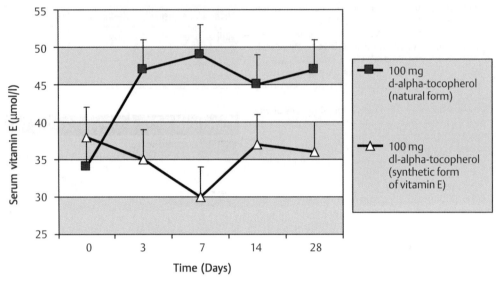

Fig. 3.**3**: **Superior bioavailability of natural compared with synthetic vitamin E.** Changes in serum concentrations of vitamin E after daily oral administration of 100 mg d-alpha-tocopherol (natural form of vitamin E) and 100 mg dl-alpha-tocopherol (synthetic form of vitamin E). Serum vitamin E levels increased 1.6-fold from baseline during administration of d-alpha-tocopherol, but did not change significantly during administration of dl-alpha-tocopherol. (Adapted from Kiyose C, et al. Am J Clin Nutr. 1997;65:785)

● Vitamin C and glutathione peroxidase (a selenium-dependent enzyme, see pp. 84) regenerate tocopherol that is oxidized during free radical scavenging, thereby recycling vitamin E for reuse by tissues. Deficiencies of vitamin C or selenium therefore sharply increase requirements for vitamin E and increase risk of deficiency.[6]

● Fat malabsorption due to liver or biliary disease, Crohn disease, chronic pancreatitis, sprue, cystic fibrosis, and abetalipoproteinemia cause poor absorption of vitamin E.

● Newborn infants, and particularly premature infants, are at high risk for deficiency due to their poor ability to absorb vitamin E and very limited tissue reserves of vitamin E.

Signs and Symptoms of Deficiency

- Decreased membrane integrity of red blood cells produces hemolysis and anemia
- Degeneration of nerve cells in the spinal cord and peripheral nerves
- Atrophy and weakness in skeletal and smooth muscles
- Cardiomyopathy with breakdown and replacement of myocardial cells with scar tissue
- Atrophy of the reproductive organs and infertility
- Possible increased risk of cancer, atherosclerosis, arthritis, and cataract

Good Dietary Sources

Food	Serving size	mg
Sunflower seeds	100 g	21
Wheat germ	100 g	12
Sweet potatoes	1, average size	7
Safflower oil	10 g	3.5
Shrimp	100 g	3.5
Salmon	100 g	2
Eggs	1, average size	0.4

almonds

Recommended Daily Intakes

Recommended daily intakes for vitamin E (mg)		
	Prevention of deficiency	
	UK RNI (1991)	USA DRI (2000)
Adult men	>4	15
Adult women*	>3	15
	Therapeutic dose range	
	Pauling (1986)	Werbach (1990/99)
Adult men	800	100–2500
Adult women*	800	100–2500

* excluding pregnant or lactating women

Preferred Form and Dosage Schedule

Natural vitamin E (d-alpha-to-copherol) is the preferred form. It is more bioavailable and more potent than synthetic vitamin E (dl-alpha-tocopherol)[1]	Take with meals

Use in Prevention and Therapy

Cardiovascular disease, incuding coronary heart disease and peripheral vascular disease. Vitamin E is beneficial in angina pectoris, peripheral claudication, and venous thrombosis. It reduces oxidation of cholesterol in low-density lipoprotein (LDL) and very low-density lipoprotein (VLDL) particles in the blood and thereby can reduce the risk of coronary heart disease.[7–9] Vitamin E may also increase levels of the "protective" high-density lipoprotein (HDL) in the blood.

Disorders of premature infants. Risk of hemolytic anemia, retrolental fibroplasia, and bronchopulmonary dysplasia is increased in newborns with vitamin E deficiency.

Anemia. Vitamin E functions as an antioxidant and stabilizes red blood cell membranes, enhancing function and durability of red cells. This may be of benefit in syndromes of hemolytic anemia and in the anemia of sickle-cell disease.

Cataract. Ample vitamin E intake may decrease oxidative damage to the lens and reduce the risk of developing cataract.

Rheumatic disorders. Vitamin E reduces joint inflammation and stiffness and is beneficial for treatment of osteoarthritis and rheumatoid arthritis. It may reduce dependence on nonsteroidal antiinflammatory drugs (NSAIDs).[10]

Cystic fibrosis, biliary atresia, and other disorders of fat malabsorption. Sequelae of vitamin E deficiency, such as hemolytic anemia and neuromuscular degeneration, often occur in disorders of fat malabsorption. Special forms of vitamin E, such as water-soluble oral forms or intramuscular injections, may be needed if fat malabsorption is severe.

Skin conditions. Vitamin E, applied topically to abrasions or burns, may reduce scar formation and contraction, and improve healing.

Protection from environmental toxins. Vitamin E helps protect the lungs against the toxic effects of air pollutants, such as ozone and nitrous oxide.[5] Vitamin E can also reduce damage to cell membranes from radiation and heavy metals, such as mercury and lead. In addition, vitamin E can protect tissues from adverse effects of certain medicines, such as paracetamol (acetaminophen).

Protection from cancer. Higher intakes of vitamin E may help reduce the risk of cancer of the skin, breast, lung, esophagus, and stomach.[11,12]

Fibrocystic breast disease. Vitamin E can be effective in reducing breast swelling and tenderness and may induce cyst regression.

Premenstrual symptoms. Vitamin E may reduce breast tenderness, fatigue, appetite cravings, depression, and insomnia associated with the menstrual cycle.[13]

Alzheimer's disease. The loss of brain function in Alzheimer's disease may be caused by oxidant damage to neurons. Vitamin E can slow progression of Alzheimer's disease and help maintain function.[14, 15]

Immunity. Vitamin E may increase resistance to viral and bacterial infections. It enhances antibody production by white blood cells and increases their ability to phagocytize (engulf and destroy) bacteria.[16] Also, by means of its antioxidant actions, vitamin E protects white blood cells from oxidant damage during their response to an infection.[16]

Diabetes. Vitamin E may protect against the oxidative damage that underlies many of the complications of diabetes. It can enhance the action of insulin and thereby reduce insulin requirements for blood sugar control.[17]

Exercise and training. Vitamin E helps protect against the damaging oxidative by-products of strenuous exercise.

Toxicity

At doses of 400–800 mg/day in healthy persons, vitamin E is nontoxic. Daily doses of 1600–3200 mg have been used for prolonged periods without significant side effects.[4] People taking anticoagulant drugs should be cautious with high doses, however. Vitamin E may enhance the effects of anticoagulants and decrease levels of vitamin K-dependent clotting factors. People with diabetes should be cautious when starting high doses of vitamin E because the vitamin may enhance the action of insulin and, rarely, produce hypoglycemia.

References

1. Kiyose C, et al. Biodiscrimination of alpha-tocopherol stereoisomers in humans after oral administration. Am J Clin Nutr. 1997;65:785.
2. Packer L. Vitamin E is nature's master antioxidant. Sci Med. 1994;1:54.
3. Steiner M. Vitamin E supplementation and platelet function. In: Bendich A, Butterworth CE, eds. Micronutrients in Health and Disease Prevention. New York: Marcel Dekker; 1991.
4. Meydani M. Vitamin E. Lancet. 1995;345:170.
5. Menzel DB. Antioxidant vitamins and prevention of lung disease. Ann NY Acad Sci. 1992;669:141
6. Kubena KS, McMurray DN. Nutrition and the immune system: a review of nutrient-nutrient interactions. J Am Diet Assoc. 1996;96:1156.
7. Jha P, et al. The antioxidant vitamins and cardiovascular disease: A critical review of the epidemiologic and clinical trial data. Ann Intern Med. 1995;123:860.
8. Stampfer M, et al. Vitamin E consumption and the risk of coronary disease in women. N Engl J Med. 1993;328:1444.
9. Stephens NG, et al. Randomised controlled trial of vitamin E in patients with coronary disease. Lancet. 1996;347:781.
10. Kohlarz G, et al. High-dose vitamin E for chronic polyarthritis. Aktuelle Rheumatol. 1990;15:233.
11. Blot W, et al. Nutrition intervention trials in Linxian, China: Supplementation with specific vitamin/mineral combinations, cancer incidence and disease-specific mortality in the general population. J Natl Cancer Inst. 1993;85:1483.
12. Trickler D, Shikler G. Prevention by vitamin E of experimental oral carcinogenesis. J Natl Cancer Inst. 1987;78:165.
13. London RS. Efficacy of alpha-tocopherol in the treatment of the premenstrual syndrome. J Reprod Med. 1987;32:400.
14. Sokol RJ. Vitamin E deficiency and neurological disorders. In: Packer L, Fuchs J, eds. Vitamin E in Health and Disease. New York: Marcel Dekker; 1993.
15. Sano M, et al.: A controlled trial of selegiline, alpha-tocopherol or both as treatment for Alzheimer's disease. New Eng J Med. 1997;336:1216.
16. Meydani SN, Beharka AA. Recent developments in vitamin E and immune response. Nutr Rev. 1996;56:S49.
17. Paolisso G, et al. Pharmacologic doses of vitamin E improve insulin action in healthy subjects and non-insulin dependent diabetic patients. Am J Clin Nutr. 1993;57:650.

Vitamin K

Vitamin K is the general term for several related compounds with vitamin K activity. There are two principal forms of vitamin K: vitamin K1 (phylloquinone) is found in plant foods and vitamin K2 (menaquinone) is derived from animal and bacterial sources.[1] Bacteria in the human colon synthesize menaquinones, which can be absorbed and partially meet requirements for vitamin K.

Functions

Blood coagulation. Vitamin K is an essential cofactor in the production of proteins that are part of the coagulation cascade in the blood. Several promote coagulation (factors II, VII, IX, X) while others slow it down (proteins C and S). Thus, activity of vitamin K balances the two opposing sides of the coagulation system in the blood.[2]

Bone metabolism. Vitamin K is a cofactor in the production of structural and regulatory proteins in bone.[3] Osteocalcin, abundant in bone, is a vitamin K-dependent protein that regulates calcium metabolism and vitamin D activity at sites of bone turnover.

Increased Risk of Deficiency

● The body stores only about 100 g of vitamin K, mainly in the liver. The liver carefully maintains this small reserve by recycling "spent" vitamin K and reusing it. If the liver is damaged or diseased, this recycling of vitamin K is impaired, sharply increasing risk of deficiency.

● Heavy alcohol consumption impairs the liver's ability to produce vitamin K-dependent coagulation factors and recycle vitamin K.

● Many drugs impair vitamin K metabolism. Broad-spectrum antibiotics destroy the colonic bacteria that produce vitamin K and can increase risk of deficiency.[4] Drugs which impair fat absorption (cholestyramine, certain antacids) can reduce absorption of vitamin K.

Coumarin anticoagulants antagonize vitamin K activity in the liver. Phenytoin and salicylates also interfere with vitamin K metabolism.

● Disorders of fat malabsorption–chronic liver or biliary disease, biliary obstruction, Crohn disease, sprue, cystic fibrosis, and pancreatitis–reduce vitamin K absorption.

● Newborn infants who are exclusively breastfed are susceptible to abnormal bleeding due to vitamin K deficiency.[4] Breast milk contains very little vitamin K and the immature liver of the newborn does not synthesize the vitamin K-dependent clotting factors efficiently. Also, because the newborn's colon is sterile for the first few days after birth, no bacterial synthesis of vitamin K occurs in the colon. To reduce the risk of vitamin K deficiency, most babies receive intramuscular vitamin K at birth.

Signs and Symptoms of Deficiency

- A tendency toward prolonged bleeding, small amounts of blood in the stool, and/or easy bruising
- Impaired normal bone mineralization and/or remodeling

Good Dietary Sources

Food	Serving size	µg
Spinach	100 g	415
Broccoli	100 g	175
Green cabbage	100 g	125
Beef liver	100 g	92
Tea, green	10 g	71
Eggs	1, average size	11
Butter	10 g	3

Recommended Daily Intake

Synthesis of vitamin K by colonic bacteria can contribute significantly to daily requirements, in some individuals supplying up to half the daily requirement.

Recommended daily intakes for vitamin K (µg)		
	Prevention of deficiency	
	UK RNI (1991)	USA RDA (1989)
Adult men	1 µg/kg body weight	60–80
Adult women *	1 µg/kg body weight	60–80
	Therapeutic dose range Werbach (1990)	
Adult men	30–100	
Adult women *	30–100	

* excluding pregnant or lactating women.

Preferred Form and Dosage Schedule

Vitamin K1 (phylloquinone)	Take with meals

Use in Prevention and Therapy

Hemorrhagic disease of newborns. To protect them from vitamin K deficiency, babies who are exclusively breastfeeding should receive an intramuscular supplement of 1 mg of vitamin K at birth.[4]

Osteoporosis. Vitamin K intake may enhance production of osteocalcin, optimize bone remodeling and mineralization, and help prevent or treat osteoporosis.[6,7]

Toxicity

Vitamin K (phylloquinone) toxicity has not been reported, even at doses as high as 4000 g/day. A vitamin K precursor, menadione, used in the past as an infant supplement, is toxic even at low doses, causing anemia and jaundice. It is no longer used as a therapeutic form of vitamin K.

References

1. Suttie JW. The importance of menaquinones in human nutrition. Ann Rev Nutr. 1995;15:399.
2. Shearer MJ. Vitamin K and vitamin K dependent proteins. Br J Hematol. 1990;75:156.
3. Binkley NC, Suttie JW. Vitamin K nutrition and osteoporosis. J Nutr. 1995;125:1812.
4. Shearer MJ. Vitamin K. Lancet. 1995;345:229.
5. Alperin JB. Coagulopathy caused by vitamin K deficiency in critically ill, hospitalized patients. JAMA. 1987;258:1916.
6. Olson RE. Osteoporosis and vitamin K intake. Am J Clin Nutr. 2000;71:1031.
7. Weber P. Management of osteoporosis: Is there a role for vitamin K? Int J Vit Nutr Res. 1997;67:350.

Thiamin (Vitamin B1)

Body reserves of thiamin (vitamin B1) are small – only about 30 mg – so a steady dietary supply of the vitamin is important to avoid deficiency. Because of its central role in energy production, most of the body's thiamin is located in muscle. Thiamin absorbed from the diet is rapidly transformed into its active form, thiamin pyrophosphate (TPP).[1]

Functions

Energy metabolism. Thiamin, as its active form TPP (combined with magnesium), is a vital coenzyme in the production of energy in cells.

Nervous system. Thiamin located in the nerve cell membrane is important for the transmission of nerve impulses in the brain and peripheral nerves.[2] Thiamin also plays an important role in the metabolism of several brain neurotransmitters (including acetylcholine and serotonin).

Protein synthesis. Thiamin is important in the synthesis of collagen (the major structural protein in the body). Thiamin deficiency is associated with decreased collagen formation and impaired wound healing.

Increased Risk of Deficiency

● Heavy alcohol consumption reduces absorption of thiamin and interferes with its conversion to TTP.

● Many processed foods that form a major part of Western diets today (e.g., sugar, white flour, white rice, oils, fats, and alcohol) have only trace amounts of thiamin. Infants who are breastfed by mothers who are thiamin deficient can rapidly develop life-threatening signs of thiamin deficiency. Also, because of poor dietary intake, the elderly are at increased risk of deficiency.[3]

● Daily consumption of coffee and black tea depletes thiamin stores in the body and may contribute to deficiency.

● Folate deficiency impairs absorption of thiamin.

● Because body reserves of thiamin are low, an increase in requirements–caused by strenuous physical exertion, fever, stress, burns, overactive thyroid, liver disease, pregnancy, lactation, or adolescence–can rapidly lead to deficiency if dietary intake is poor.[4]

● Oral contraceptive use sharply increases thiamin requirements. Several other commonly used drugs also interfere with thiamin metabolism (see Appendix I).

Most of the thiamin in cereals and grains is found in the germ. Refining of grains destroys almost all the thiamin. For example, polished white rice has only one-hundredth of the thiamin content of full-grain rice. Thiamin is fragile and easily lost in food processing and preparation. High temperatures and prolonged cooking destroy the vitamin, and because the vitamin is highly water soluble, significant amounts are lost in cooking water. Boiling vegetables can destroy up to two-thirds of their thiamin content.

Signs and Symptoms of Deficiency

Unrecognized thiamin deficiency can produce ill-defined symptoms, such as irritability, depression, fatigue, and insomnia, particularly in people with increased thiamin requirements (e.g., pregnant and breastfeeding women, women taking oral contraception, adolescents, diabetics, heavy alcohol users, the chronically ill).

- Impaired sensation, movement, and reflexes in the arms and legs
- Staggering gait, poor balance
- Mental confusion, defects in learning and memory, frequent headache, insomnia
- Personality changes (depression, irritability)
- Muscle tenderness (especially in the calf muscles) and weakness
- Cardiomyopathy, irregular heartbeat, shortness of breath, anemia
- Impaired energy production and fatigue
- Impaired protein (collagen) synthesis: poor wound healing
- Diminished antibody response to infection
- Loss of appetite, constipation

Good Dietary Sources

Food	Serving size	mg
Brewer's yeast	10 g	1.2
Pork chop	100 g	0.85
Ham	100 g	0.80
Oatmeal	100 g	0.65
Sunflower seeds	30 g	0.6
Wheat germ	30 g	0.45
Peas, green	100 g	0.32
Potato	1, average size	0.24

Recommended Daily Intakes

Recommended daily intakes for thiamin (mg)		
Prevention of deficiency		
	UK RNI (1991)	USA DRI(1998)
Adult men	0.9–1.0	1.2
Adult women*	0.8	1.1
Therapeutic dose range		
	Pauling (1986)	Werbach (1990/99)
Adult men	50–100	10–1500
Adult women*	50–100	10–1500

* excluding pregnant or lactating women

Preferred Form and Dosage Schedule

Thiamin hydrochloride	Take between or with meals, preferably with the dose divided throughout the day

Use in Prevention and Therapy

Nerve disorders. Because thiamin deficiency can reduce pain tolerance, supplemental thiamin may ease chronic pain. Thiamin may be effective in peripheral neuropathy,[5] particularly in inflammatory nerve disorders (such as trigeminal neuralgia). It may also be effective in diabetic neuropathy.

Central nervous system disorders. Thiamin may be of benefit in Alzheimer's disease,[6] anxiety, and depression (especially when associated with anxiety).

Heart failure. Particularly in the elderly, chronic heart failure that responds poorly to conventional medical therapy should raise the suspicion of thiamin deficiency. Trial thiamin supplementation may be beneficial.[7,8]

Anemia. Thiamin deficiency produces an anemia resembling that of folate or vitamin B12 deficiency (with macrocytosis) that responds to thiamin supplementation.[9]

Exercise, physical activity, and sport. Strenuous physical work or sports training increases demand for thiamin, and supplemental thiamin may improve performance if thiamin status is suboptimal.

Heavy alcohol consumption. Supplemental thiamin reduces the risk of deficiency in people who consume large amounts of alcohol.

Toxicity

Thiamin is virtually nontoxic. Doses greater than 200 mg may cause drowsiness in some people. Rare, but severe, allergic reactions have been reported when thiamin is given by injection.

References

1. Finglass PM. Thiamin. Int J Vitam Nutr Res. 1994;63:270.
2. Bettendorf L. Thiamin in excitable tissue: Reflections of a non-cofactor role. Metab Brain Dis. 1994;9:183.
3. van der Wielen RP, et al. Nutritional status of elderly female nursing home residents: The effect of supplementation with physiological doses of water-soluble vitamins. Eur J Clin Nutr. 1995;49:665.
4. Rindi G. Thiamin. In: Ziegler EE, Filer LJ, eds. Present Knowledge in Nutrition. Washington DC: ILSI Press; 1996.
5. Skelton WP, Skelton NK. Thiamine deficiency neuropathy: It's still common today. Postgrad Med. 1989;85:301.
6. Gold M, et al. Plasma and red cell thiamin deficiency in patients with dementia of the Alzheimer's type. Arch Neurol. 1995;52:1081.
7. Pfitzenmeyer P, et al. Thiamin status of elderly patients with cardiac failure, including effects of supplementation. Int J Vitam Nutr Res. 1994;64:113.
8. Shimon I, et al. Improved left ventricular function after thiamin supplementation in patients with congestive heart failure receiving long-term furosemide therapy. Am J Med. 1995;98:485–9.
9. Mandel H, et al. Thiamine-dependent beriberi in the "thiamine-responsive anemia syndrome." N Eng J Med. 1984;311:836.

Riboflavin (Vitamin B2)

Functions

Energy production. Riboflavin is an essential part of the coenzymes, flavin mononucleotide (FMN) and flavin-adenine dinucleotide (FAD). FAD and FMN play central roles in numerous metabolic pathways of carbohydrate, fatty acid, and protein metabolism. They are important in adenosine triphosphate (ATP) production through cellular respiration in mitochondria.

Antioxidant action. Riboflavin is a cofactor of glutathione reductase. This enzyme helps recycle oxidized glutathione, maintaining tissue antioxidant defenses.[1]

Increased Risk of Deficiency

● Childhood and adolescent growth, as well as pregnancy and lactation, increase demands for riboflavin.

● Malabsorption of riboflavin occurs in tropical sprue, celiac disease, resection of the small intestine, gastrointestinal and biliary obstructions, chronic diarrhea, infectious enteritis, and irritable bowel syndrome.[2]

● Thyroid hormones, oral contraceptives, phenothiazines, barbituates, and certain antibiotics can impair riboflavin status.

● Heavy alcohol consumption reduces absorption of riboflavin.[4]

● The increased metabolism and protein breakdown that occur during chronic illness, fever, cancer, and injury sharply increase metabolism of riboflavin.

Signs and Symptoms of Deficiency

- Reddened, scaly, greasy, painful, and itchy patches on the skin (especially around the nose, mouth, ears, the labia majora in females, and the scrotum in men)
- Painful fissures and cracks form at the angles of the mouth (angular stomatitis) and on the lips (cheilosis). The tongue is smooth, purplish, and painful. Swollen, sore throat
- Redness, burning, and excessive tearing of the eyes, light sensitivity. Chronic deficiency can increase risk of developing cataract
- Anemia with decreased production of red blood cells
- Lethargy, depression, personality changes. (These can sometimes appear before skin and mucous membrane changes are evident)
- Because riboflavin is important in the activation of vitamin B6 and the conversion of tryptophan to niacin, deficiency of riboflavin typically produces symptoms of vitamin B6 and niacin deficiency.[3] Pure, uncomplicated riboflavin deficiency is extremely rare; it is nearly always accompanied by multiple B-vitamin deficiencies.

Good Dietary Sources

Food	Serving size	mg
Calf liver	50 g	1.1
Mushrooms	100 g	0.45
Brewer's yeast	10 g	0.4
Spinach	100 g	0.2
Yogurt	100 g	0.18
Milk	1 large glass	0.18
Egg	1, average size	0.17
Cheddar cheese	30 g	0.15
Ground beef	100 g	0.15

Riboflavin is rapidly destroyed by exposure to bright light. Milk should be kept in opaque containers away from light to preserve its riboflavin content. Riboflavin is relatively heat resistant but, because of its high water solubility, significant amounts of riboflavin can be lost in cooking water.

Recommended Daily Intakes

Recommended daily intakes for riboflavin (mg)		
	Prevention of deficiency	
	UK RNI (1991)	USA DRI (1998)
Adult men	1.3	1.3
Adult women*	1.1	1.1
	Therapeutic dose range	
	Pauling (1986)	Werbach (1990/99)
Adult men	50–100	10–400
Adult women*	50–100	10–400

* excluding pregnant or lactating women

Preferred From and Dosage

Riboflavin	Take between or with meals, preferably with the dose divided throughout the day

Use in Prevention and Therapy

Detoxification. Riboflavin helps the liver detoxify chemicals, pesticides, and other environmental toxins.

Antioxidant functions. Riboflavin functions as an antioxidant throughout the body and may be especially important in the lens of the eye. Ample intake of riboflavin can reduce the risk of developing cataract. As a cofactor of glutathione reductase, riboflavin helps maintain the body's supply of reduced glutathione, an important antioxidant.[1]

Skin and mucous membranes. Ample riboflavin intake maintains the health of the skin and mucous membranes.[5] It may be beneficial in stomatitis, cheilosis, and skin eruptions and rashes.

Fatigue and depression. In people with increased riboflavin requirements, dietary inadequacy may produce a subclinical deficiency that causes fatigue, depression, and personality changes.[6] This may respond to riboflavin supplementation.

helps migraines in large doses

Toxicity

There are no reports of toxicity associated with riboflavin supplementation. Large doses of riboflavin will produce a harmless yellow color in the urine.

References

1. Christensen HN. Riboflavin can protect tissues from oxidative injury. Nutr Rev. 1993;51:149.
2. McCormick DB. Riboflavin. In: Shils ME, Olson JA, Shike M, Ross AC, eds. Modern Nutrition in Health and Disease. Baltimore: Williams & Wilkins; 1999.
3. McCormick DB. Two interconnected B vitamins: Riboflavin and pyridoxine. Physiol Rev. 1989;69:1170.
4. Pinto JT, et al. Mechanisms underlying the differential effects of ethanol upon the bioavailabilty of riboflavin and flavin adenine dinucleotide. J Clin Invest. 1987;79:1343.
5. Munoz N, et al. Effect of riboflavin, retinol and zinc on micronuclei of buccal mucosa and of esophagus: A randomized double-blind intervention study in China. J Natl Cancer Inst. 1987;79:687.
6. Rivlin R. Riboflavin. In: Ziegler EE, Filer LJ, eds. Present Knowledge in Nutrition. Washington DC: ILSI Press; 1996:167.

Niacin (Vitamin B3)

Two main forms of niacin are found in foods: nicotinic acid and nicotinamide. Both can be converted into active forms of niacin in the body. Niacin is unique among the vitamins in that requirements for it can be at least partially satisfied by intake of tryptophan, which is then converted by the liver into niacin. Because 60 mg of tryptophan can be converted into about 1 mg of niacin, dietary requirements for niacin are described in terms of niacin equivalents (NEs): 1 mg of niacin = 60 mg of tryptophan = 1 NE.[1]

Functions

Cellular metabolism. Niacin is required for the function of more than 200 enzymes throughout the body. It participates in biosyntheses of compounds such as fatty acids and steroids. It is vital for the breakdown of fuel molecules for energy. Niacin also plays important roles in supporting the health of the skin and mucous membranes, nervous system, and digestive system.

DNA replication and repair. Niacin is vital for synthesis of proteins (histones) that are found in cell nuclei closely bound to DNA. These proteins are important in that they aid in the repair of breaks in the DNA strand caused by oxidation, radiation, or other environmental stressors.

Antioxidant functions. Niacin plays an important role in the body's antioxidant systems,[1] particularly in the liver.

Blood sugar regulation. Niacin is a component of the glucose tolerance factor (GTF), a poorly characterized substance that, together with insulin, helps to control blood glucose.[2]

Fat and cholesterol metabolism. Nicotinic acid lowers levels of total and LDL cholesterol in the blood,[3] while increasing levels of HDL cholesterol (the healthy, protective form of cholesterol).

can cause ↑ liver enzymes
liver facial flush

Fig. 3.**4**: Treatment of hyperlipidemia with niacin.

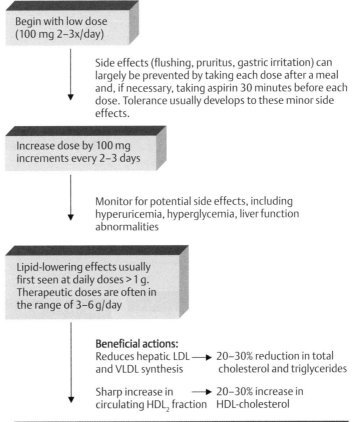

Begin with low dose (100 mg 2–3x/day)

Side effects (flushing, pruritus, gastric irritation) can largely be prevented by taking each dose after a meal and, if necessary, taking aspirin 30 minutes before each dose. Tolerance usually develops to these minor side effects.

Increase dose by 100 mg increments every 2–3 days

Monitor for potential side effects, including hyperuricemia, hyperglycemia, liver function abnormalities

Lipid-lowering effects usually first seen at daily doses > 1 g. Therapeutic doses are often in the range of 3–6 g/day

Beneficial actions:
Reduces hepatic LDL ⟶ 20–30% reduction in total
and VLDL synthesis   cholesterol and triglycerides

Sharp increase in   ⟶ 20–30% increase in
circulating HDL_2 fraction   HDL-cholesterol

10–15% reduction in mortality from coronary heart disease[1]

1. Canner P, et al. 15-year mortality in coronary drug project patients: Long term benefit with niacin. J Amer Coll Cardiol 1986; 1245.

Increased Risk of Deficiency

● Dietary deficiency can quickly deplete the body's reserves of niacin, and signs of deficiency may develop within 2 to 4 weeks. Poor intake of protein with inadequate tryptophan increases the risk of deficiency.

● Deficiencies of vitamin B6 or riboflavin impair conversion of tryptophan to niacin and reduce niacin stores in the body.[1]

● Inflammatory bowel disease and other digestive disorders cause malabsorption of niacin.[4]

● Heavy alcohol consumption interferes with absorption and metabolism of niacin.

Signs and Symptoms of Deficiency (Pellegra)

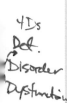

* Red, fissured, scaly, hardened patches on the skin in areas exposed to sunlight, such as elbows, knees, backs of the neck and hands, and forearms
* Inflamed, painful swollen tongue; fissures on lips
* Diminished digestive secretions, loss of appetite, bloating, flatulence, vomiting, and diarrhea
* Anxiety, apprehension, fatigue, irritability, headache, insomnia, emotional instability, confusion and disorientation
* Hallucinations, paranoia, severe depression

Good Dietary Sources

Food	Serving size (g)	mg NE
Calf liver	100	14
Peanuts	100	14
Tuna	100	10.5
Chicken, breast	100	10.5
Halibut	100	5.9
Mushrooms	100	4.7

Because most proteins contain about 1% tryptophan, a diet containing more than100 g protein/day will theoretically supply about 1 NE/day. However, not all tryptophan is converted to niacin. Dietary tryptophan is used by tissues first for protein and amino acid needs, and only then for synthesis of niacin. Niacin present in food is relatively stable during storage but will leach into water during cooking.

Recommended Daily Intakes

Recommended daily intakes for niacin (mg)		
	Prevention of deficiency	
	UK RNI (1991)	USA DRI (1998)
Adult men	16–17	16
Adult women*	12–13	14
	Therapeutic dose range	
	Pauling (1986)	Werbach (1990/99)
Adult men	300–600	100–4500
Adult women*	300–600	100–4500

* excluding pregnant or lactating women

Preferred Form and Dosage

Niacinamide or nicotinic acid	Take with meals, preferably with the dose divided throughout the day. The side effects of high doses of nicotinic acid are reduced if taken on a full stomach

Use in Prevention and Therapy

Mental illness. Niacinamide therapy may be effective in schizophrenia, particularly in conjunction with traditional medical treatment. It may be useful in the treatment of tardive dyskinesia. Niacinamide may be beneficial in obsessive-compulsive and anxiety disorders in that it may have a mild tranquilizing effect.

Atherosclerosis. Nicotinic acid improves the blood lipid profile; lowering total and LDL cholesterol and raising HDL cholesterol. It also dilates blood vessels and lowers blood pressure.[5,6] By these actions, it can reduce the risk of heart attack and stroke.

Arthritis. Niacin may be beneficial in the treatment of osteoarthritis, and particularly degenerative arthritis affecting the knee.[7]

Diabetes. Niacinamide may slow down the development of nephropathy in diabetes. Also, when given to newly diagnosed type 1 diabetics it can significantly delay the need for insulin therapy.[8]

Protection against environmental toxins. Niacin has antioxidant functions, particularly in the liver, and may help protect against damage from pesticides, chemicals, alcohol, and drugs.[1]

Headache. Nicotinic acid may be beneficial in the prevention of headaches associated with premenstrual syndrome and migraine.

Circulatory disorders. The dilation of small blood vessels by nicotinic acid can improve blood flow of nutrients and oxygen to the skin, heart, and brain and improve their function.

Toxicity

Large doses (>500 mg) of nicotinic acid (but not niacinamide) can cause dilation of capillaries, producing tingling and flushing of the skin. At doses of more than 2.5 g/day, niacin can produce hypotension and dizziness, increased uric acid in the blood, liver dysfunction, increased risk of peptic ulcer, and increased blood sugar.[9,10] These effects usually lessen in severity as the body adapts to the niacin over time and are reversible when the nicotinic acid is discontinued. Sustained-release, compared with short-acting, forms of nicotinic acid are associated with increased side effects.[10] Flushing of the skin is usually worse if nicotinic acid is taken on an empty stomach, therefore it should be taken just after meals. Niacin in the form of niacinamide does not produce these side effects.

References

1. Jacob RA, Swenseid ME. Niacin. In: Ziegler EE, Filer LJ, eds. Present Knowledge in Nutrition. Washington DC: ILSI Press; 1996.
2. Urberg M, et al Evidence for synergism between chromium and nicotinic acid in the control of glucose tolerance in elderly humans. Metabolism. 1987;38:896.
3. Luria MH. Effect of low-dose niacin on high density lipoprotein cholesterol and total cholesterol/high density lipoprotein cholesterol concentration. Arch Intern Med. 1988;148:2493.
4. Zaki I, Millard L. Pellagra complicating Crohn's disease. Postgrad Med J. 1995;71:496.
5. Holvoet P, Collen D. Lipid lowering and enhancement of fibrinolysis by niacin. Circulation. 1995;92:698.
6. Canner PL, et al. Fifteen year mortality in coronary drug project patients: Long term benefit with niacin. J Am Coll Cardiol. 1986;8:1245.
7. Hoffer A. Treatment of arthritis by nicotinic acid and nicotinamide. Can Med Assoc J. 1959;81:235.
8. Pozzilli P, et al. Meta-analysis of nicotinamide treatment in patients with recent-onset IDDM. Diabetes Care. 1996;19:1357.
9. Combs GF. The Vitamins: Fundamental Aspects of Nutrition and Health. San Diego: Academic Press; 1998.
10. Bendich A. Safety issues regarding the use of vitamin supplements. Ann NY Acad Sci. 1992;669:300.

Vitamin B6

Vitamin B6 (also called pyridoxine) from dietary sources is converted in the body to its active form of pyridoxal-5-phosphate (PLP). Activation of vitamin B6 requires adequate zinc and riboflavin. PLP is the major form of vitamin B6 circulating in the blood and is a coenzyme involved in more than 100 metabolic reactions in the body.[1] Because total body stores of vitamin B6 are low, only about 150 mg, a steady supply of vitamin B6 is essential to avoid deficiency.

Functions

Protein synthesis. PLP plays a central role in the metabolism and interconversion of amino acids and the synthesis of new proteins. For example, collagen synthesis is dependent on vitamin B6.

Maintenance of normal blood sugar levels. PLP is vital for conversion of protein and carbohydrate stores into glucose to support blood sugar between meals.[2]

Niacin formation. PLP is essential for conversion of tryptophan to niacin.

Lipid metabolism. PLP plays a central role in fat metabolism. It is important for synthesis of lipids that form the myelin sheath surrounding and protecting nerves. PLP is also vital for production of polyunsaturated fatty acids that are part of cell membranes.[3]

Red blood cell function. PLP is important in hemoglobin synthesis and oxygen transport by red blood cells.

Neurotransmitter synthesis. PLP is essential for the formation of several neurotransmitters, including serotonin (from trytophan), dopamine, and norepinephrine.

Increased Risk of Deficiency

● Rapid growth during childhood and adolesence, as well as during pregnancy and lactation, sharply increase vitamin B6 requirements.[4]

● Smoking, alcohol, and coffee all interfere with vitamin B6 metabolism.

● High intakes of protein increase vitamin B6 requirements.

● Older people tend to consume diets low in vitamin B6[5] and, compared with younger adults, absorb vitamin B6 less efficiently.[6]

● Many common drugs (including oral contraceptive pills[7]) can impair vitamin B6 status and produce deficiency (see Appendix I).

● Vitamin B6 deficiencies are common in many chronic diseases, including asthma, coronary heart disease, diabetes, kidney failure, rheumatoid arthritis, and cancer of the breast, bladder, and lymph nodes.

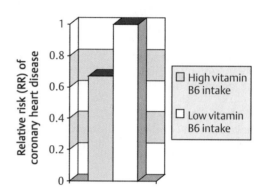

Fig. 3.**5: Vitamin B6 intake and coronary heart disease.** In 80 000 women, those with the highest intakes of vitamin B6 (median intake 4.6 mg/day) had a risk of coronary heart disease one-third lower than those with low intakes (1.1 mg/day). (From Rimm EB, et al. JAMA. 1998;279:359)

● Vitamin B6 is poorly absorbed by people with chronic digestive problems, such as diarrhea, liver problems, or irritable bowel syndrome.

Signs and Symptoms of Deficiency

• Reddened, scaly, greasy, painful, and itchy patches on the skin (especially around the nose, mouth, ears, and the genital area)
• Painful fissures and cracks at the angles of the mouth and on the lips. Smooth, purplish, painful tongue. Swollen and sore throat
• Anemia
• Weakened response of white blood cells to infection, decreased antibody production
• Abnormal brain-wave patterns, muscle twitching, convulsions
• Depression, irritability, anxiety, confusion, headache, insomnia
• Burning, tingling in hands and feet, difficulty walking
• Possible increased risk of atherosclerosis due to increased total cholesterol and LDL-cholesterol in the blood, and reduced levels of HDL-cholesterol
• Possible increased risk of calcium-oxalate kidney stones

Deficiency is usually found in conjunction with deficiencies of the other B vitamins, particularly niacin and riboflavin.

Good Dietary Sources

Food	Serving size	mg
Calf liver	100 g	0.9
Potatoes	1, average size	0.7
Banana	1, average size	0.6
Lentils	100 g	0.6
Brewer's yeast	10 g	0.44
Trout	100 g	0.35
Spinach	100 g	0.2

Vitamin B6 is sensitive to heat and light and is quicky lost into water during cooking. Modern food-processing techniques, such as dehydration and heat processing, can produce losses of 10–50% of the vitamin. High-fiber foods contain compounds that reduce the bioavailability of vitamin B6.[3] For example, the bioavailability of the vitamin contained in soybeans (rich in fiber) is less than half that of the vitamin contained in fish and meat.

Recommended Daily Intakes

Recommended daily intakes for vitamin B6 (mg)		
	Prevention of deficiency	
	UK RNI (1991)	USA DRI (1998)
Adult men	1.4	1.3–1.7
Adult women*	1.2	1.3–1.5
	Therapeutic dose range	
	Pauling (1986)	Werbach (1990/99)
Adult men	50–100	10–1500
Adult women*	50–100	10–1500

* excluding pregnant or lactating women

Preferred Form and Dosage Schedule

Pyridoxine hydrochloride is generally preferable to pyridoxal-5-phosphate (PLP) because it moves more easily through cell membranes and can cross the blood-brain barrier. However, in conditions that impair conversion of pyridoxine hydrochloride to PLP, such as liver disease and zinc or magnesium deficiency, PLP may be preferable	Take between or with meals, preferably with the dose divided throughout the day. People who have altered sleep patterns when taking vitamin B6 should take most of their daily dose in the morning.

Active form best PLP - less toxic (handwritten annotation)

Use in Prevention and Therapy

Skin disorders. Vitamin B6 may be of benefit in skin eruptions and rashes, including acne and seborrheic dermatitis.

Food allergy. Vitamin B6 can reduce sensitivity and allergy to food additives and preservatives, such as monosodium glutamate (MSG) and sulfites.

Bronchial asthma. Treatment with vitamin B6 can reduce the severity and frequency of asthmatic episodes in children and adults.

Atherosclerosis. Vitamin B6 has multiple beneficial actions in the prevention and treatment of coronary heart disease and peripheral vascular disease. It reduces the tendency for platelets to clump together, lowers LDL cholesterol and raises HDL cholesterol, and reduces levels of blood homocysteine.[8,9]

Anemia. Vitamin B6 can be beneficial in certain forms of anemia, alone or in conjunction with iron and vitamin A.

Pregnancy-associated nausea and vomiting. Vitamin B6 may reduce symptoms.

Immunity. Supplemental vitamin B6, particularly in people with marginal intakes, helps boost immunity and increase resistance to infection.[10,11]

Premenstrual syndrome (PMS). Vitamin B6 can be beneficial in the prevention of mood swings, edema, acne, and breast tenderness characteristic of PMS.[12]

Mood lability and depression. The oral contraceptive pill can induce mood lability and depression. This syndrome may be due to impaired vitamin B6 metabolism and may respond to vitamin B6 supplements.[7]

Arthritis. Certain forms of arthritis, particularly swelling and inflammation in the joints of the fingers, as well as chronic tenosynovitis, may benefit from vitamin B6 therapy.

Kidney stones. Vitamin B6 supplements reduce the amount of oxalate excreted in the urine and may help prevent kidney stones in people with hyperoxaluria.[13]

Nerve disorders. Carpal tunnel syndrome may respond to vitamin B6.[14] Other forms of nerve inflammation and neuropathy may also benefit from vitamin B6 therapy.[15]

Psychological disorders. Because of its role in neurotransmitter synthesis, especially of serotonin, vitamin B6 may be effective in depression, insomnia, nervousness, and anxiety. Certain forms of schizophrenia may respond to therapy with vitamin B6 and zinc.

Epilepsy. Vitamin B6 may be of benefit in certain forms of infant and childhood epilepsy.

Toxicity

Long-term use of very high doses of vitamin B6 (>1000 mg/day) may cause a peripheral nerve condition characterized by numbness and tingling in the hands and feet. This is thought to occur when the liver's capacity to convert vitamin B6 to PLP is exceeded. For this reason, when very high doses are used in therapy, supplements of PLP may be preferred to vitamin B6, as PLP may be associated with less toxicity. Doses of vitamin B6 not exceeding 500 mg/day, or higher doses for short periods (days to weeks), are nontoxic in healthy persons. Very high doses of vitamin B6 during lactation may reduce milk production.

References

1. Bender DA. Novel functions of vitamin B6. Proc Nutr Soc. 1994;53:625.
2. Bitsch R. Vitamin B6. Int J Vitam Nutr Res 1993;63:278.
3. Leklem JE. Vitamin B6. In: Ziegler EE, Filer LJ, eds. Present Knowledge in Nutrition. Washington DC: ILSI Press; 1996.
4. Driskell JA. Vitamin B6 requirements in humans. Nutr Res. 1994;14:293.
5. van-der Wielen RP, et al. Vitamin B6 malnutrition among elderly Europeans: The SENECA study. J Gerontol A Biol Sci Med Sci. 1996;51:B417.
6. Russell RM, Suter PM. Vitamin requirements of elderly people: An update. Am J Clin Nutr. 1993;58:4.
7. Leklem JE. Vitamin B6 requirement and oral contraceptive use–a concern? J Nutr. 1986;116:475.
8. Chasan-Taber L, et al. A prospective study of folate and vitamin B6 and risk of myocardial infarction in US physicians. J Am Coll Nutr. 1996;15;136.
9. Ellis JM, McCully KS. Prevention of myocardial infarction by vitamin B6. Res Commun Mol Pathol Pharmacol. 1995;89:208.
10. Bender DA. Non-nutritional uses of vitamin B6. Br J Nutr. 1999;81:7.
11. Rall LC, Meydani SN. Vitamin B6 and immune competence. Nutr Rev. 1993;51:217.
12. De Souza MC, et al. A synergistic effect of a daily supplement for one month of 200 mg magnesium plus 50 mg vitamin B6 for the relief of premenstrual symptoms: a randomized, double-blind crossover study. J Womens Health Gend Based Med. 2000;9:131.
13. Mitwalli A, et al. Control of hyperoxaluria with large doses of pyridoxine in patients with kidney stones. Int Urol Nephrol. 1988;20(4):353.
14. Jacobsen MD, et al. Vitamin B6 therapy for the carpal tunnel syndrome. Hand Clin. 1996;12:253.
15. Rogers KS, Mohan C. Vitamin B6 metabolism in diabetes. Bichem Med Metab Biol. 1994;52:10.

Folic Acid

Body reserves of folic acid are low–about 5–10 mg, roughly half of which is in the liver. A diet low in folate produces deficiency signs within 2–3 weeks. Most of the folate absorbed from the diet is converted to the active form, tetrahydrofolate (THF).[1]

Functions

Cell growth. Folate-containing coenzymes are essential to the production of DNA and RNA in growing and dividing cells. Because of this, cells that rapidly turn over and are re-placed, such as blood cells and cells lining the digestive tract, are particularly dependent on folate.

Protein metabolism. Folate plays a central role in the interconversion of amino acids (such as the detoxification of homocysteine to methionine) (Fig. 3.**6**) and the synthesis of structural and functional proteins.

Fetal growth and development. Folate plays a vital role in normal fetal development, par-ticularly in formation of the central nervous system.[2]

Increased Risk of Deficiency

● Folate deficiency is one of the most com-mon vitamin deficiencies.[3] Modern processed diets are low in folate and most people do not eat enough foods rich in folate, particularly vegetables and whole grains.[4]

● Many commonly used drugs impair folate status, including aspirin, antacids, oral con-traceptive pills, and antibiotics (see Appendix I).

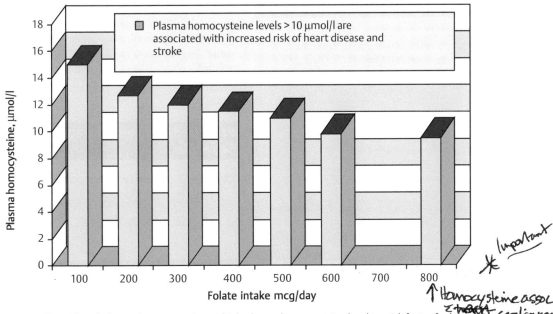

Fig. 3.**6**: **Folic acid and plasma homocysteine.** A high plasma homocysteine level is a risk factor for heart dis-ease and stroke. A strong inverse correlation between folate intake and plasma homocysteine was found in a study of 885 healthy adults. A significant dose-response relationship was evident: folate supplement users had the highest plasma folate levels and the lowest homocysteine levels.
(Source: Tucker KL, et al. JAMA. 1996;276:1879)

● Smoking lowers the body's folate levels.

● Many chronic diseases, including psoriasis, anemia, infections of the digestive or respiratory tracts, and cancer, sharply increase folate requirements. Requirements are also increased by fever, trauma, surgery, or burns. Liver disease interferes with folate metabolism and increases excretion.[1]

● Rapid growth during pregnancy, childhood, and adolescence sharply increases folate requirements. Most pregnant women are folate deficient during the second half of pregnancy.

● Heavy alcohol consumption interferes with absorption, impairs conversion to THF, and increases excretion.

● Deficiency of ascorbic acid accelerates depletion of folate reserves. Deficiency of vitamin B12 also impairs folate metabolism and produces signs of folate deficiency.

Signs and Symptoms of Deficiency

* Impaired cell growth in the digestive tract causes thinning and inflammation of tissues in the mouth, stomach, and intestine. This may cause reduced absorption of nutrients, diarrhea, sore tongue, anorexia, and weight loss
* Anemia with easy fatigue, weakness, shortness of breath, decreased ability to concentrate. Reduced production of platelets can increase risk of abnormal bleeding
* Impairments in white blood cell development reduce immune responses to infection and/or cancer
* Irritability, hostility, forgetfulness, paranoid behavior, depression
* Impaired fetal growth and development, birth defects[2]

Take folic acid + B12 together

Good Dietary Sources

Food	Serving size	μg
Wheat germ	100 g	270
Kidney beans	100 g	250
Spinach	100 g	134
Broccoli	100 g	105
Calf liver	100 g	108
Egg	1, average size	100
Soybeans	100 g	95
Brewer's yeast	10 g	92
Beets	100 g	75

Folate is highly vulnerable to destruction during food processing, storage, and preparation. For example, 50–90% of the folate in many vegetables is lost during prolonged cooking.[1]

Recommended daily intakes for folic acid (μg)

	Prevention of deficiency	
	UK RNI (1991)	USA DRI (1998)
Adult men	200	400
Adult women*	200	400

	Therapeutic dose range	
	Pauling (1986)	Werbach (1990/99)
Adult men	400–800	400–75000
Adult women*	400–800	400–75000

* excluding pregnant or lactating women

Preferred Form and Dosage Schedule

Folic acid	Take between or with meals, preferably with the dose divided throughout the day

Use in Prevention and Therapy

Birth defects. Supplemental folate (400 μg/day) during the weeks leading up to conception and during early pregnancy can reduce the risk of birth defects, particularly defects of the spine (neural tube defects) and cleft lip and palate.[5,6]

Atherosclerosis. Elevated blood homocysteine is a strong risk factor for heart disease, and supplemental folate lowers levels of homocysteine in the blood.[7] Folate supplements may help prevent atherosclerosis (heart attack, stroke, and peripheral vascular disease), particularly in people with elevated homocysteine levels.[7,8]

Psychiatric/nervous disorders. Depression, irritability, and impaired concentration may be the result of mild folate deficiency, and supplementation may be of benefit.[9] Folate may be effective as adjunctive therapy with lithium in the treatment of manic-depressive illness. Symptoms of dementia in elderly people may be improved by folic acid supplementation.[10]

Infection. Because folate deficiency impairs the immune system, supplementation may increase resistance to infection in people with low reserves of folate.

Cancer. Folate, together with vitamin A, may reduce the risk of cervical dysplasia progressing to cervical cancer.[11,12] Folate (along with vitamin B12) can reduce dysplasia in the lungs of smokers and reduce the risk of lung cancer.[13] Folate supplements may also reduce the risk of colon cancer in people with inflammatory bowel diseases.[14]

Toxicity

Folic acid is nontoxic, even at very high doses. Large doses in people with epilepsy may antagonize the actions of anticonvulsant drugs and provoke seizures. The signs of folate deficiency and vitamin B12 deficiency are similar and overlap. Although the hematologic signs of vitamin B12 deficiency respond to folate supplementation, the neurologic defects of vitamin B12 deficiency do not. Therefore, folate supplementation during vitamin B12 deficiency may partially mask the deficiency of B12 and allow the neurologic damage to progress to an irreversible stage.[7] When folate deficiency is suspected, vitamin B12 status should also be determined. If doubt exists, folate supplementation should be accompanied by vitamin B12 supplementation.

References

1. Bailey LB, Gregory JF. Folate metabolism and requirements. J Nutr. 1999;129:779.
2. Steegers-Theunissen RP. Folate metabolism and neural tube defects: A review. Eur J Obstet Gynecol Repro Biol. 1995;61:39.
3. de Bree A, et al. Folate intake in Europe: Recommended, actual and desired intake. Eur J Clin Nutr. 1997;51:643.
4. Cuskelly GJ, et al. Effect of increasing dietary folate on red cell folate: Implications for prevention of neural tube defects. Lancet. 1996;347:657.
5. Czeizel AE, et al. Prevention of the first occurrence of neural-tube defects by periconceptional vitamin supplementation. N Engl J Med. 1992;327:1832.
6. Shaw GM, et al. Risks of orofacial clefts in children born to women using multivitamins containing folic acid periconceptionally. Lancet. 1995;345:393.
7. Brattstrom L. Vitamins as homocysteine-lowering agents. J Nutr. 1996;126:S1276.
8. Boushey CJ, at al. A quantitative assessment of plasma homocysteine as a risk factor for vascular disease. Probable benefits of increasing folic acid intakes. JAMA. 1995;274:1049.
9. Alpert JE, Fava M. Nutrition and depression: the role of folate. Nutr Rev. 1997;55:145.
10. Bottiglieri T. Folate, vitamin B12 and neuropsychiatric disorders. Nutr Rev. 1996;54:382.
11. Giuliano AR, Gapstur S. Can cervical dysplasia and cancer be prevented with nutrients? Nutr Rev. 1998;56:9.
12. Butterworth C, et al. Folate deficiency and cervical dysplasia. JAMA. 1992;268:528.
13. Heimburger D, et al. Improvement in bronchial squamous metaplasia in smokers treated with folate and vitamin B12. JAMA. 1990;259:1525.
14. Lashner BA, et al. Effect of folate supplementation on the incidence of dysplasia and cancer in chronic ulcerative colitis. Gastroenterology. 1991;97:255.

Vitamin B12

Vitamin B12 is a family of related compounds that all contain a cobalt atom (another name for vitamin B12 is cobalamin). Synthetic forms of vitamin B12 are hydroxycobalamin and cyanocobalamin (these do not occur naturally in foods). The two dietary forms of vitamin

B12 are methylcobalamin (methyl-B12) and 5-deoxyadenosylcobalamin (coenzyme-B12). Our bodies contain only very small amounts of vitamin B12–about 2–5 mg, 50–90% of which is stored in the liver.[1]

Shots · Sublingual

Functions

Folate metabolism. Vitamin B12 is vital in the activation of folate to its active form (THF). In vitamin B12 deficiency, tissue stores of folate are "trapped" as inactive forms, and a functional folate deficiency results. This close interdependence of vitamin B12 and folate explains why many symptoms of folate and vitamin B12 deficiency are indistinguishable.

Amino acid metabolism. Vitamin B12 is essential for the conversion of homocysteine (a toxic amino acid) to methionine.[1]

Fat metabolism. Vitamin B12 is a coenzyme in the conversion of methylmalonate to succinate and is required for optimum fat metabolism in cells.

Cell replication. Together with folate, vitamin B12 is essential for the synthesis of nucleic acids and DNA synthesis.

Nervous system. Vitamin B12 is vital for the synthesis of myelin, the protective sheath surrounding many nerves in the periphery, spinal cord, and brain.

Antioxidant status. Vitamin B12 helps maintain glutathione in the reduced form necessary for its antioxidant functions.

Increased Risk of Deficiency

● Gastric secretion of acid and intrinsic factor is diminished in older people. Both are required for optimum vitamin B12 absorption. Therefore, many elderly people are at risk of deficiency.[2]

● Pregnancy and lactation increase vitamin B12 requirements, and if maternal intake is poor, deficiency can occur in both the mother and her baby.

● The liver is the site of vitamin B12 storage and also produces specific blood proteins important for the transport and function of the vitamin. Liver disease can thereby impair vitamin B12 status.

● In pernicious anemia, chronic gastritis with atrophy of the cells that produce intrinsic factor causes severe vitamin B12 deficiency.[3]

● Intestinal diseases, such as tropical sprue, gluten enteropathy, pancreatic disease, Crohn's disease, and chronic enteritis with diarrhea (such as that in AIDS), reduce absorption of vitamin B12.

● Strict vegetarian diets devoid of animal products, milk, and eggs contain no vitamin B12 and may produce vitamin B12 deficiency.[1]

● Heavy alcohol consumption increases the risk of vitamin B12 deficiency by damaging the gastric mucosa and liver.

● Cigarette smoking impairs vitamin B12 status and can trigger visual difficulties (dim vision and "tobacco amblyopia") in chronic smokers.

● Chronic use of para-aminosalicylic acid (PASA), colchicine, neomycin, metformin, cholestyramine, or oral contraceptive pills can increase risk of deficiency.

Signs and Symptoms of Deficiency

- Impaired cell replication leads to atrophy and inflammation of mucous membranes in the mouth and entire digestive tract, sore tongue, reduced absorption of nutrients, constipation, anorexia, and weight loss
- Anemia (megaloblastic) with easy fatigue, weakness, shortness of breath, decreased ability to concentrate
- Reduced platelet production can increase risk of abnormal bleeding
- Impaired white blood cell development reduces immune responses to infection and/or cancer

continued

- Irritability, hostility, forgetfulness, confusion, poor memory, agitation, pychosis (with delusions, hallucinations, and/or paranoid behavior), depression[4]
- Numbness and tingling in hands and feet, sensory loss, unsteady movements, poor muscular coordination, unstable gait

Good Dietary Sources

Food	Serving size	µg
Calf liver	100 g	60
Mussels	100 g	8
Salmon	100 g	3
Beef, filet	100 g	2
Egg	1, average size	1
Hard cheese	30 g	0.6
Milk	1 large glass	0.4

Plant foods, unless they are enriched with the vitamin, contain no vitamin B12. Although our intestinal bacteria synthesize small amounts of vitamin B12-like compounds, these do not contribute to nutritional needs. Therefore, the only significant dietary sources are animal products: meat, seafood, eggs, and milk products.[5] Vitamin B12 is sensitive to heat and substantial amounts can be lost during food preparation; for example, milk boiled for 2 minutes loses 30% of its vitamin B12.

Recommended Daily Intakes

Recommended daily intakes for vitamin B12 (µg)		
	Prevention of deficiency	
	UK RNI (1991)	USA DRI (1998)
Adult men	1	2.4
Adult women*	1	2.4
	Therapeutic dose range	
	Pauling (1986)	Werbach (1990/99)
Adult men	100–200	10–2000
Adult women*	100–200	10–2000

* excluding pregnant or lactating women

Preferred Form and Dosage Schedule

Hydroxycobalamin or adenosylcobalamin	Take between or with meals, preferably with the dose divided throughout the day. In older people intramuscular injection may provide better bioavailability

Use in Prevention and Therapy

Psychiatric/nervous disorders. Deficiency in the central nervous system (even with normal blood levels of vitamin B12 and without anemia[6]) may cause psychosis, depression, and/ or mania. Dementia with confusion and memory loss, particularly in the elderly, may benefit from vitamin B12.[7,8]

Appetite, vigor, and energy. Levels may improve with vitamin B12 supplementation, particularly in situations of increased stress, such as chronic illness or recovery from trauma or surgery.[9]

Atherosclerosis. Vitamin B12 is helpful in the prevention and therapy of atherosclerosis associated with high levels of blood homocysteine. Vitamin B12, together with folate, lowers blood levels by converting homocysteine to methionine.[1]

Lung cancer. Vitamin B12, together with folate, can reduce the number of smoking-induced precancerous cells in the lungs, thereby reducing risk of lung cancer.[10]

Allergic disorders. Vitamin B12 may benefit people with allergic asthma, skin allergies, and atopic eczema. It may also reduce food allergies, particularly to sulfites and other food preservatives.

Peripheral nerve disorders. Supplemental vitamin B12 may reduce the pain and symptoms of nerve disorders (such as postherpetic and trigeminal neuralgias) and accelerate healing of traumatic nerve injuries. Vitamin

B12 may also benefit diabetic patients with neuropathy.

Toxicity

There are no reports of toxicity in healthy adults, even at very high oral doses (>10 mg/day). Intravenous injection is rarely associated with allergic reactions, which can be severe (very likely caused by another component of the injected solution, not the vitamin B12).

References

1. Herbert V. Vitamin B12. In: Ziegler EE, Filer LJ, eds. Present Knowledge in Nutrition. Washington DC: ILSI Press; 1996.
2. Lindenbaum J, et al. Prevalence of cobalamin deficiency in the Framingham elderly population. Am J Clin Nutr. 1994;60:2.
3. Pruthi RK, Tefferi A. Pernicious anemia revisted. Mayo Clin Proc. 1994;69:144.
4. Oren DA, et al. A controlled trial of cyanocobalamin (vitamin B12) in the treatment of winter seasonal affective disorder. J Affect Disord. 1994;32:197.
5. Markle HV. Cobalamin. Crit Rev Clin Lab Sci. 1996;33:247.
6. Green R, Kinsella LJ. Current concepts in the diagnosis of cobalamin deficiency. Neurology. 1995;45:1435.
7. van Goor L, et al. Review: Cobalamin deficiency and mental impairment in elderly people. Age Aging. 1995;24:536.
8. Teunisse S, et al. Dementia and subclinical levels of vitamin B12: Effect of replacement therapy on dementia. J Neurol. 1996;243:522.
9. Schilling RF. Vitamin B12 deficiency: Underdiagnosed and overtreated? Hosp Prac 1995;7:47.
10. Heimburger D, et al. Improvement in bronchial squamous metaplasia in smokers treated with folate and vitamin B12. JAMA. 1990;259:1525.

Pantothenic Acid Vit B5

The biologically active form of pantothenic acid is coenzyme A (CoA). Pantothenic acid, as CoA, is an intracellular carrier for small carbon-containing groups and participates in more than 100 pathways of intermediate metabolism.[1]

Functions

Energy production. CoA transfers carbon groups formed from the breakdown of fatty acids and sugars into pathways of energy production.

Fatty acid synthesis. CoA is essential for the synthesis of fatty acids and their incorporation into cell membranes. It is also required for the synthesis of cholesterol, steroid hormones, and vitamins A and D.

Protein and amino acid synthesis. Pantothenic acid plays an important role in the synthesis of leucine, arginine, and methionine. It is essential for the formation of hemoglobin and the electron-carrying cytochrome proteins of the mitochondrial respiratory chain.[2]

Acetylcholine formation. Pantothenic acid is essential for formation of the neurotransmitter acetylcholine.

Increased Risk of Deficiency

Because pantothenic acid is widely prevalent in foods, frank deficiency in humans is very rare. Subclinical deficiency may occur, usually in conjunction with other B-vitamin deficiencies, with chronic illness, heavy alcohol consumption, or during hypocaloric dieting for weight-loss.[2]

Signs and Symptoms of Deficiency

- Vomiting and stomach pains
- Fatigue
- Headache
- Depression
- Insomnia
- Numbness and burning sensation in lower legs and feet
- Joint aches
- Anemia
- Muscle aches
- Fading of hair color
- Reduced immunity: impaired antibody response

Good Dietary sources

Food	Serving size	mg
Calf liver	100 g	7.9
Peanuts	100 g	2.6
Peas	100 g	2.1
Soybeans	100 g	1.9
Brown rice	100 g	1.7
Lobster	100 g	1.7
Watermelon	100 g	1.6
Broccoli	100 g	1.3
Egg	1, average size	0.9
Brewer's yeast	10 g	0.7

Recommended Daily Intakes

Recommended daily intakes for pantothenic acid (mg)		
	Prevention of deficiency	
	UK RNI (1991)	USA DRI (1998)
Adult men	3–7	5
Adult women*	3–7	5 _500_
	Therapeutic dose range	
	Pauling (1986)	Werbach (1990/99)
Adult men	100–200	50–1000
Adult women*	100–200	50–1000

* excluding pregnant or lactating women

Pantothenic acid supplements are often available as the salt of calcium or sodium (e.g., as calcium pantothenate) or as pantothenol, an alcohol that is readily converted by the body to pantothenic acid.

Preferred Form and Dosage Schedule

Calcium pantothenate or pantothenol	Take between or with meals, preferably with the dose divided throughout the day

Use in Prevention and Therapy

Microcytic anemia. Pantothenic acid (through its role in hemoglobin synthesis) in conjunction with iron supplementation may benefit cases of microcytic anemia, particularly if unresponsive to iron alone.

Acne. Pantothenic acid may be effective in acne.[3]

Lupus erythematosus. Lupus erythematosus and other autoimmune disorders may benefit from supplemental calcium pantothenate, alone or in conjunction with vitamin E.

Tiredness and fatigue. Subclinical pantothenic acid deficiency produces tiredness and fatigue; supplementation in people with marginal status may be of benefit. _B5 + B6 esp. important B supplement_

Arthritis. Pantothenic acid deficiencies are often found in patients with osteoarthritis and rheumatoid arthritis. Calcium pantothenate may be effective in both forms of arthritis, reducing joint pain and stiffness.[4]

Wound healing. Pantothenic acid may enhance wound healing after trauma or operation.[5]

Dyslipidemia. Pantothenic acid may be useful in the management of individuals with dyslipidemia.[6]

Toxicity

High doses of orally administered calcium pantothenate are nontoxic in humans. Doses as high as 10 g have been taken for several months without toxicity.

References

1. Tahiliani AG, Beinlich CJ. Pantothenic acid in health and disease. Vitam Hormon. 1991;46:165.
2. Plesofsky-Vig N. Pantothenic acid. In: Ziegler EE, Filer LJ, eds. Present Knowledge in Nutrition. Washington DC: ILSI Press; 1996.

3. Leung LH. Pantothenic acid deficiency as the pathogenesis of acne vulgaris. Med Hypotheses. 1995;44:490.
4. General Practitioner's Research Group. Calcium pantothenate in arthritis conditions. Practitioner. 1980;224:208.
5. Vaxman F, et al. Effect of pantothenic acid and ascorbic acid supplementation on the human skin wound healing process. Eur Surg Res. 1995;27:158.
6. Arsenio L, et al. Effectiveness of long-term treatment with pantethine in patients with dyslipidemia. Clin Therapeutics. 1986;8:537.

Biotin

Biotin is an essential part of enzyme systems that transfer CO_2 groups between molecules in the metabolism of carbohydrates, lipids, and amino acids. Body stores of biotin are small. Diets lacking biotin will produce signs of deficiency within 3–4 weeks.[1]

B like vitamin often added to B complex

Functions

Glucose synthesis. A key initial step in gluconeogenesis is dependent on a biotin-containing enzyme.

Fat metabolism. Key metabolic steps in the synthesis and breakdown of fatty acids are dependent on biotin-containing enzymes. Essential fatty acid metabolism, such as conversion of linoleic acid to various eicosanoids (see pp. 89), are dependent on biotin.

Amino acid metabolism. Biotin-containing enzymes are necessary for the breakdown of amino acids, such as threonine, isoleucine, and methionine, for use as energy.

Cell division and growth. Biotin plays an important role in DNA synthesis.

Increased Risk of Deficiency

● Biotin requirements are increased by pregnancy and lactation.

● Anticonvulsant drugs reduce absorption of biotin.[2] Oral antibiotics also increase risk of deficiency.

● Hypocaloric dieting for weight loss can produce biotin deficiency. In addition, diets that contain raw eggs can produce deficiency (raw egg white contains avidin, a biotin binder that prevents absorption).[3]

Signs and Symptoms of Deficiency

- Anorexia and nausea
- Muscle aches
- Numbness and tingling in the extremities
- Flaky, reddened patches on the skin, especially around the nose and mouth
- Hair loss and baldness
- Immunodeficiency
- Changes in mental status, depression, fatigue, anxiety
- Seizures, developmental delays (in infants with inherited defects)

Good Dietary Sources

Food	Serving size	µg
Calf liver	100 g	75
Soybeans	100 g	60
Brewer's yeast	30 g	30
Whole wheat	50 g	22
Oatmeal	100 g	20
Mushrooms	100 g	16
Egg	1, average size	12
Avocado	100 g	10
Milk	1 large glass	3.5

Small amounts of biotin are synthesized by intestinal bacteria and may contribute to nutritional requirements.[4,5]

Recommended Daily Intakes

Recommended daily intakes for biotin (µg)		
	Prevention of deficiency	
	UK RNI (1991)	USA DRI (1998)
Adult men	10–200	30
Adult women*	10–200	30
	Therapeutic dose range Werbach (1990/99)	
Adult men	300–16000	
Adult women*	300–16000	

* excluding pregnant or lactating women

Preferred Form and Dosage Schedule

Biotin	Take between or with meals, preferably with the dose divided throughout the day

Use in Prevention and Therapy

Impaired biotin metabolism. Inherited syndromes of impaired biotin metabolism in children are responsive to supplemental biotin.[1]

Anticonvulsant therapy. Biotin supplements during chronic anticonvulsant therapy reduce the risk of biotin deficiency.

Diabetes. Biotin supplements may help control blood glucose in diabetes.[6]

Dermatologic disorders. Seborrheic dermatoses and other forms of scaly skin rash may respond to biotin, particularly when taken as part of a complete vitamin B complex in conjunction with essential fatty acids (omega-6 and omega-3 fatty acids).[1] These dermatologic disorders may be due to impairments of essential fatty acid metabolism in the skin, produced by abnormal biotin metabolism or deficiency.

Hair and nail disorders. People with dry, brittle hair and fingernails may benefit from biotin.[7]

Toxicity

Biotin is nontoxic, even at chronic oral doses greater than 60 mg/day.

References

1. Mock DM. Biotin. In: Shils ME, Olson JA, Shike M, Ross AC, eds. Modern Nutrition in Health and Disease. Baltimore: Williams & Wilkins; 1999.
2. Krause KH, et al. Biotin status of epileptics. Ann NY Acad Sci. 1985;447:297.
3. Bonjour JP. Biotin. In: Machlin LJ, ed. Handbook of Vitamins. 2nd ed. New York: Marcel Dekker; 1991.
4. Mock D, et al. Serum concentrations of biotin and biotin analogs increase during acute and chronic biotin supplementation. FASEB J. 1994;8:A921.
5. Bitsch R, et al. Studies on bioavailability of oral biotin doses for humans. Int J Vitam Nutr Res. 1988;59:65.
6. Maebashi M, et al. Therapeutic evaluation of the effect of biotin on hyperglycemia in patients with non-insulin-dependent diabetes. J Clin Biochem Nutr. 1993;14:211.
7. Hochman LG, et al. Brittle nails: Response to daily biotin supplementation. Cutis. 1993:51;303.

Vitamin C (Ascorbic Acid)

Most animals are able to synthesize all the vitamin C they need from dietary sugars; humans, along with other primates, are among the few species of animals unable to synthesize the vitamin.[1] Vitamin C plays an important role in the body's ability to handle physiologic stress during infection, injury, or chronic disease. While most animals are able to increase synthesis of vitamin C during times of stress, humans' strict dependence on dietary sources of the vitamin increases risk of deficiency during stress periods.

Functions

Antioxidant function. Vitamin C is the body's primary water-soluble antioxidant.[2] It is present in the blood, body fluids, and inside all cells and helps protect against oxidation by free radicals. Vitamin C is also important in the conversion (reduction) of iron and copper to the form in which they function as cofactors in many enzyme systems, such as reduced copper in superoxide dismutase (another antioxidant).

Collagen formation. Vitamin C is an essential coenzyme in collagen synthesis. Lack of ascorbic acid results in poorly formed connective tissue in the skin, joints, muscles, and bones.

Carnitine synthesis. Ascorbic acid, together with niacin and vitamin B6, is essential for the formation of carnitine, an amino acid required for breakdown of fats for energy (see pp. 113). Lack of ascorbic acid lowers levels of carnitine and reduces energy production, producing fatigue and muscle weakness.[3]

Neurotransmitter synthesis. Ascorbic acid is essential for the production of norepinephrine and serotonin, two important neurotransmitters in the brain.

Detoxification and excretion of drugs and chemicals. Ascorbic acid helps maintain the enzyme systems in the liver that detoxify and excrete drugs and toxic environmental chemicals (such as pesticides and heavy metals).

Immunocompetence. Vitamin C is important for healthy immune function.[4] It is essential for optimum activity of white blood cells and production of the chemical mediators that direct the immune response. Lack of vitamin C sharply increases vulnerability to infection.

Cholesterol breakdown and excretion. The first key step in the breakdown of cholesterol depends on vitamin C. Cholesterol levels in the liver and blood increase if vitamin C status is impaired.

Promotion of iron absorption. Vitamin C sharply increases non-heme iron absorption from the diet or supplements.

Protection of folate and vitamin E from oxidation. Ascorbic acid protects folate and vitamin E from oxidation and helps maintain these vitamins in their active forms.

Recycles Vit E

Body and blood histamine levels. Vitamin C plays a role in controlling body and blood histamine levels, and blood histamine levels increase when vitamin C status is poor. High levels of histamine can aggravate allergies, asthma, stomach ulcers, and certain psychiatric disorders.

Hormone production. Production of epinephrine and norepinephrine, (the hormones released by the adrenal gland in response to stress) are dependent on adequate vitamin C status. *Used to make adrenaline*

Increased Risk of Deficiency

● Increased physical stress from any cause increases vitamin C requirements, particularly infection, fever, burns, surgery, trauma to soft tissues or bones, high or low temperatures, and chronic illnesses such as hyperthyroidism, rheumatoid arthritis, diabetes, alcoholism, and kidney failure.[5]

● Increased oxidant stress from chemicals, radiation, and heavy metals in the environment deplete body stores of vitamin C.[2]

● Chronic use of drugs such as aspirin and oral contraceptives (see Appendix I) impair vitamin C status.

● Older people, particularly those with chronic illness, are at high risk for vitamin C deficiency. Aging is often associated with decreasing levels of vitamin C in blood and tissues.

● Periods of rapid growth–childhood, adolescence, pregnancy, and lactation–increase vitamin C requirements.

● Regular cigarette smoking sharply increases breakdown and excretion of vitamin C and more than doubles vitamin C requirements.[6]

Signs and Symptoms of Deficiency (Scurvy)

- Impaired connective-tissue synthesis and fragility of blood vessels causes abnormal bleeding: easy bruising, inflamed and bleeding gums, joint stiffness and pain (due to bleeding into joints)
- Build-up of keratin in hair follicles producing roughened "sandpaper skin"
- Impaired wound healing
- Weakness, lassitude, fatigue (may be due to impaired carnitine synthesis)
- Psychologic/neurologic symptoms including depression and personality changes (may be due to impaired neurotransmitter synthesis)
- Impaired immunity with increased risk of infection
- Diminished antioxidant defenses may increase risk of cancer, heart disease, stroke, cataract

Good Dietary Sources

Food	Serving size	mg
Papaya	1, medium	195
Broccoli	100 g	115
Cauliflower	100 g	115
Orange	1, medium	70
Strawberries	100 g	65
Green bell peppers	1, medium	65
Grapefruit	½, medium	60
Potatoes	1, medium	28

Fruits and vegetables supply generous amounts of vitamin C. For example, a double serving of orange juice during breakfast, a mixed salad at lunch, and a generous serving of broccoli and potatoes at dinner would supply about 300 mg. However, many people's diets provide insufficient vitamin C. The main components of the modern Western diet–refined grains, sugar, meat, and milk products–are low in vitamin C. Moreover, vitamin

C is water soluble and easily and irreversibly oxidized, so that the vitamin C content of foods can be significantly reduced by cooking and loss in cooking water. A low intake of vitamin C may produce deficiency symptoms within as little as 1–2 weeks.

Recommended Daily Intakes

Recommended daily intakes for vitamin C (mg)

	Prevention of deficiency	
	UK RNI (1991)	USA DRI (2000)
Adult men	40	90
Adult women*	40	75
	Therapeutic dose range	
	Pauling (1986)	Werbach (1990/99)
Adult men	1000–18 000	50–200 000
Adult women*	1000–18 000	50–200 000

* excluding pregnant or lactating women

The body absorbs over 90% of single doses of vitamin C up to 300 mg. At greater doses absorption efficiency falls: at oral doses of 1000 mg absorption is only 20% (Fig. 3.7).[7] The metabolism of synthetic ascorbic acid is no different from that from natural sources. Body stores of vitamin C are about 1500 mg on intakes of about 100–200 mg/day.[7]

Absorbs up to 500mg in 1 dose

Preferred Form and Dosage Schedule

As ascorbic acid, calcium ascorbate, or sodium ascorbate. Sustained-release forms provide better bioavailability. Buffered forms (salts) are less acidic	Take between or with meals, preferably with the dose divided throughout the day

Vit C + Flavonoid Complex Best supplement

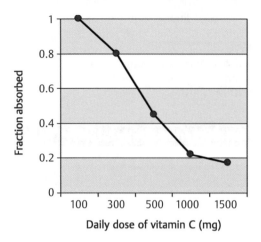

Fig. 3.7: Calculated fractional absorption of vitamin C from increasing oral doses. (Adapted from Blanchard J, et al. Am J Clin Nutr. 1997;66:1165)

Use in Prevention and Therapy

Enhanced ability to fight infection. Vitamin C, at doses of 1 g or more, increases body temperature slightly (enhancing white blood cell function), and is beneficial in lowering blood histamine. High levels of body histamine are associated with decreased immune response and increased nasal and bronchial congestion in colds and flu.[8] Vitamin C stimulates activity of white blood cells[9] and enhances their ability to destroy bacteria and viruses.

Cancer. Vitamin C plays a central role in antioxidant and immune defenses against cancer. It helps detoxify carcinogenic food additives (such as nitrates, pesticides, and other chemicals) and heavy metals. Vitamin C may reduce risk of cancer, particularly cancers of the mouth, larynx, esophagus, stomach, rectum, bladder, breast, pancreas, and uterus.[3]

At minimum 600mg/D

Atherosclerosis. Vitamin C increases breakdown and excretion of cholesterol and protects cholesterol in the body from oxidation (oxidation of cholesterol increases its atherogenicity). It can lower blood cholesterol and triglycerides, while raising HDL cholesterol. Large doses decrease platelet aggregation and may reduce risk of blood clots in the legs and lungs after surgery. In addition, vitamin C supports the strength of blood vessel walls. By these mechanisms, vitamin C may be of benefit in coronary heart disease, thrombotic stroke, and peripheral vascular disease.[10,11]

Allergic disorders. Because of its ability to lower body and blood histamine levels, vitamin C may be beneficial in bronchial asthma, exercise-induced asthma, food allergy, allergic rhinitis (hay fever), and other allergies.[12]

Heavy metal toxicity. Vitamin C plays an important role in protecting the body from heavy metals. It reduces absorption and speeds up detoxification and excretion of heavy metals.

Hemorrhoids. Supplemental vitamin C can soften the stool, strengthen the walls of the veins around the anus, and reduce swelling and tenderness.

Diabetes. Vitamin C transport and metabolism is impaired in diabetes due to high blood sugar levels.[13] Supplemental vitamin C can help speed healing of skin ulcers.

Periodontal disease. Vitamin C reduces inflammation and bleeding of the gums and helps promote healing. Ample vitamin C may reduce susceptibility to periodontal disease.

Smoking and alcohol consumption. Smokers need additional vitamin C to maintain body reserves because of increased breakdown of the vitamin with regular smoking. Vitamin C may help protect the liver from the inflammation, damage, and fat accumulation caused by heavy alcohol consumption.

Wound healing. Vitamin C can enhance the healing of wounds and fractures and be effective in burns, trauma, and surgery.[3]

Iron deficiency. Supplemental vitamin C increases iron absorption from meals and supplements and is a valuable adjunct in the treatment of iron deficiency.[3]

Male infertility. A common form of male infertility is caused by abnormal clumping together of sperm, reducing sperm motility. Supplemental vitamin C can reverse this abnormality and potentially increase fertility in this condition.[14]

Peptic ulcer disease. Vitamin C deficiency may increase risk for ulcers and subsequent hemorrhage. Supplementation may improve healing.

Eye disorders. The antioxidant actions of vitamin C may help prevent cataract.[15] High intraocular pressure due to glaucoma can be reduced with vitamin C.

Toxicity

In several large studies in which 5–10 g of vitamin C were given daily to healthy humans for several years, no adverse effects were demonstrated, other than occasional nausea, loose stools, and diarrhea.[16,17] Although reports have warned of an increased risk of kidney stones with high intakes of vitamin C (oxalate is a metabolite of ascorbic acid), large doses of vitamin C do not increase oxalate excretion into the urine and do not contribute to kidney stones in healthy people.[6] However, in pa-tients with a history of kidney stones high doses of vitamin C should be taken only under their doctor's supervision. There is no evidence to support contentions that high doses of vitamin C can cause conditioned scurvy.[17] High doses of vitamin C may decrease copper absorption, and chewable forms of vitamin C, because of their acidity, can cause erosion of dental enamel.[17]

References

1. Pauling L. Evolution and the need for ascorbic acid. Proc Natl Acad Sci USA. 1970;67:1643.
2. Frei B, et al. Ascorbate is an outstanding antioxidant in human blood plasma. Proc Nat Acad Sci. 1989;86:6377.
3. Sauerberlich HE. Pharmacology of vitamin C. Annu Rev Nutr. 1994;14:371.
4. Gershoff SN. Vitamin C: New roles, new requirements? Nutr Rev. 1993;51:313.
5. Schorah CJ, et al. Total vitamin C, ascorbic acid and dehydroascorbic acid concentrations in plasma of critically ill patients. Am J Clin Nutr. 1996;63:760.
6. Bendich A, Langseth L. The health effects of vitamin C supplementation: a review. J Am Coll Nutr. 1995;14:124.
7. Blanchard J, et al. Pharmacokinetic perspectives on megadoses of ascorbic acid. Am J Clin Nutr. 1997;66:1165.

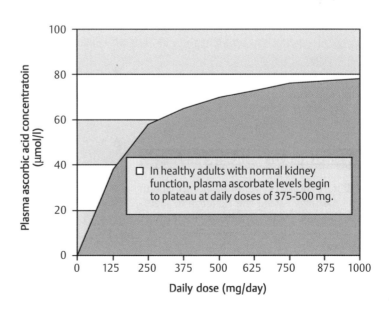

Fig. 3.**8**: Plasma concentration of ascorbic acid at different daily dosing rates. (Adapted from Blanchard J, et al. Am J Clin Nutr. 1997;66:1165)

☐ In healthy adults with normal kidney function, plasma ascorbate levels begin to plateau at daily doses of 375–500 mg.

Plasma ascorbic acid concentratoin (µmol/l)

Daily dose (mg/day)

8. Hemilia H. Vitamin C intake and susceptibility to the common cold. Br J Nutr. 1997;77:59.
9. Jeng KCG, et al. Supplementation with vitamins C and E enhances cytokine production by peripheral blood mononuclear cells in healthy adults. Am J Clin Nutr. 1996;64:960.
10. Ness AR, et al. Vitamin C status and serum lipids. Eur J Clin Nutr. 1996;50:74.
11. Simon JA. Vitamin C and cardiovascular disease: A review. J Am Coll Nutr. 1992;11:107.
12. Kodama M, Kodama T. Vitamin C and the genesis of autoimmune disease and allergy: A review. In Vivo. 1995;9:231.
13. Will JC, Byers T. Does diabetes mellitus increase the requirement for vitamin C? Nutr Rev. 1996;54:193.
14. Dawson EB, et al. Effect of ascorbic acid on male fertility. Ann N Y Acad Sci. 1987;498:312.
15. Jacques PF, et al. Long-term vitamin C supplement use and prevalence of early age-related lens opacities. Am J Clin Nutr. 1997;66:911.
16. Bendich A. Safety issues regarding the use of vitamin supplements. Ann NY Acad Sci. 1992;669:300.
17. Hathcock JN. Safety of vitamin and mineral supplements. In: Bendich A, Butterworth CE, eds. Micronutrients in Health and Disease Prevention. New York: Marcel Dekker; 1991.

Minerals and Trace Elements

Calcium

Functions

Bone and tooth structure. Calcium, together with phosphorus, forms the hydroxyapatite crystals that give strength and rigidity to bone and tooth enamel: 99% of the calcium in the body is in the skeleton.[1]

bone substance

Blood clotting. Calcium is an important component of the blood coagulation cascade.
⊇ Vit K

Muscle contraction. In skeletal and heart-muscle cells, calcium is an intracellular messenger that triggers contraction of the muscle fibers.[2]

Nerve transmission. In nerve cells calcium plays a central role in depolarization of membranes and nerve transmission.

Increased Risk of Deficiency

● If dietary intake of calcium is poor, calcium will be mobilized from the skeleton to maintain circulating levels. Low dietary intake over time can lead to demineralization of the skeleton and increase risk of osteoporosis.[3]

● Chronic use of many medications, including antacids, laxatives, and steroids, produces negative calcium balance by reducing absorption and increasing excretion.

● Malabsorption. Digestive disorders that reduce fat absorption sharply decrease the bioavailabilty of calcium from dietary sources. The unabsorbed fats bind the calcium, making it unavailable for absorption.

● Vitamin D deficiency–common among middle-aged and older adults[4,5] and in the general population during the dark winter months–reduces absorption of calcium from the diet.

● In people with atrophic gastritis (common among the elderly), loss of gastric-acid secretion reduces absorption of calcium from the diet.

● At menopause loss of estrogen accelerates loss of calcium from the skeleton and greatly increases urinary excretion. Up to 15–20% of the bone mineral density of the skeleton can be lost in the 4–6 years around menopause.

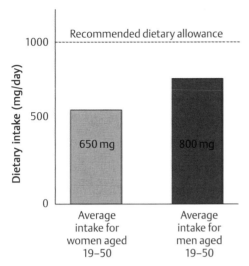

continued

Soybeans, dry	100 g	260
Cabbage	100 g	212
Yoghurt	100 g	205
Whole milk	100 dl	120
Fennel	100 g	109
Broccoli	100 g	105
Salmon	100 g	87
Orange	1, medium	80
Whole-wheat bread	100 g	63

Fig. 3.9: Calcium intake by adults in the USA. Most adults consume much less calcium than is currently recommended. Women are at higher risk of deficiency: 75–85% have inadequate intakes and 25% obtain only 200–300 mg/day.
(Sources: 1997 Dietary Reference Intakes for Calcium, Food and Nutrition Board, National Research Council; Heaney RP. Am J Clin Nutr. 1982.36;986; Human Nutrition Information Service. USDA Report 85–3, 1986)

Signs and Symptoms of Deficiency

- Osteoporosis
- Poor quality enamel predisposing to dental caries
- Muscle cramping and spasm
- Increased irritabilty of nerve cells
- Abnormal blood clotting and increased bleeding after trauma

Good Dietary Sources

Food	Serving size	mg
Cheese (hard cheeses, such as cheddar or Emmentaler, but not cottage cheese, which has little calcium)	100 g	830
Sardines (with bones)	100 g	354

Although milk products are rich sources of bioavailable calcium, they also contain high amounts of protein, phosphorus, and sodium, which can increase calcium loss from the body. Although in many of the industrialized countries more than 80% of dietary calcium comes from dairy products, it is preferable to obtain dietary calcium from a variety of foods–seeds, legumes, grains, vegetables, and calcium-rich mineral water.

Certain dietary components may interfere with absorption and/or retention of calcium 1–3:

- Protein intake >20% of total calories

- Phosphorus (milk products, meat, processed foods, colas)

- Oxalates (in spinach, rhubarb)

- Phytic acid (in whole grains and legumes)

- Sodium

- Coffee and black tea

- Alcohol

In general, the calcium bioavailabilty from milk products and most calcium supplements is approximately 25–35%. Calcium from plant sources tends to be less bioavailable because of the presence of fiber, phytic acid, and oxalates.

For every g of Protein ↑ than RDA need 5.0 mg calcium

Recommended Daily Intakes

Recommended daily intakes for calcium (mg)		
	Prevention of deficiency	
	UK RNI (1991)	USA DRI(1997)
Adult men	700	1000–1200
Adult women[*]	700	1000–1200
	Therapeutic dose range	
	Werbach (1990/99)	
Adult men	1000–3000	
Adult women[*]	1000–3000	

[*] with the exception of pregnant and lactating women

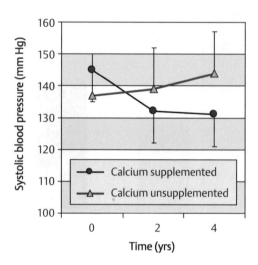

Fig. 3.**10**: **Effect on blood pressure of long-term calcium supplementation in hypertensive women.** A daily supplement of 1500 mg of calcium given to women with hypertension for 4 years produced significant and sustained lowering of systolic blood pressure. In the supplemented group mean systolic pressure fell by 13 mm Hg; in the unsupplemented group it increased by 7 mm Hg.
(Adapted from Johnson NE, et al. Am J Clin Nutr. 1985:42;12)

Preferred Form and Dosage Schedule

✳ *Need best more (double)*

Organically bound calcium (as gluconate, aspartate, citrate, or chelated forms) is generally more bioavailable than inorganic forms (carbonate, phosphate, sulfate), particularly in people with insufficient gastric acid and in many older adults	Take with meals, preferably with the dose divided throughout the day

Use in Prevention and Therapy

Colon cancer. Increased intake of calcium (together with vitamin D) may reduce the risk of developing colon cancer.[6,7] Bile salts and certain fatty acids can stimulate colonic cell proliferation; calcium may exert its protective effect by binding to these substances.

High blood pressure. Calcium can reduce blood pressure in hypertensive patients, particularly those who are salt sensitive or who have low plasma levels of renin (the kidney pressor hormone) (Fig. 3.**10**).[1,8,9] Risk of hypertensive disorders of pregnancy (preeclampsia) may be reduced by ample intake of calcium[10].

Osteoporosis. High calcium intakes during childhood and adolescence help achieve peak bone mass.[11] High intakes during adulthood can reduce or prevent loss of bone calcium associated with aging.[12]

Periodontal disease. Together with proper oral hygeine, calcium may help maintain the alveolar bone that supports the teeth.

Disorders of absorption and metabolism. In digestive disorders that produce malabsorption (such as Crohn and celiac disease) as well as in chronic renal failure, calcium may be beneficial in maintaining body stores.[1,2]

*HTN 1st Line
Calcium
Magnesium
Potassium*

Toxicity

In healthy adults, oral intakes of calcium up to 2 g per day do not have significant side effects or toxicity. People with hyperparathyroidism and people who form calcium-oxalate kidney stones should avoid high intakes of calcium. In healthy adults, high intakes of calcium do not appear to increase the risk of kidney stones. *Best to eat calcium ≈ meals*

References

1. Weaver CM, Heaney RP. Calcium. In: Shils ME, Olson JA, Shike M, Ross AC, eds. Modern Nutrition in Health and Disease. Baltimore: Williams & Wilkins; 1999.
2. Arnaud CD, Sanchez SD. Calcium and Phosphorus. In: Ziegler EE, Filer LJ, eds. Present Knowledge in Nutrition. Washington, DC: ILSI Press; 1996:245.
3. Spencer H, et al. Do protein and phosphorus cause calcium loss? J Nutr. 1988;118:657.
4. Villareal DT, et al. Subclinical vitamin D deficiency in postmenopausal women with low vertebral bone mass. J Clin Endocrinol Metab. 1991;72:628.
5. Thomas MK, et al. Hypovitaminosis D in medical inpatients. N Engl J Med. 1998;338:777.
6. Baron JA, et al. Calcium supplements for the prevention of colorectal adenomas. N Engl J Med. 1999;340:101.
7. Mobarhan S. Calcium and the colon: Recent findings. Nutr Rev. 1999;57:124.
8. Allender PS, et al. Dietary calcium and blood pressure: A meta-analysis of the randomized clinical trials. Ann Intern Med. 1996;124:825.
9. Hermansen K. Diet, blood pressure and hypertension. Br J Nutr. 2000;83:S113.
10. Bucher HC, et al. Effect of calcium supplementation on pregnancy induced hypertension and preeclampsia: A meta-analysis of randomized controlled trials. JAMA. 1996;275:1113.
11. Matkovic V. Calcium intake and peak bone mass. N Engl J Med. 1992;327:119.
12. Bronner F. Calcium and osteoporosis. Am J Clin Nutr. 1994;60:831.

Magnesium *"Great Relaxer"*

The body of an average person weighing 70 kg contains about 20–30 g of magnesium: 60% is in the skeleton and about 30% in tissues (particularly in the liver, heart, and muscle).[1] Magnesium plays an essential role in over 300 different chemical reactions in the body.

Functions

Energy metabolism. Magnesium plays a central role in energy producing reactions in cells: the breakdown and oxidation of glucose, fat, and proteins all require magnesium-dependent enzymes.[1]

Heart and muscles. Magnesium regulates calcium-triggered contraction of heart and muscle cells and is a physiologic calcium-channel clocker.[1] *Calcium contracts Magnesium relaxes*

Blood vessels. Magnesium can produce vasodilation of the coronary and peripheral arteries and lower blood pressure.[2]

Nervous system. Magnesium regulates nerve depolarization and transmission by controlling movement of ions (calcium, potassium) through ion channels in nerve membranes.

Bones and teeth. Magnesium, together with calcium and phosphorus, is important for the structure of bones and teeth.

Increased Risk of Deficiency

● Low dietary intake of magnesium is common[3] and can lead to chronic, marginal deficiency.

● Althletes in strenuous training have increased requirements.[4]

● Periods of rapid growth, such as pregnancy and lactation, as well as childhood and adolescence, increase requirements.

● Use of certain medications: diuretics (thiazides, furosemide), chemotherapy (cisplatin), cortisone preparations, and laxatives decrease magnesium retention by the body (see Appendix I).

● People with diabetes[5] and hyperparathyroidism are at increased risk of deficiency.

● Intestinal malabsorption (such as inflammatory bowel disease, chronic diarrhea, pancreatic disease) reduces absorption of dietary magnesium.

● Regular high intakes of alcohol increase loss of magnesium.

Signs and Symptoms of Deficiency[1,6]

- Muscle cramps and spasm, trembling
- Increased calcium and potassium losses leading to hypocalcemia and hypokalemia
- Personality changes: depression, irritability, difficulty concentrating
- Anorexia, nausea, and vomiting
- Possible increased risk of arrhythmias
- Increased blood triglycerides and cholesterol
- Sodium and water retention
- Impaired action of vitamin D

Good Dietary Sources

Food	Serving size	mg
Soy flour	100 g	245
Whole rice, barley	100 g	160
Wheat bran	25 g	145–150
Sunflower seeds	25 g	105
Whole-wheat bread	100 g	80–100
Lentils	100 g	75
Wheat germ	25 g	60–65
Walnuts, peanuts, almonds	50 g	65–90
Magnesium-rich mineral water	225 ml	80–120
Spinach	100 g	60

Recommended Daily Intakes

Recommended daily intakes for magnesium (mg)		
	Prevention of deficiency	
	UK RNI (1991)	USA DRI (1997)
Adult men	300	400–420
Adult women*	270–300	310–320
	Therapeutic dose range	
	Werbach (1990/99)	
Adult men	300–1000	
Adult women*	300–1000	

* with the exception of pregnant and lactating women (see pp. xx)

Preferred Form and Dosage Schedule

Organically bound forms of magnesium (orotate, gluconate, aspartate, citrate, or chelated forms) are generally more bioavailable than inorganic forms (e.g. sulfate)	Take with meals, preferably with the dose divided throughout the day

Use in Prevention and Therapy

Diabetes mellitus. Magnesium deficiency is common in both type 1 and type 2 diabetes (20–40% of diabetics are deficient) and may reduce insulin sensitivity and increase risk of high blood pressure, heart disease, and eye disease.[5]

Kidney stones. Magnesium (taken with vitamin B6) can reduce the risk of calcium-oxalate kidney stones.[7]

Heart disease. Magnesium may reduce risk of arrhythmia and angina pectoris.[8–10] It can be useful as an adjunct to digitalis, nitrates, and beta-blocker therapy and may help reduce dependence on these medications.

Hypertension. Magnesium can help control high blood pressure, particularly systolic hypertension.[2,11] Many diuretics used to treat hypertension sharply increase magnesium loss. Magnesium is also used to control hypertensive disorders of pregnancy (eclampsia).

Muscle cramps. Magnesium may reduce night-time leg cramps and cramps associated with pregnancy and menstruation.

Anxiety, irritabilty, and insomnia. These symptoms can be the result of a marginal magnesium deficiency[1] and may respond to supplementation.

Migraine headache. Magnesium may reduce frequency and severity of migraine.[12]

Premenstrual syndrome (PMS). Magnesium can help control irritabilty, menstrual cramping, and water retention.

Osteoporosis. Magnesium may be beneficial in maintaining positive calcium balance and reducing the risk of bone mineral loss and osteoporosis.[13]

Toxicity

In healthy adults magnesium is nontoxic at doses up to 1 g/day. In chronic kidney failure, magnesium cannot be excreted efficiently in the urine and supplements (or magnesium-containing antacids or laxatives) can produce high blood levels with symptoms of nausea, vomiting, low blood pressure, and arrhythmia.[1] *Non toxic to d laxative effect*

References

1. Shils M. Magnesium. In: Ziegler EE, Filer LJ, eds. Present Knowledge in Nutrition. 7th ed. Washington DC: ILSI Press; 1996.
2. Zemel PC, et al. Metabolic and hemodynamic effects of magnesium supplementation in patients with essential hypertension. Am J Clin Nutr. 1990;52:665.
3. Pennington JAT, et al. Daily intakes of nine nutritional elements: Analyzed vs. calculated values. J Am Diet Assoc. 1990;90:375.
4. Clarkson PM. Minerals: Exercise performance and supplementation in athletes. J Sports Sci. 1991;9:91.
5. Tosiello L. Hypomagnesemia and diabetes mellitus: A review of the clinical implications. Arch Intern Med. 1996;156:1143.
6. Dreosti IE. Magnesium status and health. Nutr Rev. 1995;53:S23.
7. Labeeuw M, et al. Magnesium in the physiopathology and treatment of renal calcium stones. Presse Med. 1987;16:25.
8. Antman EM. Magnesium in acute myocardial infarction: An overview of the available evidence. Am Heart J. 1996;132:487.
9. Douban S, et al. Significance of magnesium in congestive heart failure. Am Heart J. 1996;132:664.
10. Durlach J, et al. Magnesium and therapeutics. Magnes Res. 1994;7:313.
11. Nadler JL, Rude RK. Disorders of magnesium metabolism. Endocrinol Metab Clin North Am. 1995;24:623.
12. Peikert A, et al Prophylaxis of migraine with oral magnesium: Results from a prospective, multicenter, placebo-controlled and double-blind randomized study. Cephalalgia. 1996;16:257.
13. Sojka JE, Weaver CM. Magnesium supplementation and osteoporosis. Nutr Rev. 1995;53:71.

Potassium

The body contains 30–40 g of potassium; 98% is contained within cells, most of it within skeletal muscle. After calcium and phosphorus it is the third most common mineral in the body.[1]

Easier to get in food

Functions

Energy metabolism. Potassium plays a central role in energy production in cells throughout the body.

Membrane excitability and transport. All nerve transmission, muscle contraction, and hormone secretion from endocrine glands involves carefully timed shifts of cellular potassium and electrical depolarization of cell membranes.[1] For example, propagation of the electrical signal through the myocardium and contraction of the heart are dependent on the proper balance of potassium.[2]

Increased Risk of Deficiency

● Diarrhea and/or vomiting, such as in inflammatory bowel disease or gastroenteritis, increases loss of potassium.

● Chronic kidney failure sharply increases potassium excretion in urine.

● Strenuous,chronic diets for weight loss increase loss of potassium.

● Changes in body pH (both metabolic acidosis and alkalosis) cause potassium depletion.

● Many diuretics (thiazides, furosemide) increase potassium loss in urine and lead to potassium depletion.[1]

● Magnesium deficiency leads to depletion of body potassium.

Signs and Symptoms of Deficiency

- Fatigue, lethargy
- Delayed gastric emptying
- Decreased blood pressure
- Muscle weakness
- Constipation
- Cardiac arrhythmias

Good Dietary Sources

Food	Serving size	mg
Soy flour	100 g	1870
White beans	100 g	1310
Lentils	100 g	810
Bananas	200 g	790
Spinach	100 g	635
Whole-wheat and rye bread	100 g	500
Potatoes	100 g	440
Orange juice	200 ml	300–400
Vegetables	200 g	400–600
Nuts, such as almonds	50 g	225–420
Fish	100 g	300–400
Beef and chicken	100 g	280–350

Recommended Daily Intakes

The minimum daily requirement for potassium in healthy adults is approximately 2 g , and the average daily intake among the adult population is approximately 2–3 g. However, recommended daily intakes to reduce risk of high blood pressure, stroke, and heart disease, are higher–in the range of 4–5 g/day.[1,3]

Use in Prevention and Therapy

High blood pressure. Potassium can lower blood pressure in both hypertensive and normotensive people.[4] In hypertensive people it typically produces a 5–6 and 3–4 mm Hg drop in systolic and diastolic pressure, respectively.[1,5] It is particularly effective in older people and African Americans.[6] A diet containing a high potassium/sodium ratio may help reduce high blood pressure and risk of stroke.[7] *Magnesium & potassium go hand in hand*

Constipation. Regular intake of laxatives to treat constipation may actually worsen symptoms by causing depletion of body potassium. Reducing laxative use, increasing dietary potassium and fiber intake, and increasing exercise can produce more regular bowel habits.

Chronic diarrhea. Potassium-rich diets and potassium supplements may be useful to replace potassium losses in chronic diarrhea.

Cardiac arrhythmias. Potassium depletion (often together with magnesium depletion) produced by diuretic therapy and/or low dietary intake can increase the risk of arrhythmias. People with heart disease and those taking thiazide or 'loop' diuretics should be sure to obtain adequate dietary potassium.

Exercise. Prolonged strenuous exercise or physical activity, particularly in hot weather, may produce loss of potassium in sweat of up to 10 g/day. Potassium depletion can increase muscle fatigue, reduce performance, and cause muscle cramping and spasms.

Used to get 12-16x more Potassium than Sodium; now 3-4x more Sodium

Toxicity

Too much potassium can produce cardiac arrhythmias, weakness and fatigue, nausea, and a fall in blood pressure. In healthy adults daily intakes exceeding 8 g can produce hyperkalemia.[1] In kidney and/or heart disease the daily dose that is toxic is lower; potassium supplements should only be taken under the supervision of a physician.

References

1. Luft K. Potassium and its regulation. In: Ziegler EE, Filer LJ, eds. Present Knowledge in Nutrition. 7th ed. Washington DC: ILSI Press; 1996.
2. Surawicz B. Arrhythmias and electrolyte disturbances. Bull NY Acad Med. 1967;43:1160.
3. National Research Council. Recommended Dietary Allowances, 10th ed. Washington DC: National Academy Press; 1989.
4. Krishna GG, Miller E, Kapoor S. Increased blood pressure during potassium depletion in normotensive men. N Engl J Med. 1989;320:1177.
5. Capuccio FP, Macgregor GA. Does potassium supplementation lower blood pressure? A metaanalysis of published trials. J Hypertens. 1991;9:465.
6. Brancati FL, et al. Effect of potassium supplementation on blood pressure in African Americans on a low potassium diet. A randomized, double blind, controlled trial. Arch Intern Med. 1996;156:61.
7. Khaw KT, et al. Dietary potassium and stroke-associated mortality: A 12-year prospective population study. N Engl J Med. 1987;316:235.

Iron

The average adult man has about 3.8 g of body iron, the average woman 2.3 g.[1] About two-thirds of body iron is in a functional form, circulating in the blood as hemoglobin and in muscle cells as myoglobin. The remainder is stored, primarily in the bone marrow and liver. Because iron is a powerful oxidant and potentially harmful, it is stored and transported carefully bound to protective proteins and surrounded by antioxidants.

Functions

Oxygen transport. Iron plays a critical role in transferring oxygen from the lungs to tissues; 60% of body iron is in red blood cells as hemoglobin.

Muscle function. About 10% of body iron is in the form of myoglobin in muscle cells.[1] Myoglobin stores oxygen within muscle cells and releases it to provide energy during physical activity.

Energy production. Iron is an essential part of the mitochondrial cytochromes that serve as electron carriers in the production of energy as adenosine triphosphate (ATP).[2]

Enzyme function. Iron is an essential cofactor for several important enzyme systems. These include the cytochrome P450 system in liver that breaks down chemicals and toxins, as well as the antioxidant peroxidases and catalases that protect against free radicals.[1,2] Other iron-containing enzymes play roles in the production of brain neurotransmitters and thyroid hormone.

Increased Risk of Deficiency

● Iron deficiency is one of the most common nutritional deficiencies and is particularly prevalent in women and children. It is estimated that 50–70% of young, healthy women have some degree of iron deficiency and that 6–10% of children are iron deficient (Fig. 3.**12**).[2]

● Growth during childhood and adolescence sharply increases the need for iron. Iron requirements during pregnancy double.[2] These high requirements may be difficult to cover unless the diet emphasizes iron-rich foods.

● Iron-poor diets are a comon cause of deficiency in infants and young children (milk has very little iron)[3] and in vegetarians. Plant-based diets contain iron of very low bioavailability. Drinking large amounts of coffee or tea with meals can sharply reduce iron absorption.[4]

● Stomach conditions that reduce gastric-acid secretion sharply reduce the body's ability to absorb iron. These include atrophic gastritis (common among the elderly, see pp. 148), stomach surgery, and chronic use of antacids.

● Heavy menstrual bleeding is a common cause of iron deficiency in women. Chronic, small losses of blood from the gastrointestinal tract can go unnoticed but gradually produce iron deficiency. This can be due to bleeding from hemorrhoids, small ulcers, irritation from aspirin or other NSAIDs, steroid use, or heavy alcohol intake.[1] Frequent blood donation can also produce iron deficiency.

● Iron deficiency is common among long-distance runners and swimmers.[2] This appears to be the result of increased iron turnover and iron loss from the digestive tract.

● Chronic illness reduces the body's ability to mobilize iron from stores, thereby reducing iron supply to the bone marrow for hemoglobin synthesis.

● Deficiencies of vitamin A, vitamin B6, and copper reduce the body's ability to mobilize and transfer body stores of iron.

Signs and Symptoms of Deficiency[2,5]

- Anemia; pallor; dry skin; poorly-formed, up-turned nails; brittle hair
- Quick fatigue, weakness, lack of energy
- Loss of appetite
- Inability to maintain body warmth when exposed to cold
- Learning difficulties, impaired memory and concentration
- Impaired mental and motor development during childhood[6]
- Inflammation of the oral mucosa
- Increased susceptibility to infection[7]
- Increased uptake and vulnerability to environmental lead and cadmium
- In athletes: reduced performance, early fatigue, increased lactic acid production in muscles, and muscle cramping *restless leg syndrome*

continued

- In pregnancy: increased risk of premature birth and of delivering a low birthweight infant

Good Dietary Sources

Food	Serving size (g)	mg
Liver (pork)	100	20
Oysters	100	13
Soy flour, millet	100	9
Liver (beef, veal)	100	7–8
Lentils	100	7
White beans	100	6
Oatmeal, rye	100	5
Whole rice, dried figs and apricots	100	3–4
Meat (beef, veal, pork, chicken), eggs, whole-wheat bread, carrots, zuchini, dried dates	100	2

Cast Iron Pans

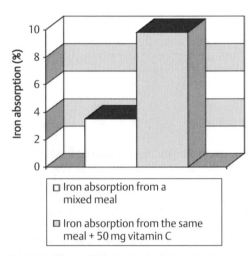

Fig. 3.**11**: **Effect of supplemental vitamin C on iron absorption.** Vitamin C is a potent enhancer of non-heme iron absorption from foods. From a simple meal of corn, rice, and black beans, a 50 mg supplement of vitamin C increases nonheme iron absorption about three-fold. (Adapted from Hallberg L, et al. Am J Clin Nutr. 1984;39:577)

The bioavailability of iron from foods varies greatly, ranging from less than 2% in certain plant foods, to 15–20% from meats, to nearly 50% from human-breast milk.[1,4] Iron is poorly absorbed from foods high in phytates, such as spinach and lentils. It is better absorbed from carrots, potatoes, soybeans and broccoli. Iron absorption is highest from meals including meat, poultry, or fish. Vitamin C is a strong promoter of iron absorption, and when vitamin C-rich foods are combined with iron-containing foods, bioavailability of the iron is substantially increased (Fig. 3.**11**).[4]

Recommended daily intakes for iron (mg)		
	Prevention of deficiency	
	UK RNI (1991)	USA RDA (1989)
Adult men	8.7	10
Adult women*	8.7–14.8	10–15
	Therapeutic dose range	
	Werbach (1990/99)	
Adult men	10–200	
Adult women*	10–200	

* with the exception of pregnant and lactating women

Recommended Daily Intakes

Iron supplements are generally twice as well absorbed when taken between meals.[1] Absorption is decreased by taking the iron with tea, coffee, or milk and increased by taking the iron with fruit juice or a vitamin C supplement.[4] Slow-release preparations may decrease gastrointestinal side effects (abdominal pain, nausea). Absorption of iron from a multimineral preparation will be impaired if the preparation also contains large amounts of calcium (>250 mg).[1]

Ferritin test – used to check for iron def.

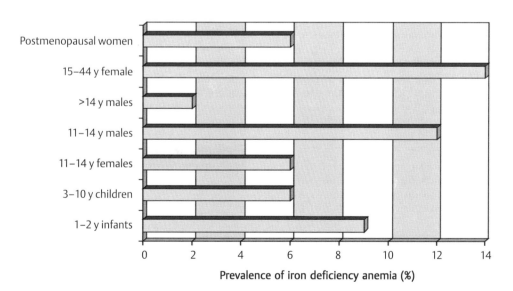

Fig. 3.**12**: **Prevalence of iron-deficiency anemia.** Iron-deficiency anemia is common among many age groups, particularly infants, adolescents, and young women. Without iron supplements more than 60% of pregnant women develop iron-deficiency anemia in the second half of pregnancy.
(Sources: Taylor PG, et al. J Am Diet Assoc. 1988;88:45; Herbert V. Am J Clin Nutr. 1987;45:679)

Preferred Form and Dosage Schedule

Iron fumarate may be more bioavailable than iron gluconate and iron sulfate. Elemental iron is poorly absorbed.	Iron supplements should usually be taken between meals. However, gastrointestinal side effects are more common when iron is taken on an empty stomach. If abdominal pain or nausea occur, taking the iron with meals may reduce these side effects

↑GI SE

Use in Prevention and Therapy

Anemia. High doses of supplemental iron, together with vitamin C, are used to treat iron-deficiency anemia.

Fatigue and lack of energy. Moderate to severe iron deficiency produces clear signs of anemia. However, "subclinical" chronic iron deficiency (reduced iron stores), without signs of anemia, is much more subtle and common. It produces nonspecific symptoms of fatigue, lack of energy, headache, and difficulty concentrating. Supplemental iron together with vitamin C replenishes depleted iron stores and can eliminate these symptoms.

Learning difficulties in children and adolescents. Subclinical iron deficiency can impair learning and concentration.[8] Increased intake of iron-rich foods together with supplemental vitamin C can be beneficial.

Infections. Recurrent infections in childhood (frequent colds, flu, ear infections) may be a sign of lowered immune resistance due to iron deficiency.[7]

Pregnancy. Iron supplementation is usually needed to prevent iron-deficiency anemia during pregnancy.[1,2,9]

Exercise and sport. Regular long-distance running and swimming often lead to depletion of iron stores and reduced performance. Replenishing low iron stores will increase maximal oxygen consumption and endurance.[10]

Toxicity

Acute iron poisoning in young children can be fatal. A lethal dose of iron is about 2–2.5 g in a 10 kg child.[1] Iron supplements must be kept out of reach of children. To treat anemia, iron is often given in high doses of 30–60 mg/day. At this level, particularly on an empty stomach, supplements can cause abdominal pain, nausea, and vomiting.

Just as too little iron can seriously impair health, too much iron can also be harmful. In healthy adults body regulation of iron balance usually maintains tissue stores at normal levels.[11] However, in hereditary hemochromatosis (HH), a common inherited defect in the regulation of iron absorption, risk of iron overload and chronic toxicity is sharply increased. About 1 in 10 people are heterozygous for this disorder and may be vulnerable to damage from excess iron.[1,12] Over many years excessive accumulation of body iron can gradually overload tissue storage capacity. Iron is a powerful oxidant, and iron overload can do widespread damage. In the liver it produces chronic inflammation and injury, which increases risk of liver cancer.[13] Iron overload may also increase risk of coronary heart disease.[14] Screening for HH, by measuring transferrin saturation, can detect the disorder before clinical signs of overload occur.[1]

References

1. Yip R, Dallman PR. Iron. In: Ziegler EE, Filer LJ, eds. Present Knowledge in Nutrition. Washington DC: ILSI Press; 1996.
2. Fairbanks V. Iron in medicine and nutrition. In: Shils ME, Olson JA, Shike M, Ross AC, eds. Modern Nutrition in Health and Disease. Baltimore: Williams & Wilkins;1999.
3. Oski F. Iron deficiency in infancy and childhood. N Engl J Med. 1993;329:190.
4. Hurrell RF. Bioavailabilty of iron. Eur J Clin Nutr. 1997;51:S4.
5. Beard JL, et al. Iron metabolism: A comprehensive review. Nutr Rev. 1996;54:295.

6. Idjradinata P, Pollitt E. Reversal of developmental delays in iron-deficient infants treated with iron. Lancet. 1993;341:1.
7. Dallman PR. Iron deficiency and the immune response. Am J Clin Nutr. 1987;46;329.
8. Bruner AB, et al. Randomised study of cognitive effects of iron supplementation in non-anemic iron-deficient girls. Lancet. 1996:348;992.
9. Yip R. Iron supplementation during pregnancy: Is it effective? Am J Clin Nutr. 1996;63:853.
10. Armstrong LA, Maresh CM: Vitamin and mineral supplements as nutritional aids to exercise performance and health. Nutr Rev. 1996;54:S149.
11. Mascotti DP, et al. Regulation of iron metabolism. Annu Rev Nutr. 1995;15:239.
12. Lynch SR. Iron overload: Prevalence and impact on health. Nutr Rev. 1995;53:255.
13. Yip R, et al. Is there an association between iron status and risk of cancer? Am J Clin Nutr. 1991;53:30.
14. Sempos CT, et al. Serum ferritin and death from all causes and cardiovascular disease. The NHANES II mortality study. Ann Epidemiol. 2000;10:441–8.

Zinc

The zinc content of a healthy 70 kg adult is 1.5–2.5 g.[1] Zinc is ubiquitously distributed among cells in the body and is the most abundant intracellular trace element. It has important enzymatic, structural, immune, and regulatory functions.

Functions

Enzyme function. More than 200 zinc-dependent enzymes have broad and diverse functions throughout the body. The RNA polymerases essential for the synthesis of new proteins require zinc.[1] Another prominent example is alcohol dehydrogenase, the liver enzyme that metabolizes ethanol. Zinc-dependent enzymes play an important role in DNA synthesis, neurotransmitter metabolism, free-radical deactivation, and metabolism of a variety of hormones (growth, thyroid, and sex hormones and insulin).

Structure and function of proteins. Zinc, as part of "zinc finger" proteins, plays an important role in cell growth and differentiation and intracellular signaling.[1]

Immune function. Zinc is important in production and regulation of the cellular and humoral immune response.[2,3]

Cytoprotection. Zinc provides protection against various toxic componds, including organic toxins, heavy metals, radiation, and endotoxins produced by pathogenic bacteria.[1]

Antioxidant function. Zinc is an essential part of the structure of the important antioxidant enzyme copper/zinc superoxide dismutase (Cu/Zn SOD). This enzyme is particularly important in the protection of cell lipids from peroxidation and breakdown (Fig. 3.**13**).[1,4]

Increased Risk of Deficiency

● Mild zinc deficiency is common, particularly among children, adolescents, pregnant and lactating women, and the elderly.[5–8] Vegetarian and semivegetarian diets are low in bioavailable zinc. Chronic dieting for weight loss often leads to zinc deficiency.

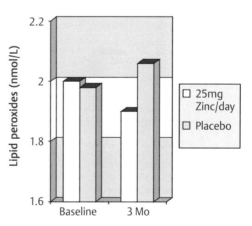

Fig. 3.**13**: **Effect of zinc supplementation on oxidation of plasma lipids.** A 25-mg zinc supplement given to 118 older adults for 3 months significantly decreased plasma lipid peroxides. The ability of zinc to reduce lipid oxidation could play an important role in the prevention and/or modulation of chronic disease in older people. (Adapted from Fortes C, et al. Eur J Clin Nutr. 1997;51:97)

● Malabsorption of zinc occurs in a variety of digestive disorders, including pancreatic insufficiency, inflammatory bowel diseases, and chronic diarrhea. The rare, inherited disorder acrodermatitis enteropathica is characterized by impaired zinc absorption and profound zinc deficiency.[8]

● High-dose calcium supplements may increase zinc loss and zinc requirements (Fig. 3.**14**).[9]

● Heavy consumption of alcohol reduces absorption and increases loss of zinc.[1]

● Liver and kidney disease increase zinc requirements.

● Poorly controlled diabetes mellitus increases urinary zinc loss and can lead to deficiency.[10]

● Chronic infection or inflammatory disease (such as rheumatoid arthritis) increase zinc requirements.[11]

Signs and Symptoms of Deficiency

- Dermatitis, inflammatory acne, reduced wound healing, white spots on the nails, hair thinning and loss
- Reduced sense of smell and taste (often accompanied by anorexia). Night blindness due to impaired vitamin A metabolism in the retina
- Slow growth; stunted, delayed sexual development and late puberty
- Impaired enzyme function and neurotransmitter metabolism may produce depression, irritability, poor concentration, and learning difficulties in children
- Weakened antioxidant defenses. Reduced resistance to environmental pollutants and radiation. Increased lipid peroxidation
- Impaired testicular and ovarian function. Poor sperm production, disordered ovulation, reduced fertility in both males and females
- Weakened immune response. Increased infections, including the common cold, flu, urinary-tract infections. Reduction in cellular immune defenses to environmental agents and cancer

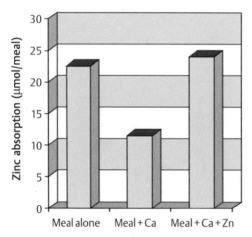

Fig. 3.**14**: **Effect of high-dose calcium supplementation on zinc absorption.** In 10 adults zinc absorption from a test meal containing 112 µmol of zinc was 22.5 µmol. When a 600-mg calcium supplement was taken with the meal, zinc absorption decreased significantly to 11.5 µmol. However, when an 8-mg zinc supplement was given along with the calcium, total zinc absorption from the meal was restored to 24.6 µmol. High-dose calcium supplements should not be taken with meals because they may interfere with trace mineral absorption.
(Adapted from Wood RJ, et al. Am J Clin Nutr. 1997;65:1803)

Good Dietary Sources

Food	Serving size	mg
Calf liver	100 g	6–8
Oysters	100 g	>7
Lentils	100 g	5
Green peas	100 g	4
Whole-wheat bread	100 g	2–4
White beans	100 g	3
Meat (beef, veal, chicken)	100 g	3
Wheat bran	25 g	3
Corn	100 g	2.5
Oatmeal	50 g	2
Eggs	1, medium	1.5

Overall, absorption of zinc from foods is approximately 33%,[1] but absorption varies from 5% to 50% depending on the fiber, phytate, and calcium content (all of which decrease bioavailability).[12] In general, zinc bioavailability from plant sources is low, (often about 10–15%). Meat, liver, and oysters contain large amounts of zinc that is three to four times more bioavailable than zinc from plant foods.[1]

Recommended Daily Intakes

Recommended daily intakes for zinc (mg)		
	Prevention of deficiency	
	UK RNI (1991)	USA RDA (1989)
Adult men	9.5	15
Adult women*	7	12
	Therapeutic dose range	
	Werbach (1990/99)	
Adult men	20–150	
Adult women*	20–150	

* with the exception of pregnant and lactating women

Preferred Form and Dosage Schedule

Organically bound forms (zinc gluconate, orotate, protein hydrolysate, and chelated forms) generally have greater bioavailability than zinc sulfate	Zinc supplements should usually be taken between meals. If gastrointestinal side effects occur, taking zinc with meals may reduce these

The average dietary intake of zinc in the adult population of many of the industrialized countries is lower than recommended[6–8]: in women it is about 10 mg, in men 12 mg. Chronic, marginal zinc deficiency appears to be common, even in otherwise healthy adults.[6–8,13]

Use in Prevention and Therapy

Eye disease. Zinc may be beneficial in the prevention and treatment of macular degeneration, a common cause of visual impairment in the elderly.[14]

Trauma, burns, surgery. Zinc helps regulate the inflammatory and immune response to injury and enhances protein synthesis and wound healing.[15]

Infectious disease. Zinc can reduce risk of infections and enhance immune response to vaccinations. In lozenge form it can be used to treat the common cold.[16] Zinc reduces the duration and severity of acute diarrheal disease in young children.[17]

Growth in childhood. Even subtle, marginal zinc deficiencys impairs growth in children and interferes with skeleton formation.[18] Supplements can help children reach their genetically programmed full height.[19]

Male fertility. Zinc may improve sperm quality and, in some cases, increase fertility.[20]

Skin diseases. Conditions such as acne, eczema, and psoriasis may respond to zinc, particularly in people who are zinc deficient.[21]

Heavy alcohol consumption. Zinc can enhance metabolism of alcohol and reduce the toxic effects (lipid peroxidation) of alcohol on the liver.

Rheumatic diseases. Rheumatoid and psoriatic arthritis may cause marginal zinc deficiency, due to chronic inflammation and use of medication (steroids, NSAIDs including aspirin, and penicillamine).[11] In such cases, zinc may help modify the inflammatory process and reduce pain and swelling.[22,23] Zinc may also help reduce the oxidant stress of chronic rheumatic disorders.[4]

Toxicity

Zinc is nontoxic at moderate supplementation levels (<100 mg /day).[1] At doses higher than

150 mg zinc may cause nausea and vomiting and may interfere with copper absorption.[7] At very high doses (>300 mg/day), zinc may impair immune function and decrease HDL cholesterol levels in the blood.[24]

10-15 zinc to 1 copper

References

1. Cousins RJ. Zinc. In: Ziegler EE, Filer LJ, eds. Present Knowledge in Nutrition. Washington DC: ILSI Press; 1996.
2. Shankar AH, Prasad AS. Zinc and immune function: the biological basis of altered resistance to infection. Am J Clin Nutr. 1998;68:447S.
3. Beck FWJ, et al. Changes in cytokine production and T cell subpopulations in experimentally-induced zinc deficiency in humans. Am J Physiol. 1997;227:E1002.
4. Fortes P, et al. Zinc supplementation and plasma lipid peroxides in an elderly population. Eur J Clin Nutr. 1997;51:97.
5. Prasad AS. Zinc deficiency in women, infants and children. J Am Coll Nutr. 1996;15:113.
6. Sandstead HH. Is zinc deficiency a public health problem? Nutrition. 1995;11:S87.
7. Prasad AS. Zinc: The biology and therapeutics of an ion. Ann Intern Med. 1996;125:142.
8. Aggett PJ, Comerford JG: Zinc and human health. Nutr Rev. 1995;53:S16.
9. Wood R, Jheng J. Calcium supplementation reduces intestinal zinc absorption and balance in humans. FASEB J. 1995;9:A283.
10. Thompson KH, Godin DV. Micronutrients and antioxidants in the progression of diabetes. Nutr Res. 1995;15:1377.
11. Honkanen VEA, et al. Plasma zinc and copper concentrations in rheumatoid arthritis: Influence of dietary factors and disease activity. Am J Clin Nutr. 1991;54:1082.
12. Fairweather-Tait S, Hurrell RF. Bioavailabilty of minerals and trace elements. Nutr Res Rev. 1996;9:295.
13. Lee DY, et al. Homeostasis of zinc in marginal zinc deficiency: role of absorption and endogenous excretion of zinc. J Lab Clin Med. 1993;122:549.
14. Newsome DA, et al. Oral zinc in macular degeneration. Arch Ophthalmol. 1988;106:192.
15. Lansdown AB. Zinc in the healing wound. Lancet. 1996;347:706.
16. Prasad AS, et al. Duration of symptoms and plasma cytokine levels in patients with the common cold treated with zinc acetate. A randomized, double-blind, placebo-controlled trial Ann Intern Med. 2000;133:245.
17. Sazawal S, et al. Zinc supplementation in young children with acute diarrhea in India. 1995;333:839.
18. King J. Does poor zinc nutriture retard skeletal growth and mineralization in adolescents? Am J Clin Nutr. 1996;64:375.
19. Walravens PA, et al. Linear growth of low income preschool children receiving a zinc supplement. Am J Clin Nutr. 1983;38:195.
20. Piesse J. Zinc and human male infertility. Int Clin Nutr Rev. 1983;3:4.
21. Pohit J, et al. Zinc status of acne vulgaris patients. J Appl Nutr. 1985;37:18.
22. Peretz A, et al. Effects of zinc supplementation on the phagocytic functions of polymorphonuclears in patients with inflammatory rheumatic diseases. J Trace Elem Electrolytes Health Dis. 1994;8:189.
23. Lally EV, Crowley JP. An element of uncertainty: The clinical significance of zinc deficiency in rheumatoid arthritis. Intern Med. 1987;8:98.
24. Hathcock JN. Safety of vitamin and mineral supplements. In: Bendich A, Butterworth CE, eds. Micronutrients in Health and Disease Prevention. New York: Marcel Dekker; 1991.

Manganese

The average adult has between 200 and 400 μmol of total body manganese, most of it in the bone, kidney, pancreas, and liver.[1] Manganese concentrations are high in mitochondria, where it plays an important role as an antioxidant.

Functions

Carbohydrate metabolism. The synthesis of new glucose from pyruvate is dependent on manganese-containing enzymes.[1] Maintenance of blood sugar levels between meals is therefore dependent on manganese.

Insulin production. Manganese is essential for normal insulin synthesis and secretion by the pancreas.[1]

Antioxidant protection. Manganese superoxide dismutase (SOD) is an important antioxidant enzyme that helps protect cells against damage from free radicals, particularly lipid peroxidation in mitochondria.[2]

Protein metabolism. Manganese plays an essential role in the breakdown and excretion of excess nitrogen from dietary sources and from normal protein turnover. Manganese deficiency increases potentially toxic ammonia levels in blood and decreases production of urea.[1]

Bone and cartilage synthesis. The synthesis of proteoglycans, important components of the connective tissues, cartilage, and bone, is dependent on manganese.[1,3]

Enzyme activation. Manganese plays a role in the nonspecific activation of many enzymes, including those that are important in breakdown of histamine, regulation of neurotransmitters in the brain, production of prothrombin in blood clotting, and lipid metabolism.[1]

Increased Risk of Deficiency

● Manganese intakes in many people are below recommended levels, with teenage girls and adult women particularly at risk.[1] Diets high in refined carbohydrates and processed foods tend to be low in manganese; refining of grains reduces the manganese content by more than 50%. Diets that emphasize animal products, such as milk products, eggs, and meat, are low in manganese.

● Increased oxidant stress from environmental sources (chemicals, drugs, and alcohol) may increase manganese requirements. For example, high alcohol intake increases the need for manganese in the liver, to protect liver cells from toxicity.[4]

● Taking high amounts of iron (60 mg/day) to treat iron-deficiency anemia sharply decreases manganese bioavailabilty.[5]

Signs and Symptoms of Deficiency[1,3,6]

- Reduction in HDL cholesterol and total cholesterol in the blood, increased liver fat concentrations
- Impaired insulin secretion, glucose intolerance
- Decreased appetite and weight loss
- Impaired bone production (possible increased risk of osteoporosis) and cartilage production. Possible increased bone turnover and increased levels of serum calcium and phosphorus. Deficiency during growth produces skeletal malformations
- Increased vulnerability to oxidative damage from free radicals
- Dermatitis and reduced hair and nail growth. Reddening of hair

Good Dietary Sources

Food	Serving size	mg
Oatmeal	100 g	5
Soy flour	100 g	4
Whole-wheat flour	100 g	3.5
Hazelnuts	50 g	3
Whole-wheat bread	100 g	2.5
Wheat germ	25 g	2.5
White beans	100 g	2
Dried fruit (apricots, figs)	100 g	2
Walnuts, almonds	50 g	1
Whole rice	100 g	1
Black tea and coffee	100 ml	1–2

The bioavailability of manganese from foods ranges from 1–25%. High dietary levels of iron[4] and phytate[7] (in foods such as beans and lentils) may reduce absorption of manganese. In general, meat, milk products, and eggs contain very low amounts, vegetables intermediate amounts, and nuts and whole grains higher amounts of manganese.

Coffe and tea contain relatively high levels of manganese, and these sources may account for up to 10% of daily intake for some people.[1] The typical highly refined modern diet that emphasizes meat and milk products contains only about 0.4–1.8 mg/day, less than half recommended levels.[8]

Recommended Daily Intakes

Recommended daily intakes for manganese (mg)		
	Prevention of deficiency	
	UK Safe intake level (1991)	USA ESADDI (1989)
Adult men	1.4	2–5
Adult women	1.4	2–5
	Therapeutic dose range Werbach (1990/99)	
Adult men	2–190	
Adult women	2–190	

Preferred Form and Dosage Schedule

Organically bound forms (manganese gluconate or chelates) generally have greater bioavailability than manganese sulfate	Take with meals, preferably with the dose divided throughout the day

Use in Prevention and Therapy

Osteoporosis. Women with osteoporosis tend to have low blood manganese levels. Supplementation may improve bone health in postmenopausal women.[9]

Diabetes mellitus. Manganese deficiency may reduce glucose tolerance, insulin secretion, and ability to control blood sugar. In diabetics who are manganese deficient supplementation may improve glucose metabolism.[10,11]

Epilepsy. Epileptics are at increased risk of low blood manganese levels.[12]

Asthma. Low levels of manganese have been found in the bronchi of asthmatics.[13]

Premenstrual syndrome. Manganese (together with calcium) may be beneficial in PMS.[14]

Toxicity

Manganese supplements in the range of 2 to 50 mg/day appear to be safe in healthy adults. Maganese toxicity can occur as a result of exposure to high amounts of environmental manganese (industrial workers) and to very high oral doses of manganese. Toxicity produces abnormalities of the central nervous system, including psychosis with hyperirritabilty and violence, lack of coordination, dementia, and symptoms similar to those of Parkinson disease.[15]

References

1. Keen CL, Zidenberg-Cherr S. Manganese. In: Ziegler EE, Filer LJ, eds. Present Knowledge in Nutrition. Washington DC: ILSI Press: 1996.
2. Coassin, et al. Antioxidant effect of manganese. Arch Biochem Biophys. 1992;299:330.
3. Klimis-Tavantzis DJ, ed. Manganese in Health and Disease. Boca Raton: CRC Press; 1994.
4. Davis CD, Greger JL. Longitudinal changes in manganese superoxide dismutase and other indices of manganese and iron status in women. Am J Clin Nutr. 1992;55:747.
5. Halsted C, Keen CL. Alcoholism and micronutrient metabolism and deficiencies. Eur J Gastroenterol Hepatol. 1990;2:399.
6. Friedman BJ, et al. Manganese balance and clinical observations in young men fed a manganese-deficient diet. J Nutr. 1987;117:133.
7. Davidsson L, et al. Manganese absorption in humans: The effect of phytic acid and ascorbic acid in soy formula. Am J Clin Nutr. 1995;62:984.
8. Nielsen FH. Ultratrace minerals. In: Shils ME, Olson JA, Shike M, Ross AC, eds. Modern Nutrition in Health and Disease. Baltimore: Williams & Wilkins; 1999.
9. Strause L, et al. Spinal bone loss in postmenopausal women supplemented with calcium and trace minerals. J Nutr. 1994;124:1060.
10. Walter RM, et al. Acute oral manganese administration does not consistently affect glucose tolerance in non-diabetic and type II diabetic humans. J Trace Elem Exp Med. 1991;4:73.

11. Rubenstein AH, et al. Manganese-induced hypoglycemia. Lancet. 1962;2:1348.
12. Carl GF, et al. Association of low blood manganese levels with epilepsy. Neurology. 1986;36:1584.
13. Campbell MJ, et al. Low levels of manganese in bronchial biopsies from asthmatic subjects. J Allergy Clin Immunol. 1992;89:342.
14. Penland JC. Dietary calcium and manganese effect on menstrual cycle symptoms. Am J Obst Gynecol. 1993;168:1417.
15. Keen Cl, et al. Nutritional and toxicological aspects of manganese intake: An overview. In: Mertz W et al, eds. Risk Assessment of Essential Trace Elements. Washington DC: ILSI Press; 1994.

Copper

The average human adult contains 60–120 mg of total body copper. Highest concentrations are found in the kidney, liver, brain, and heart.[1] Copper-containing enzymes play an important role in energy production, iron metabolism, connective-tissue synthesis, and antioxidant protection.

Functions

Energy production. Copper is found in the mitochondria of all cells. It is essential for energy production and, as a cofactor of cytochrome c oxidase, catalyzes the final step of the electron transport chain.[1]

Iron metabolism. Copper is required for normal mobilization and transfer of iron from storage sites to the bone marrow for erythropoesis.[2]

Connective-tissue synthesis. Synthesis of collagen and elastin in connective tissue requires the copper-containing enzyme, lysyl oxidase. Thus, wound healing and the integrity of blood vessel walls is dependent on copper.[3]

Antioxidant protection. Several copper-containing enzymes play an important role in antioxidant defense. Zn/Cu superoxide dismutase (SOD) is an important antioxidant within cells and works together with selenium-dependent glutathione peroxidase. Ceruloplasmin, a protein containing a cluster of copper atoms, circulates in the blood and is a potent scavenger of free radicals.[1,3]

Pigment production. Synthesis of melanin, the pigment that helps protect the skin from sun damage and colors the hair and eyes, is dependent on copper.

Metabolism of hormones and neurotransmitters. Copper-containing enzymes are required for the synthesis of epinephrine and norepinephrine in the adrenal and nervous system. Other copper-dependent enzymes catalyze the breakdown of serotonin, histamine, and dopamine.[3]

Increased Risk of Deficiency

● Although overt copper deficiency is rare, long-term consumption of diets marginal in copper (about 1 mg/day) may produce marginal copper deficiency[4] accompanied by subtle, nonspecific symptoms (elevated blood cholesterol, arthritis, glucose intolerance).[4,5]

● High intakes of supplemental iron (30–60 mg/day), molybdenum, or zinc[6] may interefere with copper bioavailability.

● Infants who are fed only cow's milk (milk is very low in copper) may develop copper deficiency.

● Prolonged use of antacids may reduce absorption of copper and contribute to deficiency.

● Gastrointestinal disorders–chronic diarrhea, celiac disease, active inflammatory bowel disease–may reduce absorption and increase loss from the digestive tract.

● Because copper plays a central role in antioxidant defenses, turnover and loss of copper may be accelerated during times of increased oxidative stress. For example, cigarette smoking, exposure to environmental chemicals, and chronic illness such as rheumatoid arthritis,[7] may increase copper requirements.

Signs and Symptoms of Deficiency[1,3,4]

- Anemia resembling iron-deficiency anemia but not completely responding to iron, accompanied by leukopenia and neutropenia
- Abnormal skeletal growth, osteoporosis
- Changes and loss of hair and skin pigmentation and vitiligo
- Weakness and fatigue
- Increased vulnerability to oxidative damage (low activity of ceruloplasmin and Cu/Zn SOD)
- Hypercholesterolemia, hypertriglyceridemia, and glucose intolerance
- Possible increase in fragility of blood vessel walls and increased risk of aneurysm
- Possible weakening of immune responses and impaired activation of T cells

Good Dietary Sources

Food	Serving size	mg
Liver (calf)	100 g	3.5–5.5
Certain ports and sherry	50 ml	3–10
Oysters	100 g	2.5
Lentils, chick peas, kidney beans	100 g	0.7–0.8
Sunflower seeds	25 g	0.7
Hazelnuts, walnuts, almonds	50 g	0.5
Hard cheeses	50 g	0.5
Dried apricots	50 g	0.3
Chicken, beef, lamb	100 g	0.3
Fish	100 g	0.2

Copper from dietary sources and supplements is efficiently absorbed; values for absorption range from 55% to 75%.[3]

Recommended Daily Intakes

Recommended daily intakes for copper (mg)		
	Prevention of deficiency	
	UK RNI (1991)	USA ESADDI (1989)
Adult men	1.2	1.5–3
Adult women	1.2	1.5–3
	Therapeutic dose range	
	Werbach (1990/99)	
Adult men	2–10	
Adult women	2–10	

Preferred Form and Dosage Schedule

Although copper sulfate is the most common supplemental form, organically bound forms of copper (orotate, chelates) may be more bioavailable	Take between meals, preferably with the dose divided throughout the day

Use in Prevention and Therapy

Anemia. Malnourishment with marginal or deficient copper intakes may lead to mild normocytic or microcytic anemia. Moreover, in cases of iron-deficiency anemia treated with high-dose iron supplementation, copper supplements may help maintain copper status (iron decreases the absorption of copper) and may enhance iron supply to the bone marrow.[2]

Rheumatoid arthritis. Copper, particularly in those with long-standing disease and marginal dietary intakes of copper, may be beneficial in helping reduce pain and inflammation.[7]

Cardiovascular disease. Chronic low intakes of copper may increase risk of cardiovascular disease by simultaneously elevating blood cholesterol and triglycerides[5,8] while weakening the vascular wall (elastin and collagen synthesis are copper dependent) and impairing vascular function.[9]

Immune function. Even mild copper deficiency may reduce immune function by reducing T-cell activation[10] and causing neutropenia.[11] In malnourishment caused by chronic infection, copper may be beneficial in helping to maintain immune strength.

Zinc therapy. Because long-term, high doses of zinc can reduce bioavailabilty of dietary copper,[6] copper intake should be increased to maintain copper balance.

Toxicity

Copper is generally well tolerated and safe at doses of up to 5 mg/day in healthy adults. In adults doses higher than 7 mg/day may produce abdominal pain, nausea, vomiting, and diarrhea,[6] and liver damage.

Wilson's disease is a rare inherited disorder of copper storage (affecting 1 in 200 000 people), in which biliary excretion of copper is impaired.[12] This results in accumulation of copper in the liver and brain that can lead to cirrhosis, liver failure, and neurologic damage. If diagnosed early and treated with regular copper chelation (using penicillamine together with zinc), damage can be avoided.

References

1. Linder MC, et al. Copper: Biochemistry and molecular biology. Am J Clin Nutr. 1996;63:S797.
2. Hirase N, et al. Anemia and neutropenia in a case of copper deficiency: Role of copper in normal hematopoesis. Acta Haematol. 1990;87:195.
3. Lindner M. Copper. In: Ziegler EE, Filer LJ, eds. Present Knowledge in Nutrition. Washington DC: ILSI Press; 1996.
4. Prohaska JR. Biochemical changes in copper deficiency. J Nutr Biochem. 1990;1:452.
5. Klevay LM. Decreased glucose tolerance in two men during experimental copper depletion. Nutr Rep Int. 1986;33:371.
6. Turnland JR. Copper. In: Shils ME, Olson JA, Shike M,

Ross AC, eds. Modern Nutrition in Health and Disease. Williams & Wilkins: Baltimore; 1999.
7. Honkanen VEA, et al. Plasma zinc and copper concentrations in rheumatoid arthritis: Influence of dietary factors and disease activity. Am J Clin Nutr. 1991;54:1082.
8. Reiser S, et al. Effect of copper intake on blood cholesterol and its lipoprotein distribution in men. Nutr Rep Int. 1987;36:641.
9. Schuschke DA. Dietary copper in the physiology of the microcirculation. J Nutr. 1997;127:2274.
10. Failla ML, Hokins RG. Is low copper status immunosuppressive? Nutr Rev. 1998;56:S59.
11. Percival SS. Neutropenia caused by copper deficiency: Possible mechanisms of action. Nutr Rev. 1995;53:59.
12. Petruhkin K, Gilliam TC. Genetic disorders of copper metabolism: A review. Curr Opin Pediatr. 1994;6:698.

Molybdenum

The total body content of molybdenum in the average adult is approximately 10 mg, with 60% in the skeleton and 20% in the liver. Molybdenum is an essential cofactor in several enzyme systems that are important for metabolism, detoxification, and excretion of potentially harmful compounds.[1,2]

Functions

Antioxidant effects. Molybdenum is a cofactor of the enzyme xanthine oxidase.[1] Xanthine oxidase catalyzes formation of uric acid, an important antioxidant in the bloodstream that helps protect against free radical damage.

Protection from toxic effects of chemicals and drugs. A group of molybdenum-dependent enzymes, the molybdenum hydroxylases, are important for detoxification and excretion of foreign compounds by the liver.[2]

Iron metabolism. Molybdenum appears to be important for optimum transport and storage of iron in tissues.

Sulfur metabolism. The molybdenum-containing enzyme, sulfite oxidase, is essential for the metabolism and breakdown of sulfur-containing amino acids (e.g., cysteine, methionine, taurine, homocysteine) and for conversion of sulfite (a toxic compound) to sulfate.[1]

Increased Risk of Deficiency

● Modern, affluent diets high in refined carbohydrates, fats and oils, and meat products tend to be low in molybdenum. Refining of grains reduces their molybdenum content by more than 40%. The daily intake of molybdenum of most adults in the industrialized countries is only about 50–100 µg,[3,4] compared with recommended daily requirements of 75–250 µg.[5]

● Regular exposure to drugs and chemicals that increase oxidant stress and require detoxification by the liver may increase molybdenum requirements.[1,2]

● Digestive disorders that produce diarrhea and malabsorption can increase molybdenum loss and sharply increase needs. For example, in patients with active Crohn's disease, daily losses of molybdenum can be higher than 400 µg/day.

Signs and Symptoms of Deficiency[1,5,6]

- Decreased uric-acid production and reduced antioxidant protection
- Impaired metabolism of potentially toxic sulfur-containing amino acids (methionine, homocysteine), which can result in mental disturbances and, if severe, coma[7]
- Increased sensitivity to sulfites in the environment (air pollution) and in the diet (used as preservatives on salad bars, in dried fruits and wine)
- Hair loss
- Fatigue
- Possible increased risk of cancer (particularly cancer of the esophagus)
- Possible increased risk of kidney stones (xanthine stones)

Good Dietary Sources

Food	Serving size	µg
Soy flour	100 g	180
Red cabbage	100 g	120
White beans	100 g	100
Potatoes	100 g	5–85
Whole rice	100 g	80
Green peas	100 g	70
Spinach	100 g	50
Eggs	1, medium	49
Green beans	100 g	43
Whole-wheat bread	100 g	31
Wheat germ	25 g	25

Approximately 80–90% of molybdenum in the diet is absorbed by healthy adults.[8]

Recommended Daily Intakes

Recommended daily intakes for molybdenum (µg)		
	Prevention of deficiency	
	UK Safe intake level (1991)	USA ESADDI (1989)
Adult men	50–400	75–250
Adult women	50–400	75–250
	Therapeutic dose range	
	Werbach (1990/99)	
Adult men	100–2000	
Adult women	100–2000	

Preferred Form and Dosage Schedule

Sodium molybdenate	Take with meals, preferably with the dose divided throughout the day

B12, Molybdenum – Sulfite Sensitivity

Use in Prevention and Therapy

Reduction of sulfite sensitivity. A diet low in molybdenum may increase sensitivity to sulfites. Sulfites are produced by industrial emissions and car exhausts and may also be added to certain foods as preservatives (salad and vegetables, dried fruit, wine). Sulfite sensitivity can produce a range of symptoms including wheezing and shortness of breath, dermatitis, itching and hives, swelling around the eyes, hands, and feet, as well as dizziness, nausea, and vomiting.

Protection from adverse effects of environmental chemicals and drugs. Molybdenum is a cofactor in enzymes that provide antioxidant protection and help the liver detoxify foreign compounds. Thus, increasing molybdenum intake may help protect against damage during exposure to environmental chemicals and drugs.[1,2]

Cancer. Molybdenum may help reduce risk of cancer, particularly cancer of the esophagus.[9]

Toxicity

Molybdenum, at doses lower than 1 mg/day, appears to be nontoxic in healthy adults. At very high doses (10 to 20 times higher than found in normal diets), molybdenum may increase production of uric acid and precipitate gout.

References

1. Nielsen FH. Trace elements. In: Ziegler EE, Filer LJ, eds. Present Knowledge in Nutrition. Washington DC: ILSI Press; 1996.
2. Beedham C. Molybdenum hydroxylases as drug metabolizing enzymes. Drug Metab Rev. 1985;16:119.
3. Pennington JAT. Molybdenum, nickel, cobalt, vanadium and strontium in total diets. J Am Diet Assoc. 1987;87:1644.
4. Glei M, et al. Molybdenum intake and balance in German adults. In: Defizite und Überschüsse an Mengen- und Spurenelementen in der Ernährung. Leipzig: Verlag Harald Schubert; 1994:251–6.
5. Rajagopalan KV. Molybdenum: An essential trace element. Nutr Rev. 1987;45:321.
6. World Health Organization. Molybdenum. In: Trace elements in human nutrition and health. Geneva: WHO; 1996.
7. Abumrad NN, et al. Amino acid intolerance during prolonged total parenteral nutrition reversed by molybdate therapy. Am J Clin Nutr. 1981;34:2551.
8. Turnland J, et al. Molybdenum absorption, excretion and retention studied with stable isotopes in young men a five intakes of dietary molybdenum. Am J Clin Nutr. 1995;62:790.
9. Taylor PR, et al. Prevention of esophageal cancer: The nutrition intervention trials in Linxan, China. Cancer Res. 1994;54:2029S.

Chromium

Chromium is an essential trace element that is the active component of the "glucose tolerance factor" (GTF).[1–3] GTF enhances insulin action and helps regulate carbohydrate, lipid, and protein metabolism. Chromium is widely distributed throughout the body in low concentrations: for example, the liver contains only about 1 µg/100 g dry weight.[4]

Functions

Carbohydrate metabolism. As the active component of GTF (together with niacin and the amino acids glycine, glutamic acid, and cysteine), chromium potentiates insulin action. Chromium can improve glucose tolerance after meals and helps maintain a steady blood level of glucose between meals. The mechanism of this effect appears to be enhancement of insulin binding to its receptor.[3]

Lipid metabolism. Chromium, particularly in hyperlipidemia, may decrease total and LDL-cholesterol levels in blood while increasing HDL-cholesterol levels.[1,3,5]

Protein metabolism. Through its potentiation of insulin action, chromium may increase uptake of amino acids into muscle, heart, and liver and enhance protein synthesis.

Cell division and growth. Chromium binds to DNA and may enhance RNA synthesis. Chromium may thereby play a role in regulation of cell growth.[3]

Increased Risk of Deficiency

● Modern diets in the industrialized countries that are high in fat and refined carbohydrates contain only low amounts of chromium.[3] High intake of sugars increases chromium loss in the urine.[6] Refining grains reduces the chromium content dramatically: whole wheat contains 10 times the amount of chromium found in white flour. Studies have repeatedly found that chromium intakes from typical modern diets provide only 25–50 µg/day of chromium, far below recommended requirements of 50–200 µg/day.[1,3]

● Increased stress–from strenuous exercise, physical activity, infection, trauma, or illness–sharply increases chromium loss in the urine, elevates chromium requirements, and may exacerbate a deficiency.[3]

● Pregnancy may increase needs for chromium.[3]

● In older people intakes of chromium are often below recommended levels. Chromium levels in serum, hair, and sweat decrease with age.[7] This may increase the risk for age-associated hypercholesterolemia and glucose intolerance.[5]

Signs and Symptoms of Deficiency[1–3]

- Impaired glucose tolerance and reduced insulin action
- Weight loss
- Elevated cholesterol and triglyceride levels in blood
- Peripheral neuropathy

Good Dietary Sources

Food	Serving size (g)	µg
Lentils	100	70
Whole-wheat bread	100	49
Molasses	30	36
Chicken	100	26
Brewer's yeast	10	20

Stainless-steel cookware typically contains 11–30% chromium. Chromium can leach from stainless steel into cooked foods (especially acidic foods like tomato sauce) and contribute to chromium intake.[8] However, intestinal absorption of inorganic chromium is only 0.5–3%. Chromium in an organic form (as GTF in brewer's yeast, or a chelate with an amino acid) is much better absorbed (about 10%). Ascorbic acid markedly promotes chromium absorption. For example, absorption of 1 mg of chromium chloride given with 100 mg vitamin C is two to three times higher than when taken without vitamin C.[9]

Recommended Daily Intakes

Recommended daily intakes for chromium (µg)		
	Prevention of deficiency	
	UK Safe intake level (1991)	USA ESADDI (1989)
Adult men	25	50–200
Adult women*	25	50–200
	Therapeutic dose range	
	Werbach (1990/99)	
Adult men	200–3000	
Adult women*	200–3000	

* with the exception of pregnant and lactating women

Preferred Form and Dosage Schedule

Organic forms of chromium (high chromium yeast, chromium GTF, chromium aspartate, picolinate, and nicotinate) are preferable. Chromium chloride is very poorly absorbed (<1%)	Take between meals, preferably with the dose divided throughout the day

Use in Prevention and Therapy

Impaired glucose tolerance and diabetes. In impaired glucose tolerance and type 2 diabetes chromium can improve insulin action, reduce postmeal glucose levels, and help control blood glucose (Fig. **3.15**).[1,3,10,11] It may also reduce hypertriglyceridemia in type 2 diabetes.[12]

Hyperlipidemia and atherosclerosis. Chromium can improve the lipid profile in hyperlipidemia by decreasing total and LDL cholesterol, lowering triglycerides, and raising HDL cholesterol.[1,3,5,9] In coronary heart disease blood chromium levels are five to eight times lower than healthy controls.[13]

Metabolic stress. During recovery from trauma, surgery, or illness chromium loss is accelerated. Increased chromium turnover may be a response to the insulin resistance that typically develops during recovery.[3]

Toxicity

Chronic daily intake of trivalent chromium (Cr^{+3}) and chromium in brewer's yeast in the range of 100 to 300 µg is considered safe.[1,3] Supplementation of up to 1000 µg of chromium picolinate for several months in adults has produced no adverse effects.[11] Heavy chronic exposure to airborne hexavalent chromium (Cr^{+6}), produced in metalworking industries, can be toxic.[14] Symptoms include dermatitis and increased risk of lung cancer.

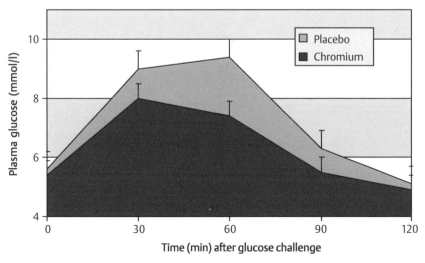

Fig. **3.15**: Effects of supplemental chromium (200 µg/ day) vs. placebo on a standard glucose tolerance test in 17 adults with impaired glucose tolerance. Plasma glucose and insulin (not shown) were significantly lower in the supplemented group.
(Adapted from Anderson RA, et al. Am J Clin Nutr. 1991;54:909)

References

1. Mertz W. Chromium in human nutrition: A review. J Nutr. 1993;123:626.
2. Ducros V. Chromium metabolism: A literature review. Biol Trace Elem Res. 1992;32:65.
3. Stoecker BJ. Chromium. In: Ziegler EE, Filer LJ, eds. Present Knowledge in Nutrition. Washington DC: ILSI Press; 1996.
4. Vuori E, Kumpulainen J. A new low level of chromium in human liver and spleen. Trace Elem Med. 1987;4:88.
5. Hermann J, et al. Effect of chromium supplementation on plasma lipids, apolipoproteins and glucose in elderly subjects. Nutr Res. 1994;14:671.
6. Kozlovsky AS, et al. Effects of diets high in simple sugars on urinary chromium losses. Metabolism. 1986;35:515.
7. Davis S, et al. Age-related decreases in chromium levels in 51,665 hair, sweat and serum samples from 40,872 patients: Implications for the prevention of cardiovascular disease and type II diabetes. Metabolism. 1997;46:469.
8. Kuligowski J, Halperin KM. Stainless steel cookware as a significant source of nickel, chromium and iron. Arch Environ Contam Toxicol. 1992;23:211.
9. Offenbacher EG. Promotion of chromium absorption by ascorbic acid. Trace Elem Electrolytes. 1994;11:178.
10. Abraham AS, et al. The effects of chromium supplementation on serum glucose and lipids in patients with and without non-insulin-dependent diabetes. Metabolism. 1992;41:768.
11. Anderson R, et al. Chromium supplementation in type II diabetes. Diabetes. 1997;46:1786.
12. Lee NA, Reasner CA. Beneficial effect of chromium supplementation on serum triglyceride levels in NIDDM. Diabetes care. 1994;17:1449.
13. Newman HAI, et al. Serum chromium and angiographically determined coronary artery disease. Clin Chem. 1978;24:541.
14. Anderson RA. Nutritional and toxicological aspects of chromium intake: An overview. In: Mertz W, et al., eds. Risk Assessment of Essential Trace Elements. Washington DC: ILSI Press; 1994.

Iodine

Iodine deficiency is one of the most common nutritional deficiencies. Worldwide, it is estimated that nearly 1 billion people are at risk of iodine deficiency disorders (IDD).[1] Iodine deficiency, both in utero and during early childhood, can impair mental development and is the most prevalent cause of preventable mental retardation in the world.[2] Despite widespread efforts to iodize salt, IDD continues to be severe in regions of Africa, Southeast Asia, and Latin America. IDD also remains a common problem in Central and Southern Europe: it is estimated that 10–15% of the German population is iodine deficient and up to 50% of the adolescent and adult populations of Spain and Italy.[3]

Functions

Thyroid hormone synthesis. The only known function of iodine in the body is as an essential component of the thyroid hormones.[2,4] The thyroid gland removes iodine from the blood and attaches it to tyrosine-containing proteins to form the thyroid hormones, thyroxine (T_4) and triiodothyronine (T_3). The thyroid hormones are then secreted into the bloodstream and are important regulators of cell activity and growth, both in utero and throughout life. Although they affect all tissues, they are particularly important in the development of the nervous and skeletal systems.

Increased Risk of Deficiency

● In coastal areas the environment and food supply is rich in iodine because of the proximity of the ocean (sea water contains 50–60 µg iodide/l). However, in many inland areas of the world the soil is deficient in iodine. The iodine content is especially low in regions where the iodine has been leached from the soil by glacial run-off (mountain regions) and in flood plains. In these areas, plants grown on iodine-deficient soils and the animals that graze on them are iodine deficient and the human food supply lacks iodine.

● Iodine requirements increase during pregnancy and lactation, and maternal deficiency during these periods can have profound adverse effects on the growth and development of the infant.[2,4]

● Although a diet low in iodine is the primary cause of goiter and IDD, other dietary factors can exacerbate the deficiency. These so-called "goitrogens" block uptake and/or use of iodine. They include substances in cassava, millet, sweet potatoes, and certain beans, as well as several industrial pollutants (resorcinol, phthalic acid) that may contaminate food and water.[2,5]

Signs and Symptoms of Deficiency[2,4]

- In the fetus: increased abortion, stillbirths, and congential defects. Cretinism (mental retardation, deafness, spasticity)
- Increased infant mortality, psychomotor and mental impairment, hypothyroidism
- In children and adolescents: goiter (enlargement of the thyroid gland), hypothyroidism, impaired mental function, impaired physical growth
- In adults: goiter, hypothyroidism, impaired mental function

The signs and symptoms of hypothyroidism include weight gain, edema, fatigue, lack of energy, slow heart rate, low blood pressure, hair loss, and dry skin.

Good Dietary Sources

Food	Serving size (g)	µg
Mussels, clams, salmon	100	200–250
Shrimp, cod	100	120–130
Mackerel, tuna, herring, halibut	100	50–75
Iodized salt	1	15–25

In most inland areas adequate iodine intake to prevent deficiency is difficult to obtain from usual diets (except those rich in fish and other seafood). Therefore, daily use of iodized salt (both at home and by the food industry) is critical to prevent IDD. Especially during pregnancy, lactation, and childhood, use of iodized salt for home food preparation is important. If needed, iodine can also be obtained in the form of kelp supplements.

Recommended Daily Intakes

Recommended daily intakes for iodine (µg)		
	Prevention of deficiency	
	UK RNI (1991)	USA RDA (1989)
Adult men	140	150
Adult women*	140	150
	Therapeutic dose range Werbach (1990)	
Adult men	100–230000	
Adult women*	100–230000	

* with the exception of pregnant and lactating women

Even in areas where iodized salt is available, iodine intake may be low. For example, in areas of Spain, Germany, Belgium,[6] Italy, and New Zealand[7] average adult iodine intake is estimated to be only 20–80 µg/day.[3] Several European countries are in the process of increasing the level of iodine in salt in an attempt to maintain adequate levels of intake.

Preferred Form and Dosage Schedule

Kelp (sea algae), or potassium iodide	Take with or between meals

Use in Prevention and Therapy

IDD. Ample intake of iodine (from seafood, iodized salt, or kelp supplements), especially during pregnancy, lactation, and childhood, will maintain production of thyroid hormone and prevent IDD. Inadequate iodine intake during childhood can impair learning ability and school performance.[2]

Hypothyroidism. If the iodine content of the diet is marginal or low, borderline hypothyroidism may produce symptoms of fatigue, lassitude, and poor concentration. Replenishing thyroid stores of iodine can be beneficial.

Toxicity

Iodine intake at levels of 100–500 µg/day are essentially nontoxic. Although iodine can occasionally precipitate acne in susceptible individuals, high levels of intake (up to 1 mg/day) are well tolerated in most healthy adults. However, very high daily intake (>2 mg/day) may impair thyroid hormone production. Moreover, in cases of long-standing iodine deficiency and goiter, abruptly increasing iodine intake may cause hyperthyroidism and, rarely, thyrotoxicosis.[2]

References

1. WHO/UNICEF/ICCIDD. Indicators for assessing iodine deficiency disorders and their control through salt iodization. Geneva; WHO: 1994.
2. Stanbury JB. Iodine deficiency and the iodine deficiency disorders. In: Ziegler EE, Filer LJ, eds. Present Knowledge in Nutrition. Washington DC: ILSI Press; 1996.
3. Delange F, Bürgi H. Iodine deficiency disorders in Europe. WHO Bull. 1989;67:317.
4. Delange F. Disorders induced by iodine deficiency. Thyroid. 1994;4:107.
5. Hurrell RF. Bioavailability of iodine. Eur J Clin Nutr. 1997;51:S9.
6. Bourdoux PP. Borderline iodine deficiency in Belgium. J Endocrinol Invest. 1990;13:77.
7. Thomson CD, et al. Iodine status of New Zealand residents as assessed by urinary iodide excretion and thyroid hormones. Br J Nutr. 1997;78:901.

Selenium

Selenium is an essential trace element that is a component of several enzyme systems. Selenium is found in all human tissues at an average concentration of about 20 µg/100 g.[1] The liver and kidney contain particularly high amounts.

Functions

Antioxidant protection. Selenium is an essential component of a family of four enzymes, the glutathione peroxidases 1–4.[2] They catalyze reduction and deactivation of free radicals and other potential oxidants using glutathione as the electron donor. They are present in the blood, extracellular fluid, and inside cells and play a central role in the body's antioxidant defense system.

Immune modulation. Selenium plays an important role in the immune system.[3,4] It may help regulate production of immunoglobulins (such as IgG) and tumor necrosis factor (TNF) and may enhance activity of certain white blood cells, the natural killer (NK) cells.

Thyroid hormone metabolism. The thyroid gland secretes mainly thyroxine (T_4). This is converted to triiodothyronine (T_3) in the liver and kidney by a selenium-containing enzyme type-I-iodothyronine-deiodinase.[5] This conversion increases the potency of thyroid hormone and is important in enhancing its peripheral activity.

Increased Risk of Deficiency

● The selenium concentration of soil varies widely around the world. Selenium concentrations of plants and animals grown or kept on different soils can differ up to a thousand fold. The most extreme example is in China. Corn and rice grown in regions with selenium-rich soils have selenium contents of 8 and 4 µg/g; the same crops grown in selenium-poor areas have contents of 0.005 and 0.007 µg/g, respectively.[6] This produces large variations in dietary selenium intake. In Scandinavia, Central Europe, New Zealand, Africa and parts of China large populations are at risk of low selenium intake.

● Because selenium is an essential component of the glutathione peroxidases, turnover and loss of selenium are accelerated during times of increased oxidative stress. For example, strenuous exercise or physical activity, cigarette smoking, increased exposure to environmental chemicals, mercury, or radiation, and chronic illness (such as rheumatoid arthitis[7]) may increase selenium needs.

● Malabsorption may be caused by certain digestive disorders. Pancreatic disorders, cystic fibrosis, and the inflammatory bowel diseases all may decrease selenium bioavailability and increase needs.

Signs and Symptoms of Deficiency[1,6]

- Decreased resistance to oxidative damage
- Childhood osteoarthritis (Kashin-Beck disease)
- Muscle weakness
- Possible increased risk of cancer
- Cardiomyopathy and heart failure (Keshan disease)
- Possible weakening of the immune system and increased risk of infection

Good Dietary Sources

Food	Serving size (g)	µg
Herring, Tuna	100	120–140
Sardines	100	80–100
Liver (calf)	100	50–70
Soy beans	100	50–70
Whole-wheat bread	100	30–60
Beef	100	30–40
Pork	100	25–35
Salmon, cod	100	20–30
White beans	100	10–25
Milk products	100	4–10

In general, high amounts of selenium are found in organ meats and seafood, intermediate amounts in meats and grains, and low amounts in milk products, fruit, and vegetables.[1,6]

Recommended Daily Intakes

Recommended daily intakes for selenium (µg)		
	Prevention of deficiency	
	UK RNI (1991)	USA DRI (2000)
Adult men		60
Adult women*		60
	Therapeutic dose range	
	Werbach (1990)	
Adult men	200–1000	
Adult women*	200–1000	

* with the exception of pregnant and lactating women

Preferred Form and Dosage Schedule

Organic forms of selenium (selenomethionine, selenocysteine, selenium-rich yeast, and selenium aspartate) are preferable. Sodium selenite is less bioavailable	Take with meals, preferably with the dose divided throughout the day

Depending on the selenium content of soil, intake of selenium in the industrialized countries varies: from low levels in Scandinavia, New Zealand, and Germany (20–50 µg/day) to higher intakes in the UK and USA (60–110 µg/day).[1,6]

Use in Prevention and Therapy

Cancer. Selenium has anticancer properties, possibly through its effects on the immune system or its antioxidant actions (Fig. 3.**16**). Regions of the USA with the highest intakes of selenium tend to have lower rates of cancer,[8,9] and higher blood levels of selenium are associated with lower risk of cancer.[8,9] Supplementation in older men can reduce risk of lung, colon, and prostate cancer by nearly 50%.[9]

Fig. 3.**16**: **Role of selenium in primary prevention of cancer.** In an intervention trial including nearly 30 000 adults, 7500 received an antioxidant supplement containing 50 µg selenium (along with 30 mg vitamin E and 15 mg beta-carotene) for 5 years. The supplemented group had a significant 13% reduction in cancer mortality, compared with those not receiving the supplement. (Adapted from Blot WJ, et al. J Nat Cancer Inst. 1993;85:148)

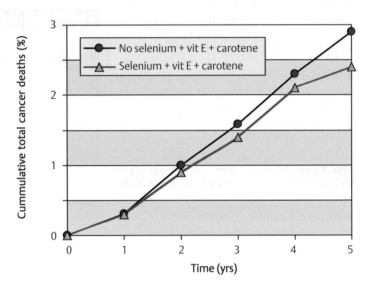

Chronic inflammatory disorders. Diseases such as rheumatoid arthritis[7] and inflammatory bowel disease may benefit from increased intake of selenium.

Infectious disease. Selenium deficiency appears to increase susceptibility to, and severity of, viral infections.[3,4] Selenium deficiency is associated with a sharply higher risk of mortality from AIDS.[10]

Heart disease. Severe selenium deficiency, possibly exacerbated by concomitant vitamin E deficiency and viral infection, produces cardiomyopathy and heart failure (Keshan disease).[1,6] This disorder is found mainly in adolescents and young women. Decreased selenium levels in blood have been found in patients with coronary heart disease.[11] In heart disease patients, particularly those with low selenium intakes, increasing selenium intake may be beneficial.

Hypothyroidism. Selenium deficiency may reduce peripheral activation of thyroid hormones and may trigger or exacerbate hypothyroidism.[5]

Childhood osteoarthritis. Severe selenium deficiency may contribute to cases of juvenile osteoarthritis (Kashin-Beck disease).[1,6]

Heavy body burden of heavy metals. Selenium may help prevent chronic accumulation of lead and mercury from environmental contamination of the food and water supply.

Toxicity

Daily intakes of up to 500 µg/day appear to be safe in healthy adults.[1,12] Chronic intakes higher than 900 µg/day are associated with nausea, vomiting, hair loss, nail changes, fatigue, and peripheral neuropathy.[12]

References

1. Rayman MP. The importance of selenium to human health. Lancet. 2000;356:233.
2. Foster LH, Sumar S. Selenium in health and disease: A review. Crit Rev Food Sci Nutr. 1997;37:211.
3. Kubena KS, McMurray DN. Nutrition and the immune system: A review of nutrient-nutrient interactions. J Am Diet Assoc. 1996;96:1156.
4. Look MP, et al. Serum selenium, plasma glutathione and erythrocyte glutathione peroxidase levels in asymptomatic vs. symptomatic HIV infection. Eur J Clin Nutr. 1997;51:266.
5. Olivieri O, et al. Selenium, zinc, and thyroid hormones in healthy subjects: Low T3/T4 ratio in the elderly is related to impaired selenium status. Biol Trace Elem Res. 1996;51:31.

6. Levander OA, Burk RF. Selenium. In: Ziegler EE, Filer LJ, eds. Present Knowledge in Nutrition. Washington DC: ILSI Press; 1996.
7. Tarp U. Selenium and rheumatoid arthritis: A review. Analyst. 1995;120:877.
8. Garland M, et al. The epidemiology of selenium and human cancer. In: Frei B, ed. Natural antioxidants in human health and disease. San Diego: Academic Press; 1994:263.
9. Clark LC, et al. Effects of selenium supplementation for cancer prevention in patients with carcinoma of the skin. JAMA. 1996;276:1957.
10. Baum MK, et al. High risk of HIV-related mortality is associated with selenium deficiency. J Acquir Immune Def Syndr Hum Retrovirol. 1997;15:370.
11. Kok FJ, et al. Decreased selenium levels in acute myocardial infarction. JAMA. 1989;261:1161.
12. Levander O. Human selenium nutrition and toxicity. In: Mertz W, et al., eds. Risk Assessment of Essential Trace Elements. Washington DC: ILSI Press; 1994.

Fluoride

Fluoride is naturally found in minute amounts in all foods. Although fluoride was once considered an essential nutrient, it is no longer considered essential but rather "beneficial" for human health. Its benefits are a sharp reduction in prevalence and severity of dental caries in both children and adults when an optimum dose is ingested (about 0.05 mg/kg body weight/day).[1] However, the range of fluoride intake compatible with human health is narrow: toxicity may appear at levels of intake only two to five times the dose needed to help prevent dental caries.[2,3]

Functions

Tooth structure. Fluoride can be incorporated into the crystalline structure of the dental enamel. It reduces the solubility of the enamel crystals, increasing their resistance to acid formed by oral bacteria. It can also enhance remineralization of damaged enamel.[4,5]

Bone metabolism. Fluoride can enhance bone formation by stimulating osteoblast activity.[6]

Signs and Symptoms of Deficiency

Increased susceptibility to dental caries

Good to have in toothpaste

Good Dietary Sources[7,8]

Food	Serving size	mg
Fluoridated water*	1 l	0.7–1.2
Canned sardines (including bones)	100 g	0.2–0.4
Tea (brewed with non-fluoridated water)	100 ml	0.01–0.42
Fluoridated salt	1 g	0.25
Chicken	100 g	0.06–0.1

* natural fluoride levels in water range from 0.01–2 mg/100 ml

Many children obtain additional fluoride by ingesting fluoride-containing toothpastes that usually contain about 1–1.5 mg/g.[7]

Recommended Daily Intakes[9]

Age (years)	mg
0–0.5	0.01
0.5–1	0.5
1–3	0.7
4–8	1.0
9–13	2.0
14–18	3.0
>18	3–4

Recommended fluoride supplement dose (mg/day) at different concentrations of fluoride in drinking water[10]

Age	<0.3 mg/l	0.3–0.6 mg/l	>0.7 mg/l
0–6 months	0	0	0
6 months to 3 years	0.25	0	0
3–6 years	0.5	0.25	0
6–16 years	1	0.5	0

Preferred Form and Dosage Schedule

As sodium fluoride	At bedtime, after brushing teeth[11]

Use in Prevention and Therapy

Caries prevention. Optimum fluoride intake sharply reduces the prevalence and severity of dental caries.[2,4] Low-level fluoride supplementation (through water, salt, or supplements) can reduce risk of caries in children by more than two-thirds.[4] In areas where water or salt is fluoridated, supplementation by other means, such as fluoride mouthwashes or tablets, is unnecessary.

Osteoporosis. Fluoride can stimulate osteoblastic activity and new bone formation, but its role in osteoporosis remains unclear.[6,14] Although one study found a decrease in vertebral fractures with intermittent fluoride and calcium therapy,[12] another found that skeletal fragility and fracture rates were increased by daily supplementation with fluoride and calcium.[13] Overall, it appears fluoride has little beneficial effect in osteoporosis.[14]

Toxicity

Chronic intakes of up to 5 mg fluoride/day in healthy adults appear to be safe. As intakes rise above this level, toxicity occurs. The first sign is dental fluorosis, in which the excess fluoride interferes with mineralization of the enamel and produces weakened, stained, and pitted enamel. Ingestion of more than 8–10 mg fluoride/day may produce skeletal deformities, osteoporosis, and osteomalacia, along with secondary hyperparathyroidism and calcification of soft tissues.[2,3]

References

1. Burt BA. The changing patterns of systemic fluoride intake. J Dent Res. 1992;71:1228.
2. National Research Council. Health effects of ingested fluoride. Washington, DC: National Academy Press; 1993.
3. Whitford GM. The metabolism and toxicity of fluoride. Monographs in Oral Science. Vol. 16. Basel: Karger; 1996.
4. Richmond VL. Thirty years of fluoridation: A review. Am J Clin Nutr. 1985;41:129.
5. Horowitz HS. Commentary on and recommendations for the proper uses of fluoride. J Public Health. 1995;55:57.
6. Kleerekorper M. Fluoride and the skeleton. Crit Rev Clin Lab Sci. 1996;33:139.
7. Phipps KR. Fluoride. In: Ziegler EE, Filer LJ, eds. Present Knowledge in Nutrition. Washington DC: ILSI Press; 1996.
8. Levy SM. Sources of fluoride intake in children. J Public Health Dent. 1995;55:39.
9. Institute of Medicine, Food and Nutrition Board. Dietary Reference Intakes for Calcium, Phosphorus, Magnesium, Vitamin D and Fluoride. Washington DC: National Academy Press; 1997.
10. American Academy of Pediatrics. Fluoride supplementation for children. Pediatrics. 1995;95:777.
11. Ismail AI. Fluoride supplements: current effectiveness, side effects and recommendations. Comm Dent Oral Epidemiol. 1994;22:164.
12. Riggs BL, et al. Effect of fluoride treatment on the fracture rate in postmenopausal women with osteoporosis. N Engl J Med. 1990;322:802.
13. Pak CYC, et al. Treatment of postmenopausal osteoporosis with slow release sodium fluoride: Final report of a randomized controlled trial. Ann Intern Med. 1995;123:401.
14. Eastell R. Treatment of postmenopausal osteoporosis. N Engl J Med. 1998;338:736.

Fats and Fat-Related Compounds

Essential Fatty Acids: Omega-3 and Omega-6 Fatty Acids

The two essential fatty acids for humans are linoleic and linolenic acid. Because mammalian cells lack the enzymes necessary for their synthesis, these two polyunsaturated fats must be obtained from dietary sources and are therefore termed essential fatty acids (EFAs). Linoleic acid is a member of the omega-6 fatty acid family, whereas linolenic acid is part of the omega-3 fatty acid group. The omega-3 or omega-6 designation (n-3 and n-6 notation is also used) refers to the distance of the first unsaturated bond from the methyl end of the fatty acid.

Functions

Cell membrane structure. EFAs are used to build and maintain cell membranes. Incorpor-

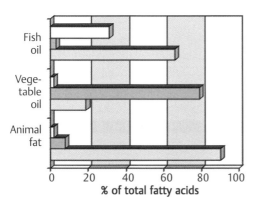

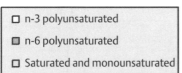

Fig. 3.**17**: **Fatty acid composition of the common fats and oils in the human diet.** Fish oils contain approximately 30% omega-3 polyunsaturated fats. They are the richest natural source of omega-3 fatty acids.

ation of EFAs into membranes increases membrane fluidity and enhances cell function. Membranes containing fatty acids derived from linoleic and linolenic acid are more fluid and resilient. If the diet is low in EFAs but high in saturated fats from animal foods, saturated fatty acids will replace EFAs in cell membranes, decreasing membrane fluidity, cell responsiveness, and function.

Eicosanoid formation. Both linoleic and linolenic acid are precursors in the synthesis of eicosanoids. Eicosanoids are hormonelike substances that have wide-ranging functions. Produced throughout the body, they are potent regulators of cell growth, blood pressure, platelet aggregation, and inflammation.[1] They also coordinate physiologic interactions among cells. The three major types of eicosanoids are prostaglandins, thromboxanes. and leukotrienes.

● **n-6 eicosanoids.** Dietary linoleic acid can be converted into gamma-linolenic acid (GLA) in the body. GLA can then be further metabolized to form the n-6 group of eicosanoids. One of the most important is the prostaglandin PGE1, which regulates and reduces the inflammatory response and inhibits platelet aggregation. Consuming generous amounts of linoleic acid or GLA can increase production of PGE1 in tissues. This can be beneficial in inflammatory disorders, such as rheumatoid arthritis and eczema, and in reducing thrombosis.[2,3] While many plant, seed, and nut oils are rich in linoleic acid, GLA is found preformed in only a few natural sources, such as borage seed oil and evening primrose oil.

● **n-3 eicosanoids.** In a similar way, dietary linolenic acid can be desaturated and elongated by cells to form the omega-3 fatty acids, eicosapentanoic acid (EPA) and docosahexanoic acid (DHA). These fats are then metabolized into prostaglandins that tend to reduce inflammation, dilate blood vessels and decrease platelet aggregation.[4] Increasing consumption of the omega-3 fatty acids can therefore be beneficial in disorders such as high blood pressure, atherosclerosis, and arthritis.[5,6] However, omega-3 fatty acids are only found in a few foods. Fatty fish from cold waters, such as salmon and mackerel, are the richest dietary source.

In humans, the conversion of linoleic acid to GLA and linolenic acid to EPA and DHA is through metabolic pathways of limited capacity. Intense competition exists for the enzyme systems in these pathways: high intakes of arachidonic acid (from meat and animal products) will saturate these pathways and inhibit production of GLA, DHA and EPA. Moreover,

these metabolic pathways can be impaired by chronic illness, high intake of saturated fat and alcohol, and poor nutritional status.[7] Deficiencies of vitamin B6, zinc, or magnesium impair the production of GLA, EPA, and DHA.

The typical diet in the industrialized countries is high in alcohol and animal products (rich in saturated fat and arachidonic acid) but low in fish, plant oils, zinc, and magnesium. This reduces production of beneficial eicosanoids from GLA, EPA, and DHA and favors production of proinflammatory and proaggregatory

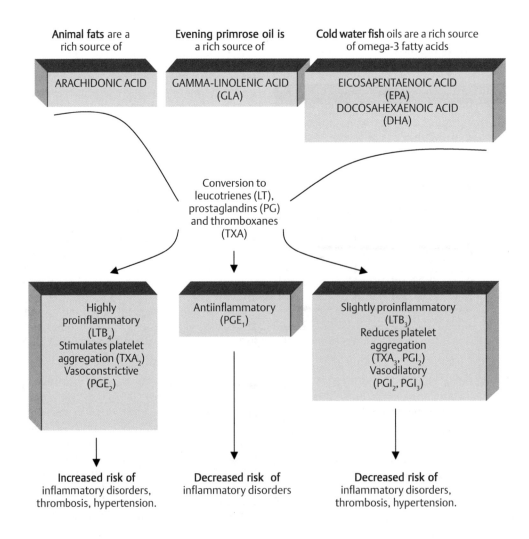

eicosanoids from arachidonic acid.[4] Reducing intake of animal products and alcohol while increasing intake of whole grains and high-quality, cold-pressed plant oils may provide significant health benefits. Another effective way to increase body stores of GLA, EPA, and DHA, especially when requirements are increased, is to obtain them directly from high-quality supplements. Fish-oil capsules contain about 30% EPA and DHA, while evening primrose oil contains about 10% GLA and 70% linoleic acid.

Increased Risk of Deficiency

Until recently EFA deficiency was regarded as a rarity, the reason being that clinical signs traditionally used for detection of deficiency (skin and hair changes) become visible only when deficiency is well advanced. However, with the development of more sensitive methods of diagnosis, subclinical EFA deficiency has been found to be much more common.[8]

● Diets rich in red meat, eggs, and milk but low in plant oils, fish, and seafood reduce body stores of GLA, EPA, and DHA.

● Deficiencies of zinc, magnesium, and vitamin B6 impair production of GLA, EPA, and DHA from dietary EFAs.

● Elderly people are less able to convert dietary EFAs to GLA, EPA, and DHA.

● Disorders of fat malabsorption, such as liver or biliary disease, Crohn disease, chronic pancreatitis, sprue, and cystic fibrosis reduce absorption of EFAs.

● Major physiologic stress due to injury, chronic illness, or surgery[8] increases requirements for EFAs and their metabolites.

● EFA requirements are elevated during periods of rapid growth, such as in pregnancy, childhood and adolescence.

Signs and Symptoms of Deficiency

- Dry, scaly skin
- Hair loss
- Impaired wound healing
- Impaired vision
- In childhood, reduced growth and impaired brain and eye development
- Male and female infertility
- Kidney damage, hematuria
- Possible increased risk of high blood pressure
- Reduced liver function
- Increased fragility of red blood cells
- Reduced immune function; increased vulnerability to infections
- Possible increased risk of atherosclerosis and venous thrombosis
- Possible increased risk of inflammatory disorders, such as rheumatoid arthritis

Good Dietary Sources

Linoleic acid	GLA
Vegetable oils (corn, safflower, soybean, sesame, sunflower)	Evening primrose oil, borage oil, blackcurrant oil

Linolenic acid	EPA and DHA
Soybeans, walnuts, wheat germ, linseeds, and their oils	Fish and shellfish (see next table), wild game

Marine sources of the omega-3 fatty acids (mg/100 g fish)

	EPA	DHA
Herring	2700	450
Tuna	1070	2280
Salmon	700	2140
Mackerel	690	1300
Halibut	190	500
Brook trout	150	335
Lobster	280	130
Shrimp	215	150

To obtain an optimum balance of fatty acids in the diet, the following dietary recommendations should be followed:

● Saturated fat intake should be reduced by eating fewer meat and whole-fat milk products

● High-quality, cold-pressed soybean, walnut, linseed, or wheat-germ oil should be used for salad dressings

● Intake of fish should be increased (two to three meals of cold-water fish per week)

● Intake of vegetables and wild game (such as venison and rabbit) should be increased

Recommended Daily Intakes

Recommended daily intakes for EFAs		
	Prevention of deficiency	
	UK (1991)	European PRI (1992)
n-3 fatty acids	0.2% of total calories	0.5% of total calories
n-6 fatty acids	1% of total calories	2% of total calories
	Therapeutic dose range Various authors	
n-3 fatty acids	1–10 g EPA + DHA (3–30 g fish oil)	
n-6 fatty acids	100–600 mg GLA (1–6 g evening primrose oil)	

Recommended intake of EPA and DHA varies according to the indication:
1. As a daily supplement in healthy people who rarely eat fish, to maintain a balanced intake of fats, fish-oil supplements are usually taken in the 0.5–1.0 g/day range.
2. For people with chronic ailments that may benefit from increasing omega-3 intake, supplements are usually in the range of 2–4 g/day.
3. For high-dose, acute therapy for serious illness or recovery from injury or major surgery, fish oil supplements are given in the range of 3–30 g/day.

Preferred Forms and Dosage Schedule

Omega-3 fatty acids	As fish oil capsules containing vitamin E as an antioxidant	Take with meals, preferably with the dose divided throughout the day
Omega-6 fatty acids	Although borage oil has a higher concentration of GLA, evening primrose oil is generally preferable in that it contains a better range of fatty acids. Capsules of evening primrose oil should contain vitamin E as an antioxidant	Take with meals, preferably with the dose divided throughout the day

High doses of GLA, EPA, and DHA should always be taken with additional vitamin E. As body stores of these polyunsaturated fats increase, additional vitamin E antioxidant protection is required. When taking omega-3 and omega-6 fatty-acid supplements, additional vitamin E (30–100 mg) and selenium (50–100 µg) is recommended.

Use in Prevention and Therapy

Gamma-linolenic Acid (GLA)

Atopic eczema. In families with an allergic predisposition (atopy), the conversion of linoleic acid to GLA is often poor, reducing levels of GLA and its product PGE1.[9] Supplementation with GLA (as evening primrose oil) can be beneficial in reducing the intensity of the allergic response as well as the scaling, itching, and skin sensitivity.[2,3]

Rheumatoid arthritis. Supplementation with GLA enhances PGE1 formation and may reduce inflammation and joint stiffness.[10,11]

Psoriasis. GLA can reduce skin inflammation, redness, and scaling.[12]

Diabetes. Diabetics have impaired ability to convert linoleic acid to GLA. Supplementation with GLA can be of benefit in reducing hyperlipidemia and improving motor and sensory nerve function in diabetic neuropathy.[13]

PMS. GLA may improve symptoms of PMS, including depression and irritability, breast tenderness, and fluid retention.

Hyperactivity. Children with hyperactivity (attention-deficit hyperactivity disorder) are at higher risk of EFA deficiency and may benefit from GLA supplementation.[14]

Hyperlipidemia. GLA may reduce plasma total cholesterol.[13,15]

Omega-3 Fatty Acids (EPA and DHA)

Coronary heart disease, heart attack, and stroke. Omega-3 fatty acids are beneficial in the prevention and treatment of atherosclerosis. They can reduce the tendency for platelet aggregation, blood clot formation, and cardiac arrhythmia.[16,17]

High blood pressure. Omega-3 fatty acids can lower blood pressure in hypertension.[6]

High blood lipids. Omega-3 fatty acids lower levels of triglycerides (and, to a lesser extent, total cholesterol), while increasing HDL cholesterol.[16,18]

Bronchial asthma. Omega-3 fatty acids can reduce chronic inflammation and the frequency and severity of asthma.[19]

Diabetes. Omega-3 fatty acids can reduce high levels of triglycerides, reduce blood pressure, and reduce leakage of proteins from small blood vessels. However, in some

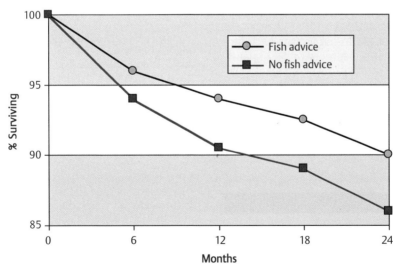

Fig. 3.**19: Fish consumption in patients with coronary heart disease.** 2000 adults with coronary disease and history of a myocardial infarction were randomized to three groups: one group was told to increase their fiber intake, the second to reduce their intake of saturated fat, the third to eat at least two portions of fish rich in omega-3 fatty acids each week. After 2 years the trial was stopped because the group advised to eat fish had a significant 29% reduction in all-cause mortality and a 33% reduction in deaths from heart disease. (Adapted from Burr ML, et al. Lancet. 1989;2:757)

diabetics, omega-3 fatty acids may also have adverse effects, such as reducing insulin action and increasing blood sugar.

Osteoarthritis. Omega-3 fatty acids may reduce pain and ease movement.

Migraine headache. Omega-3 fatty acids can reduce migraine frequency and intensity.

Autoimmune, rheumatic, and inflammatory disorders. In rheumatoid arthritis supplemental omega-3 fatty acids may reduce pain, inflammation, and joint stiffness.[20] Other disorders, such as Crohn disease[21] and ulcerative colitis[22] can also benefit from omega-3 fatty acids.

Skin disorders. Omega-3 fatty acids may reduce skin inflammation, redness, and scaling in patients with psoriasis and/or atopic eczema.[23]

Toxicity

High doses of EFAs without additional vitamin E intake can deplete body stores of vitamin E. In diabetics high doses of omega-3 fatty acids can sometimes reduce insulin action and elevate blood sugar. In individuals with rare inherited bleeding disorders or taking anticoagulant drugs, high-dose omega-3 supplementation may increase risk of abnormal bleeding. GLA should be used with caution in epilepsy or manic-depressive disorder. Rarely, high-dose supplementation may aggravate these disorders.

References

1. Hansen HS. New biological and clinical roles for the n-6 and n-3 fatty acids. Nutr Rev. 1994;52:162.
2. Fan Y, Chapkin RS. Importance of dietary gamma-linolenic acid in human health and nutrition. J Nutr. 1998;128:1411–4.
3. Horrobin DF. Nutritional and metabolic importance of gamma-linolenic acid. Prog Lipid Res. 1992;31:163.
4. Simopoulos AP. Essential fatty acids in health and chronic disease. Am J Clin Nutr. 1999;70:560S-69S.
5. Sassen LM, et al. Fish oil and the prevention and regression of atherosclerosis. Cardiovasc Drugs Ther. 1994;8:179.
6. Bonaa KH, et al. Effect of EPA and DHA on blood pressure in hypertension. N Engl J Med. 1990;322:795.
7. Brenner RR. Nutritional and hormonal factors influencing fatty acid desaturation of essential fatty acids. Prog Lipid Res. 1981;20:41.
8. Linscheer WG, et al. Lipids. In: Shils ME, Olson JA, Shike M, eds. Modern nutrition in health and disease. Philadelphia: Lea & Febiger; 1994.
9. Melnik BC, Plewig G. Is the origin of atopy linked to deficient conversion of omega-6-fatty acids to prostaglandin E1? J Am Acad Dermatol. 1989;21:557.
10. Joe LA, Hart LL. Evening primrose oil in rheumatoid arthritis. Ann Pharmacother. 1993;27:1475.
11. Zurier RB, et al. Gamma-linolenic acid treatment of rheumatoid arthritis. A randomized, placebo-controlled trial. Arthritis Rhem. 1996;39:1808–17.
12. Oliwiecki S, Burton JL. Evening primrose oil and marine oil in the treatment of psoriaisis. Clin Exp Dermatol. 1994;19:127.
13. The Gamma-linolenic Acid Multicenter Trial Group. Treatment of diabetic neuropathy with gamma-linolenic acid. Diabetes Care. 1993;16:8.
14. Stevens LJ. Essential fatty acid metabolism in boys with attention-deficit hyperactivity disorder. Am J Clin Nutr. 1995;62:761.
15. Horrobin DF, Manku MS. How do polyunsaturated fatty acids lower plasma cholesterol levels. Lipids. 1983;18:588.
16. Minnis RC, et al. Oily fish and fish oil supplements in the prevention of coronary heart disease. J Hum Nutr Diet. 1998;11:13.
17. Nair SSD, et al. Prevention of cardiac arrhythmia by dietary (n-3) PUFAs and their mechanism of action. J Nutr. 1997;127:383.
18. Harris WS. n-3 fatty acids and serum lipoproteins: Human studies. Am J Clin Nutr. 1997;65:1645S.
19. Broughton KS, et al. Reduced asthma symptoms with n-3 fatty acid ingestion are related to 5-series leukotriene production. Am J Clin Nutr. 1997;65:1011.
20. Belch JJF, et al. Effects of altering dietary essential fatty acids on requirements for non-steroidal anti-inflammatory drugs in patients with rheumatoid arthritis: A double-blind placebo controlled study. Ann Rheum Dis. 1988;47:96.
21. Belluzzi A, et al. Effect of an enteric coated fish oil preparation on relapses in Crohn disease. N Engl J med. 1996;334:1557.
22. Sanders TAB. Polyunsaturated fatty acids and inflammatory bowel disease. Am J Clin Nutr. 2000;71:339S-42S.
23. Ziboh VA. Essential fatty acids/eicosanoid biosynthesis in the skin: Biological significance. Proc Soc Exp Biol Med. 1994;205:1.

Choline and Lecithin

Choline is an essential component of the phospholipids found in cell membranes throughout the body. Choline is widely distributed in foods and can also be synthesized in limited amounts in the liver. However, this synthetic pathway alone cannot meet the body's needs, especially during times of increased physiologic stress. Diets low in choline may result in low body stores of choline and liver dysfunction,[1] thus ample dietary intake is important.

The term "lecithin" is used in two ways. In chemistry, lecithin is another name for phosphatidylcholine, which contains about 13% choline by weight, and is the major form of choline in foods. The term "lecithin" is more commonly used in nutrition to mean a substance typically derived from soybeans that contains a mixture of phosphatidylcholine (usually about 25%), myoinositol, and other phospholipids.

Functions

Formation of cell membranes and myelin. Choline is required to form cell membranes and the myelin sheath surrounding nerves.

Synthesis of acetylcholine in the peripheral and central nervous systems. Acetylcholine is one of the principal neurotransmitters mediating emotion and behavior in the brain.[2]

Liver metabolism of triglycerides and fats. The metabolism of triglycerides and other fats in the liver in preparation for circulation to peripheral tissues is dependent on choline. Phosphatidylcholine is an essential component of VLDL. Poor choline status is associated with fat accumulation in liver cells that can impair liver function and increase risk of hepatocarcinogenesis.[1]

Increased Risk of Deficiency

● Regular alcohol intake increases turnover of choline in the liver and can lead to depletion of body stores.

● A low dietary intake of folate sharply increases choline requirements. Risk of choline deficiency is increased in conditions of impaired folate status, including use of many common drugs (antibiotics, aspirin, oral contraceptive pills), chronic illnesses (liver disease, alcoholism, anemia), and vitamin B12 deficiency.

● Pancreatic or intestinal disorders cause poor absorption of dietary choline and may lead to deficiency.

● AIDS increases risk of choline deficiency.

Signs and Symptoms of Deficiency

- Fat accumulation in the liver leading to liver damage
- Impaired kidney function
- Infertility
- Decreased hematopoesis
- Hypertension
- Abnormal growth
- Impairments in learning and memory
- Impairment in carnitine metabolism
- Possible increased risk of liver cancer

Good Dietary Sources

Food	Serving size	mg
Calf liver	100 g	520
Eggs	1, medium size	270
Peanuts	100 g	95
Beef, filet	100 g	66
Cauliflower	100 g	42
Iceberg lettuce	100 g	31
Whole-wheat bread	100 g	13

Choline is found in many foods, though usual daily consumption of choline in Western Europe and the USA tends to be low, ranging from 0.2–1.0 g/day.[3] Lecithin supplements are particularly rich sources of choline, usually containing about 20–25% phosphatidylcholine. Therefore, 5 g of lecithin contain about 1 g of phosphatidlycholine.

Recommended Daily Intakes

The US DRI (1998) for choline is 425 mg for women and 450 mg for men. Dietary supplementation with choline is usually in the 0.5–1.5 g/day range, while supplementation with lecithin is in the 2–10 g/day range.

Lecithin	Take with meals

Use in Prevention and Therapy

Cardiovascular disease. Supplemental lecithin may lower triglycerides and LDL cholesterol in the blood and at the same time increase HDL cholesterol levels. These actions may reduce risk of atherosclerosis.

Memory. Supplemental choline and/or lecithin can increase levels of acetylcholine in the brain. Acetylcholine is involved in memory storage and retrieval, and choline and lecithin supplements may improve memory, particularly in the elderly.[1,4]

Alzheimer disease. Alzheimer's disease is characterized by low brain acetylcholine levels. Choline and lecithin may be effective in Alzheimer's disease and other forms of dementia by increasing acetylcholine levels in the brain.[5,6]

Movement disorders. Abnormalities in the acetylcholine system in the brain may produce motor disturbances. Therefore, choline and lecithin supplements may benefit people with Parkinson disease, Huntington disease, and other nervous disorders characterized by abnormal movements.[7] Choline and lecithin may also be beneficial in reducing tardive dyskinesia associated with antipsychotic drug use.[1]

Mania. Supplements can benefit people with mania, even cases resistant to traditional therapy with lithium.[8]

Pregnancy. Choline requirements are sharply increased during pregnancy. Pregnant women who do not obtain adequate dietary choline may develop fatty changes in the liver.[1] Supplemental choline can replace depleted choline stores and protect the liver.

Heavy alcohol consumption. Chronic alcohol consumption lowers blood and liver levels of choline and produces fatty liver and liver damage. Supplemental choline can reduce damage from alcohol and accelerate healing of the liver.

Hepatitis. Choline and lecithin reduce the symptoms and duration of viral hepatitis and may help prevent relapses.

Gallstones. Lecithin may prevent cholesterol from precipitating as stones in the gallbladder.

Toxicity

Very high doses of choline (>20 g/day for several weeks) may produce nausea, vomiting, dizziness, and a fishy body odor. Lower doses (1–10 g) of choline have not been reported to cause toxicity. High doses of choline may produce depression in rare individuals.

References

1. Canty DJ, Zeisel SH. Lecithin and cholin in human health and disease. Nutr Rev. 1994;52:327.
2. Zeisel SH. Choline and phosphatidylcholine. In: ME Shils, JA Olson, M Shike, AC Ross, eds. Modern Nutrition in Health and Disease. Baltimore: Williams & Wilkins; 1999.
3. Zeisel SH, et al. Normal plasma choline responses to ingested lecithin. Neurology. 1980;30:1226.
4. Cohen BM, et al. Decreased brain choline uptake in older adults.JAMA. 1995;274:902.
5. Bierer LM, et al. Neurochemical correlates of dementia severity in Alzheimer's disease relative importance of cholnergic deficits. J Neurochem. 1995;64:749.

6. Little A, et al. A double-blind, placeco-controlled trial of high dose lecithin in Alzheimer's disease. J Neurol Neurosurg Psychiatry. 1985;48:736.
7. Growdon JH. Use of phosphatidylcholine in brain diseases: An overview. In: Hanin I, Ansell GB, eds. Lecithin: Technological, Biological and Therapeutic Aspects. New York: Plenum Press; 1987.
8. Cohen BM, et al. Lecithin in the treatment of mania: Double-blind, placebo-controlled trials. Am J Psychiatry. 1982;139:1162.

Amino Acids

Branched-Chain Amino Acids: Leucine, Isoleucine, and Valine

The branched-chain amino acids (BCAAs), leucine, isoleucine, and valine are essential amino acids whose chemical structure is distinguished by a branch point. BCAAs are found in high amounts in skeletal muscle and are often referred to as the "stress" amino acids because they play important roles in energy metabolism and the body's response to stress.[1]

Functions

Energy metabolism in muscle. In contrast to other amino acids that are metabolized by the liver after intestinal absorption, BCAAs bypass the liver and circulate directly to the muscles. They can be taken up by muscle cells and used as an energy source.[2]

Protein synthesis and breakdown. During times of increased physiologic stress, such as injury, illness, or surgery, the body begins to break down protein at high rates. In these conditions, supplemental BCAAs help decrease protein breakdown and encourage protein conservation and synthesis.[3]

Reduced synthesis of neurotransmitters. BCAAs are transported into the brain by the same carrier that transports the amino acids phenylalanine, tyrosine, and tryptophan. Therefore, by competing for uptake, supplemental BCAAs can lower brain levels of these amino acids. Since phenylalanine, tyrosine, and tryptophan are precursors for certain neurotransmitters (including serotonin and dopamine), BCAAs can reduce activity of these neurotransmitters in the brain.[4]

Good Dietary Sources

BCAAs are richly supplied by many foods; they make up about half of the essential amino acids in the average diet.

Food	Serving size	Valine (mg)	Leucine (mg)	Isoleucine (mg)
Peanuts	100 g	1450	2030	1230
Tuna	100 g	1420	2170	1210
Salmon	100 g	1390	1770	1160
Beef, filet	100 g	1150	1700	1090
Veal, filet	100 g	1120	1660	1110
Chickpeas	100 g	980	1460	1140
Wheat germ	50 g	840	1085	660
Cottage cheese	100 g	825	1230	790
Brown rice	100 g	500	690	340
Milk	1 large glass	230	350	210

Recommended Daily Intakes

In healthy people the daily requirement for BCAAs to replace losses from normal protein metabolism and turnover are as follows[5]:

Valine	10 mg/kg body weight
Isoleucine	10 mg/kg body weight
Leucine	14 mg/kg body weight

In situations of increased physiologic stress, requirements for BCAAs sharply increase to levels of 5–10 g/day. Supplemental BCAAs are usually given in the range of 1–10 g/day. Intravenous doses range from 0.5–1.5 mg/kg body weight/day.

Preferred Form and Dosage Schedule

As a salt of L-valine, L-leucine, or L-isoleucine	Take in divided doses between meals

Use in Prevention and Therapy

Stress. During increased physiologic stress, body requirements for BCAAs are greatly increased relative to other amino acids. Supplemental BCAAs are important in conserving body stores of protein in chronic illness, anorexia nervosa, very low-calorie diets, injury, surgery, burns, or infection.[3]

Sports. Strenuous physical activity and athletic training sharply increase requirements for BCAAs. Supplemental BCAAs supply energy for working muscle and may improve performance in athletic events, particularly in endurance events such as long-distance running or cycling.[6] Because BCAAs enhance protein synthesis and reduce protein breakdown during strenuous exercise,[7,8] they may also be helpful in increasing muscle mass in weightlifting and other sports.

Liver disease. Severe liver disease often causes impaired brain function (encephalopathy) due to very high levels of tyrosine and tryptophan in the brain. Because BCAAs compete with these amino acids for transport into the brain, supplemental BCAAs (taken orally or intravenously), in conjunction with vitamin B6, lower brain levels of tyrosine and tryptophan and may improve mentation.[4,9]

Anorexia. Appetite and food intake are increased when serotonin levels in the brain are low. By reducing brain uptake of tryptophan (the precursor of serotonin), BCAAs may increase appetite and food intake in disorders where appetite is lost (chronic infection, AIDS, cancer).

Neuromuscular disorders. Combined supplementation with valine, leucine, and isoleucine may be of benefit in amyotrophic lateral sclerosis (ALS).[10] Huntington chorea is characterized by low levels of circulating BCAAs, and supplemental BCAAs may also be beneficial in this disorder.

Toxicity

High doses of BCAAs may reduce transport of tryptophan (the precursor to serotonin) into the brain. In conditions that may be aggravated if serotonin levels are lowered (insomnia, depression, migraine), caution should be exercised with high doses of BCAAs.

References

1. Harper AE, et al. Branched chain amino acid metabolism. Ann Rev Nutr. 1984;4:409.
2. Harris RA, et al. Regulation of branched-chain amino acid catabolism. J Nutr. 1994;124:1499S.
3. Cerra FB, et al. Branched chains support postoperative protein synthesis. Surgery. 1982;92:192.
4. Anonymous. Branched-chain amino acids reverse hepatic encephalopathy. Intern Med News. 1985;18:5.
5. World Health Organization. Energy and protein requirements. Tech Rep Series. 1985;724.
6. Blomstrand E, et al. Administration of branched-chain amino acids during prolonged exercise: effects on performance and on plasma concentrations of some amino acids. Eur J Appl Physiol. 1991;63:83.
7. Blomstrand E, et al. Effect of branched-chain amino acid and carbohydrate supplementation on the

exercise-induced change in plasma and muscle concentration of amino acids in human subjects. Acta Physiol Scand. 1995;153:87.

8. MacLean DA, et al. Branched-chain amino acids augment ammonia metabolism while attenuating protein breakdown during exercise. Am J Physiol. 1994;267:E1010.

9. Morgan MY, et al. Plasma ratio of valine, leucine and isoleucine to phenylalanine and tyrosine in liver disease. Gut. 1978;19:1068.

10. Plaitakas A, et al. Pilot trial of branched-chain amino acids in amyotrophic lateral sclerosis. Lancet. 1988;1:1015.

Arginine

The body's supply of arginine is derived from both dietary protein and endogenous synthesis by the liver. Because the liver's ability to synthesize arginine is limited, a generous dietary supply becomes critical in situations of increased need.[1] Rapid growth (e.g., in pregnancy, infancy, and childhood), strenuous physical exercise, stress, surgery, trauma, or chronic illness all sharply increase arginine requirements.

Functions

Hormone release. Arginine stimulates the release of several important hormones: growth hormone from the pituitary gland, insulin from the pancreas, and norepinephrine from the adrenal gland.[2]

Blood-cell production. Arginine stimulates production of white blood cells.[3]

Cancer prevention. Arginine may reduce tumor growth and thereby have anti-cancer properties.

Nitric-oxide production. Arginine plays an essential role in production of nitric oxide.[4] Nitric oxide helps control white blood-cell function, dilation of blood vessels, and neurotransmission in the brain.

Component of the urea cycle. Arginine is a key component of the urea cycle in the liver, the metabolic pathway that rids the body of excess nitrogen.[5]

Polyamine synthesis. Arginine plays an important role in the synthesis of polyamines (spermine, spermidine) required for cell division and growth.

Good Dietary Sources

Food	Serving size	mg
Peanuts	100 g	3460
Soybeans	100 g	2200
Hazelnuts	100 g	2030
Shrimps	100 g	1740
Lamb, filet	100 g	1400
Chicken, breast	100 g	1350
Tuna	100 g	1250
Wheat germ	50 g	1150
Oatmeal	100 g	870
Eggs	1, average size	450

Recommended Daily Intakes

Supplemental L-arginine is typically available in 500-mg doses. Recommended doses for arginine supplementation range from 1.5 to 6 g/day. Because the absorption of single high doses (>3 g) is poor, arginine supplements should be divided through the day. Because lysine competes with arginine for absorption and metabolism in the body, a diet low in lysine can enhance the effects of arginine supplementation.

Preferred Form and Dosage Schedule

As a salt of L-arginine	Take in divided doses between meals

Use in Prevention and Therapy

Immunity. Supplemental arginine strengthens the immune system by stimulating production of more active and effective white blood cells.[6,7]

Diabetes. Arginine supports the actions of insulin and helps maintain normal levels of blood glucose and triglycerides. Arginine also reduces platelet aggregation and can improve blood flow in diabetic eye, kidney, and foot disease.

Stress. Injury, surgery, or chronic illness often leads to rapid and destructive breakdown of body protein. Supplemental arginine reduces protein catabolism and helps maintain protein stores.[8,9] In situations of acute stress arginine enhances the release of the stress hormones norepinephrine and epinephrine from the adrenal gland.

Wound healing. Supplemental arginine may enhance wound healing and tissue repair by improving collagen deposition at the healing site.

Male fertility. Normal semen is rich in arginine, and arginine can be of benefit in treatment of male infertility. In cases of low sperm counts supplementation may increase sperm count and sperm motility.

Atherosclerosis. Low arginine levels at sites of atherosclerosis may constrict blood vessels around the atherosclerotic plaque, reducing blood flow. Supplemental arginine may increase nitric-oxide production and dilate blood vessels.[10]

Toxicity

Doses of 1–6 g/day of arginine are generally well tolerated by healthy adults. High-dose arginine supplementation may produce diarrhea, which is likely due to poor absorption of the arginine.

References

1. Abcouwer SF, Souba WW. Glutamine and arginine. In: ME Shils, JA Olson, M Shike, AC Ross, eds. Modern Nutrition in Health and Disease. Baltimore: Williams & Wilkins; 1999.
2. Hurson M, et al. Metabolic effects of arginine in a healthy elderly population. JPEN. 1995;19:227.
3. Moriguchi S, et al. Functional changes in human lymphocytes and monocytes after in vitro incubation with arginine. Nutr Res. 1987;7:719.
4. Castillo L, et al. Plasma arginine, citrulline and ornithine kinetics in adults, with observations on nitric oxide synthesis. Am J Physiol. 1995;268:E360.
5. Visek WJ. Arginine needs, physiological state and usual diets. J Nutr. 1986;116:36.
6. Mendez C, et al. Effects of supplemental dietary arginine, canola oil and trace elements on cellular immune function in critically injured patients. Shock. 1996;6:7.
7. Wu CW, et al. Can daily dietary arginine supplements affect the function and subpopulation of lymphocytes in patients with advanced gastric cancer? Digestion. 1993;54:118.
8. Daly JM, et al. Immune and metabolic effects of arginine in the surgical patient. Ann Surg. 1988;208:512.
9. Cynober L. Can arginine and ornithine support gut functions? Gut. 1994;35:S42.
10.. Boger RH, Bode-Borger SM. The clinical pharmacology of arginine. Ann Rev Rev Pharmacol Toxicol 2001;41:79.

Lysine

Lysine is an essential amino acid. Diets deficient in lysine can impair growth in children and reduce immune function.

Functions

Lysine plays an important role in maintenance of the immune system and has antiviral activity.[1]

Lysine is a precursor of carnitine,[2] and supplemental lysine can enhance carnitine synthesis.

Good Dietary Sources

Food	Serving size (g)	mg
Tuna	100	2210
Pork loin	100	2120
Shrimps	100	2020
Beef, filet	100	2020
Soybeans	100	1900
Lentils	100	1890
Chicken, breast	100	1790
Peanuts	100	1100
Parmesan cheese	30	950
Wheat germ	50	950

Recommended Daily Intakes

In healthy adults the daily requirement needed to replace losses from normal protein metabolism are as follows[3]:

Lysine	14 mg/kg body weight

Lysine requirements of children per kg body weight are three times higher than those of adults. Recommendations for 10–12-year-olds are for 44 mg/kg body weight.[3] Lysine supplements are best absorbed if taken on an empty stomach and not in combination with other amino acids. Usual doses of lysine supplementation range from 0.5 to 4 g/day.

Lysine and arginine share a common transport system for intestinal absorption and uptake into cells of the body and brain. Because arginine competes for uptake with lysine, a high ratio of lysine/arginine in the diet can enhance the effects of lysine supplementation.[4]

Preferred Form and Dosage Schedule

As a salt of L-lysine	Take in divided doses between meals

Use in Prevention and Therapy

Herpes simplex and other viral infections. Lysine helps prevent and treat herpes simplex infections (labial and genital).[1,5].

Immunity. Lysine deficiency weakens the immune system. Supplementation, may improve immune system function.

Carnitine metabolism. In conditions where carnitine stores in the body are low (see pp. 114) lysine can enhance carnitine synthesis and help rebuild body stores.[2]

Toxicity

There are no reports of toxicity in healthy adults consuming lysine in the 1–4 g/day range.

References

1. Griffith RS, et al. Success of L-lysine therapy in frequently recurrent herpes simplex infection. Dermatologica. 1987;175:183.
2. Rebouche CJ, et al. Utilization of dietary precursors for carnitine synthesis in human adults. J Nutr. 1989;119:1907.
3. World Health Organization. Energy and protein requirements. Tech Rep Series. 1985;724.
4. Algert SJ, et al. Assessment of dietary intake of lysine and arginine in pateints with herpes simplex. J Am Diet Assoc. 1987;87:1560.
5. Wright EF. Clinical effectiveness of lysine in treating recurrent apthous ulcers and herpes labialis. Gen Dent. 1994;42:40.

Glutamine

Glutamine is the most abundant amino acid in tissues and the blood.[1] It is important as an energy source and as a precursor to glutathione. Glutamine can be taken up by the brain and converted to gamma-aminobutyric acid (GABA), an inhibitory neurotransmitter.

Functions

Energy metabolism. Glutamine is broken down to produce energy in many tissues in the body. It is especially important as an energy source for the cells lining the digestive tract and the white blood cells. Glutamine can be taken up by the liver and converted to glucose to maintain blood sugar levels.[2]

Glutathione synthesis. Glutamine, together with cysteine, serves as the precursor in the synthesis of glutathione, an important antioxidant[1] (see pp. 105).

Conversion to GABA. Glutamine is readily taken up by the brain and converted to GABA. GABA is an important inhibitory neurotransmitter with tranquilizing, calming effects.[3] Valium and other benzodiazepine drugs exert their calming effects by enhancing the actions of GABA in the brain.

Good Dietary Sources

Food	Serving size	mg
Ham	100 g	2860
Cheddar cheese	30 g	1600
Turkey, breast	100 g	1330
Chicken, breast	100 g	990
Milk	1 large glass	820
Egg	1, average size	800

Many high-protein foods are rich in glutamic acid, which is converted in the body to glutamine.

Recommended Daily Intakes

Oral glutamine supplements are normally taken in the range of 2–12 g/day. To enhance glutathione synthesis and antioxidant protection, glutamine should be taken with cysteine and selenium.[1]

Preferred Form and Dosage Schedule

As a salt of L-glutamine	Take in divided doses between meals

Use in Prevention and Therapy

Stress situations. During times of increased physiologic stress, glutamine requirements in the intestine, the immune system, and liver increase sharply (Fig. 3.**20**). During these periods, glutamine synthesis may not be sufficient and glutamine becomes an essential amino acid. Supplemental glutamine can be beneficial in injuries, major operations, burns, and chronic illness.[4]

Disorders of the gastrointestinal tract. Because glutamine is a principal energy source for intestinal cells, glutamine is important when the intestine needs to maintain or repair itself during and after damage from drugs, surgery, or chronic illness.[5] Glutamine may be effective in inflammatory diseases of

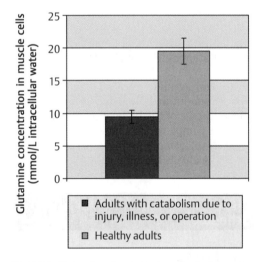

Fig. 3.**20**: **Glutamine levels in muscle during catabolic illness.** Glutamine levels in muscle during recovery from serious illness, injury, or surgery are about 50% lower than those in healthy individuals. (Adapted from Stehle P, et al. Ernähr Umschau. 1996;43:318)

the intestine (e.g., Crohn's disease, ulcerative colitis, infectious diarrhea) and during intestinal surgery. Glutamine also helps repair damage to the digestive-tract lining caused by peptic ulcer disease or gastritis from aspirin or alcohol.

Immune system. Glutamine supports the immune system and enhances white blood-cell function.[6]

Antioxidant system. Glutamine increases levels of glutathione in the liver and intestine, enhancing the antioxidant defenses of these tissues.[1]

Sedative effects. Because GABA has mild sedative and calming effects,[7] supplemental glutamine taken up and converted to GABA may benefit those suffering from irritability, nervousness, anxiety, and, in some cases, affective disorders. [8]

Toxicity

Very high doses of glutamine may increase levels of glutamate in the brain,[1] which may worsen mania or epilepsy. Large doses of glutamine should be avoided in these disorders.

References

1. Shou J. Glutamine. In: G Zaloga, ed. Nutrition in Critical Care. St. Louis: Mosby; 1994.
2. Curthoys NP, Watford M. Regulation of glutaminase activity and glutamine metabolism. Annu Rev Nutr. 1995;15:134.
3. Hertz L, et al., ed. Glutamine, Glutamate and GABA in the Central Nervous System. New York: Alan Liss; 1983.
4. Hall JC, et al. Glutamine. Br J Surg. 1996;83:305.
5. Moskovitz B, et al. Glutamine metabolism and utilization: relevance to major problems in health care. Pharmacol Res. 1994;30:61.
6. Parry-Billings M, et al. Does glutamine contribute to immunosupression after major burns? Lancet. 1990;336:523.
7. De-Deyn PP, et al. Epilepsy and the GABA-hypothesis: A brief review and some examples. Acta Neurol Belg. 1990;90:65.
8. Petty F. GABA and mood disorders: A brief review and hypothesis. J Affect Disord. 1995;34:275.

Methionine

Methionine is an essential amino acid. It is the dietary precursor to both cysteine and taurine. Like cysteine and taurine, it is distinctive in that it contains a sulfur group.

Functions

Protein and nucleic-acid metabolism. The active form of methionine is S-adenosylmethionine (SAM). SAM plays a central role in the synthesis of many important body compounds, including carnitine, choline, epinephrine, melatonin, and nucleic acids. It is particularly active in the brain. Low levels of SAM in the brain can produce lethargy and depression and, when severe, psychiatric disorders.[1]

Amino-acid synthesis. Methionine is the sole dietary precursor to both cysteine and taurine.

Good Dietary Sources (Methionine and Cysteine*)

Food	serving size	mg
Salmon	100 g	700
Shrimp	100 g	670
Turkey, breast	100 g	630
Soybeans	100 g	580
Beef, filet	100 g	570
Cashew nuts	100 g	330
Wheat germ	50 g	280
Hard cheeses	30 g	250
Egg	1, average size	240

* Food content of the sulfur-containing amino acids methionine and cysteine is usually measured together.

Recommended Daily Intakes

In healthy adults the daily requirement needed to replace losses from normal protein metabolism is as follows[2]:

Methionine + cysteine	13 mg/kg body weight

Supplementation of methionine is normally in the range of 0.5 to 5.0 g and should be taken with vitamin B6.[3]

Preferred Form and Dosage Schedule

As a salt of L-methionine	Take in divided doses between meals

Use in Prevention and Therapy

Depression. Methionine readily passes into the brain, where it is activated to SAM. Methionine supplementation may be beneficial in depression, elevating mood and leading to an increased feeling of well-being (Fig. 3.**21**).[4-6]

Parkinson disease. L-dopa therapy (used to treat Parkinson disease) lowers levels of SAM in the brain. Used alongside L-dopa, methionine supplementation maintains SAM levels in the brain. It can ease movement, increase activity levels, reduce tremor, and improve sleep and mood.

Detoxification. Methionine, together with zinc, can enhance detoxification and excretion of chemicals, drugs, and lead.[7]

Urinary tract infections. Methione helps prevent chronic urinary tract infections. It acidifys the urine, discouraging growth of pathogenic bacteria.

Toxicity

Large doses of methionine can be metabolized to homocysteine, a toxic metabolite. However, production of homocysteine is minimized by taking vitamin B6 along with methionine. High doses of methionine increase urinary excretion of calcium and should be avoided by women with, or at high risk of, osteoporosis. Very high doses in patients with schizophrenia may exacerbate hallucinations.

Fig. 3.**21**: **S-adenosylmethionine (SAM) and mood improvement in depression.** As measured by the Hamilton Rating Scale for Depression (HRSD), SAM given for 3 weeks in oral doses of 1600 mg/day produced significant improvement in subjects with depression.
(From: Friedel HA. Drugs. 1989;38:389)

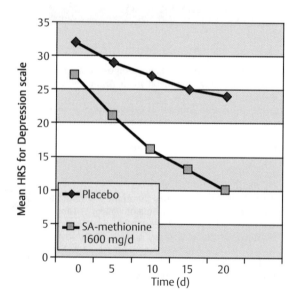

References

1. Reynolds EH, et al. Methylation and mood. Lancet. 1984;1:196.
2. World Health Organization. Energy and protein requirements. Tech Rep Series. 1985;724.
3. Stegink LD, et al. Plasma methionine levels in normal adult subjects after oral loading with L-methionine and N-acetyl-L-methionine. J Nutr. 1980;110:42.
4. Fava M, et al. Rapidity of onset of the antidepressant effect of S-adenosyl-methionine. Psychiatr Res. 1995;56:295.
5. Bressa GM. S-adenosyl-methionine as an antidepressant: Meta analysis of clinical studies. Acta Neurol Scand Suppl. 1994;154:7.
6. Young SN. The use of diet and dietary components in the study of factors controlling affect in humans: A review. J Psychiatr Neurosci. 1993;18:235.
7. Crome P, et al. Oral methionine in the treatment of severe paracetamol overdose. Lancet. 1976;2:829.

Cysteine and Glutathione

The amino acid cysteine contains a sulfur group that allows it to function as an important antioxidant. Cysteine can function independently as an antioxidant, or it can be combined with glutamic acid and glycine in liver cells to form glutathione. Glutathione is a principal water-soluble antioxidant in cells and the blood.[1] The dietary supply of cysteine is a primary determinant of how much glutathione is synthesized in the body, and supplements of cysteine can boost tissue levels of glutathione.

Functions

Antioxidant and detoxification function. Cysteine, alone or as part of glutathione, is a potent antioxidant, protecting against free radical damage.[2] Glutathione, working with the enzyme glutathione peroxidase (a selenium-containing enzyme), detoxifies free radicals, drugs, and toxic chemicals. It also recycles oxidized vitamin E and vitamin C, conserving body stores of these antioxidants.[3]

Cell-membrane synthesis and repair. Cysteine (working together with pantothenic acid) plays a central role in the synthesis of important fatty acids used in production of cell membranes and the myelin sheath surrounding nerve cells. Glutathione plays an important role in the health of red blood cells, maintaining the integrity of the red cell membranes.

Connective-tissue synthesis. In connective tissue, muscle, and bone two molecules of cysteine are joined by their sulfur groups in a "disulfide bridge." These bridges impart strength and stiffness to connective tissue.

Leukotriene synthesis. Glutathione plays an important role in the production of leukotrienes. Leukotrienes are important chemical messengers. They modulate the activity of white blood cells in inflammatory and immune responses.

Good Dietary Sources

Because cysteine content of foods is difficult to measure and methionine is the precursor of cysteine, food content of these two sulfur-containing amino acids is usually measured together. The best sources of these amino acids is shown on pages 103.

Recommended Daily Intakes

In healthy adults, the daily requirement needed to replace losses from normal protein metabolism is as follows[4]:

Cysteine + methionine	13 mg/kg body weight

Recommended doses for L-cysteine are in the range of 500–1500 mg/day. If the primary aim of therapy is increasing glutathione levels, cysteine should be supplemented with glutamine and selenium. Selenium supports optimum functioning of the glutathione detoxification system[5].

The glutathione that is oxidized during detoxification reactions is reconverted to active glutathione by enzymes requiring vitamin B2 (riboflavin) and vitamin B12. Thus, riboflavin or vitamin B12 deficiency reduces glutathione activity in tissues.

Preferred Form and Dosage Schedule

As a salt of L-cysteine. Because the absorption of glutathione supplements is unpredictable, cysteine supplements are the preferred method of increasing glutathione levels in the body.	Take in divided doses between meals

Use in Prevention and Therapy

Bronchitis. Cysteine (in the form N-acetylcysteine) can benefit patients with bronchitis and asthma by loosening and thinning mucus that accumulates in the bronchi, allowing it to be more easily removed by coughing.

Chronic diseases and the aging process. Cysteine and glutathione (by protecting DNA from free-radical damage) may help slow down aging changes[6]. The amount of glutathione in cells tends to decrease with age. Elderly people may benefit from supplements of cysteine or glutathione to maintain optimum glutathione activity.

Pollution and other environmental hazards. Cysteine and glutathione help protect against toxins and pollutants, including drugs, bacterial toxins, peroxidized fats, heavy metals (lead, cadmium, arsenic, etc.), air pollutants, automobile exhaust fumes, food additives, and pesticides.[7] Cysteine helps protect the lungs of smokers from the toxic effects of formaldehyde and acetaldehyde, two of the many toxic ingredients in cigarette smoke. Cysteine can be important in cancer chemotherapy, reducing toxicity from agents such as cyclophosphamide and doxorubicin.

Heavy alcohol consumption. Cysteine and glutathione may help protect the liver and other tissues from damage from heavy alcohol consumption by detoxifying acetaldehyde, the major toxic metabolite of ethanol.

Immune support. Cysteine, through glutathione, strengthens the immune system by enhancing production of important immunoregulators (leukotrienes) and maintaining white blood-cell function.

Gastritis and ulcers. The cells of the gastric lining are rich in glutathione, which helps protect the stomach wall against damage from gastric acid. Cysteine or glutathione supplementation enhances this protective function and may be beneficial in gastritis and ulcers.

Cataracts. During aging the glutathione content of the lens gradually decreases. This increases vulnerability of the lens to oxidative damage from ultraviolet light that contributes to cataract. Glutathione and cysteine, through their antioxidant actions, (together with riboflavin) may play a central role in the prevention of cataracts.[8]

Exercise. Vigorous exercise may deplete the body of glutathione. This increases the risk of oxidative damage in overworked skeletal muscle. Supplemental cysteine can help maintain glutathione stores during exercise.[9]

Toxicity

Supplements of L-cystine (formed by joining two cysteine molecules) should be avoided because they provide none of the antioxidant effects of cysteine and may increase risk of kidney stones. High doses of cysteine may be converted to cystine and precipitate formation of kidney and bladder stones. Ample vitamin C intake helps prevent conversion of cysteine to cystine and reduces the risk of this side effect. Large doses of supplemental cysteine may interfere with the action of insulin and thereby worsen blood-sugar control in diabetes; diabetics should consult their physician before taking large doses of cysteine. There are no reports of toxicity from glutathione supplements.

References

1. Lomaestro BM, Malone M. Glutathione in health and disease: Pharmacotherapeutic issues. Ann Pharmacol. 1995;29:1263.
2. Bray TM, Taylor CG. Tissue glutathione, nutrition and oxidative stress. Can J Physiol Pharmacol. 1993;71:746.
3. Kubena KS, McMurray DN. Nutrition and the immune system: A review of nutrient-nutrient interactions. J Am Diet Assoc. 1996;96:1156.
4. World Health Organization. Energy and protein requirements. Tech Rep Series. 1985;724.
5. Neve J. Human selenium supplementation as assessed by changes in blood selenium and glutathione peroxidase activity. J Trace Elem Med Biol. 1995;9:65.
6. Kretzschmar M, Muller D. Aging, training and exercise. A review of effects of plasma glutathione and lipid peroxides. Sports Med. 1993;15:196.
7. Smith TK. Dietary modulation of the glutathione detoxification pathway and the potential for altered xenobiotic metabolism. Adv Exp Med Biol. 1991;289:165.
8. Reddy VN. Glutathione and its function in the lens—an overview. Exp Eye Res. 1990;50:71.
9. Sastre J, et al. Exhaustive physical exercise causes oxidation of glutathione status in blood: Prevention by antioxidant administration. Am J Physiol. 1992;263:R992.

Phenylalanine and Tyrosine

The essential amino acid phenylalanine (PA) can be converted to tyrosine in the liver. Both amino acids play important roles in the metabolism of hormones and neurotransmitters. In certain conditions, such as severe infection or liver disease, the ability of the liver to convert PA to tyrosine is impaired and tyrosine becomes a dietary essential amino acid.

Functions

Neurotransmitter synthesis. PA and tyrosine can readily cross from the blood into the brain and are precursors in the synthesis of the neurotransmitters dopamine, norepinephrine, and epinephrine.

Enkephalin metabolism. PA slows the breakdown of brain chemicals called enkephalins that have opiate-like, pain-reducing properties.[1]

Hormone synthesis. Tyrosine is an essential precursor in production of the thyroid hormones.

Good Dietary Sources (Phenylalanine)

Food	Serving size	mg
Soybeans	100 g	1970
Peanuts	100 g	1540
Almonds	100 g	1140
Tuna	100 g	1050
Beef, filet	100 g	930
Trout	100 g	920
Cottage cheese	100 g	635
Wheat germ	50 g	600
Hard cheese	30 g	540
Egg	1, average size	400

Recommended Daily Intakes

In healthy people the daily requirement needed to replace losses from normal protein metabolism is as follows[2]:

Supplemental PA is usually given in daily doses ranging from 200 mg to 8 g. Supplemental tyrosine is given in doses ranging from 200 mg to 6 g. PA and tyrosine should generally not be given concurrently, as the risk of side effects may be increased. Conversion of these amino acids to neurotransmitters in the brain can be enhanced if they are given together with vitamin B6.

Phenylalanine plus tyrosine	14 mg/kg body weight

Preferred Form and Dosage Schedule

As a salt of L-tyrosine or L-phenylalanine. Supplemental amino acids should nearly always be given as the L form (the naturally occurring isomer), but because the D form of PA has unique actions on pain pathways in the brain, supplements of PA taken for this purpose should be in the form of D, L-phenylalanine. For treatment of conditions other than chronic pain, the L-phenylalanine form is preferable and effective	Take in divided doses between meals

Use in Prevention and Therapy

Pain modulation. The D-isomer of PA is an effective pain reliever.[1] It is found in supplements of D,L-phenylalanine (DLPA). It can enhance the activity of brain enkephalins and the pain-reducing effects of acupuncture and transcutaneous electrical nerve stimulation (TENS). DLPA may reduce headaches and peripheral aches associated with PMS.

Depression. Patients with depression may benefit from tyrosine[4,5] (Fig. 3.**22**) and/or PA.[6,7] Supplements increase brain levels of the norepinephrine and epinephrine, which can improve mood.[8,9]

Parkinson disease. In Parkinson disease the cells that produce dopamine in certain areas of the brain are lost. PA and tyrosine, as precursors to dopamine, may be helpful in increasing dopamine levels and reducing symptoms.

Hyperactivity in children. Tyrosine supplements may sometimes be beneficial in hyperactive children, improving concentration and behavior.[10]

Cocaine addiction. Supplemental tyrosine, in conjunction with tryptophan, is of benefit in the treatment of cocaine abuse. Tyrosine and tryptophan blunt the feelings of the cocaine "high" and reduce the depression caused by withdrawal of the drug.

Benefits of PA/Tyrosine Restriction in Certain Disorders

Low PA diets are used in the treatment of phenylketonuria, an inherited disorder occurring in approximately one out of every 20–40000 live births.[3] In PKU, because of a lack of the liver enzyme that converts PA to tyrosine, very high levels (>400 times normal) of PA are found in the blood and tissues; these can damage the brain, cause seizures, and produce mental retardation. A special diet very low in PA prevents the rise in blood PA and damage to the brain.

Very high levels of PA and tyrosine are found in the blood of patients with severe liver disease and may contribute to mental impairment (encephalopathy) and coma in these patients. Low PA/tyrosine diets combined with high amounts of BCAAs–BCAAs compete with PA and tyrosine for transport into the brain–can improve mental functioning in these patients (see pp. 98).[11]

Toxicity

Supplemental phenylalanine and tyrosine may cause headache, anxiety, or high blood pressure in rare individuals. They should not be used by pregnant or lactating women, in severe liver disease or PKU. PA and tyrosine supplements should be avoided by patients receiving MAO inhibitor-type antidepressants. PA and tyrosine supplements should also be avoided by schizophrenics, particularly those with high dopamine levels, as supplements may further increase brain dopamine and worsen the condition.

Fig. 3.**22**: **Tyrosine supplements and depression.** In a crossover trial of tyrosine in depression, a woman unable to tolerate standard antidepressant therapy was given 100 mg/kg of tyrosine in 3 daily doses for 2 weeks, a placebo for 18 days, then tyrosine again for a further 5 weeks. During treatment with tyrosine (both periods) depression was significantly alleviated (as measured by both the Hamilton and Zung Scales), compared with both baseline and the placebo period.
(Adapted from Gelenberg AJ, et al. Am J Psychiat. 1980;137:622)

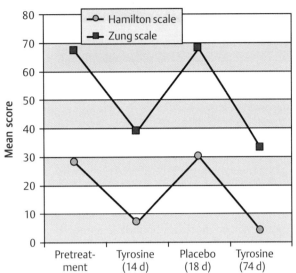

References

1. Walsh NE, et al. Analgesic effectiveness of D-phenylalanine in chronic pain patients. Arch Phys Med Rehab. 1986;67:436.
2. World Health Organization. Energy and protein requirements. Tech Rep Series. 1985;724.
3. Lindner MC. Nutrition and metabolism of proteins. In: MC Lindner, ed. Nutritional Biochemistry and Metabolism. New York: Elsevier; 1991.
4. Gelenberg AJ, et al. Tyrosine for depression: A double blind trial. J Affect Disord. 1990;19:125.
5. Mouret J, et al. L-Tyrosine cures immediate and long term, dopamine dependent depressions. Clinical and polygraphic studies. Coll R Acad Sci III. 1988;306:93.
6. Beckman V, Ludoph E. DL-phenylalanine as antidepressant. Arzneimit Forschung. 1978;28:1283.
7. Kravitz HM, et al. Dietary supplements of phenylalanine and other amino acid precursors of brain neuroamines in the treatment of depressive disorders. J Am Osteo Assoc. 1984;84:119.
8. Crowdon JM. Neuro-transmitter precursors in the diet: their use in the treatment of brain diseases. In. Wurtman RJ, Wurtman JJ, eds. Nutrition and the Brain. Vol 3. New York: Raven Press; 1979.
9. Young SN. The use of diet and dietary components in the study of factors controlling affect in humans: A review. J Psychiatr Neurosci. 1993;18:235–44.
10. Reimherr RW, et al. An open trial of L-tyrosine in the treatment of attention deficit disorders, residual type. Am J Psychiatry. 1987;144:1071.
11. Morgan MY, et al. Plasma ratio of valine, leucine and isoleucine to phenylalanine and tyrosine in liver disease. Gut. 1978;19:1068.

Tryptophan

Tryptophan is an essential amino acid. It is used to build cell proteins and is a precursor of two important compounds, serotonin (a neurotransmitter) and niacin (vitamin B3).

Functions

Neurotransmitter synthesis. Serotonin is a neurotransmitter that is formed from tryptophan. Increased dietary intake of tryptophan increases levels of serotonin in the brain and can cause mild drowsiness, improve mood, and reduce appetite.[1]

Niacin metabolism. Niacin (vitamin B3) can be formed from tryptophan when dietary intake of preformed niacin is low. About 60 mg of tryptophan is required to synthesize 1 mg of niacin.[2]

Good Dietary Sources

Food	Serving size	mg
Cashew nuts	100 g	450
Veal, filet	100 g	350
Sunflower seeds	100 g	310
Tuna	100 g	300
Chicken, breast	100 g	270
Beef, filet	100 g	260
Oatmeal	100 g	190
Eggs	1, average size	165
Wheat germ	50 g	165
Hard cheese	30 g	150

Tryptophan is the least abundant essential amino acid in the food supply. Because dietary levels of tryptophan are low relative to other amino acids, supplementation with even 1 g is a substantial dietary increase.

Recommended Daily Intakes

In healthy adults the daily requirement needed to replace losses from normal protein metabolism is as follows[3]:

Tryptophan	3.5 mg/kg body weight

Oral supplementation with tryptophan is generally in the range of 500 mg to 3 g. Five other amino acids–phenylalanine, tyrosine, leucine, isoleucine, and valine–all compete with tryptophan for uptake into the brain. By reducing intake of these amino acids, brain uptake of tryptophan can be increased.[4] The ability of tryptophan to raise brain serotonin levels is enhanced by concurrent ingestion of a small amount of carbohydrate (the insulin released in response to the carbohydrate will remove valine, leucine, and isoleucine from the blood into muscle, so competition for brain tryptophan uptake will be reduced). Ample vitamin B6 and riboflavin is required for production of serotonin (or niacin) from tryptophan.[1]

Preferred Form and Dosage Schedule

As a salt of L-tryptophan	Take in divided doses between meals

Use in Prevention and Therapy

Sleep disorders. Tryptophan is effective in treating insomnia, significantly reducing the time needed to fall asleep.[5]

Depression and mania. Lack of serotonin in the brain contributes to some forms of depression.[6] Therefore, depression, especially when marked by agitation and suicidal tendencies, may benefit from tryptophan and vitamin B6 supplementation.[7,8] Mania has also been successfully treated with tryptophan.

Aggressivity. Supplemental tryptophan, together with vitamin B6, has a calming effect and can decrease aggressive behavior.[8]

Schizophrenia. Tryptophan can be effective by enhancing serotonin production to balance the excess of dopamine found in some forms of schizophrenia.[9]

Oral contraceptive pills. The pill can interfere with tryptophan metabolism to serotonin (possibly by impairing vitamin B6 status). The depression and moodiness associated with use of oral contraceptive pills may improve with tryptophan supplementation.

Appetite. Increasing tryptophan intake can enhance production of serotonin in the brain, thereby reducing appetite and carbohydrate craving.

Toxicity

Use of certain tryptophan supplements in the 1980s was associated with the eosinophilia-myalgia syndrome (EMS).[10] This syndrome is characterized by abnormal accumulation of eosinophils in connective tissues, muscle and joint pains, and excessive deposition of collagen in skin. In severe cases, EMS resulted in impaired brain function, disability, and death. The tryptophan that caused EMS originated from a single manufacturer. It appears that the manufacturing process produced altered compounds, including abnormal forms of tryptophan that may have been responsible for causing the syndrome. It is very unlikely that pure tryptophan can cause EMS, but tryptophan supplements remain unavailable in many countries.

References

1. Lindner MC. Nutrition and metabolism of proteins. In: MC Lindner, ed. Nutritional Biochemistry and Metabolism. New York: Elsevier; 1991.
2. Jacob RA, Swenseid ME. Niacin. In: Ziegler EE, Filer LJ., eds. Present Knowledge in Nutrition. Washington DC: ILSI Press; 1996.
3. World Health Organization. Energy and protein requirements. Tech Rep Series. 1985;724.
4. Lucini V, et al. Predictive value of tryptophan/large neutral amino acids ratio to antidepressant response. J Affect Disord. 1996;36:129.
5. Schneider-Helmert D, Spinweber CL. Evaluation of L-tryptophan for treatment of insomnia: A review. Psychopharmacology Berl. 1986;89:1.
6. Cowen PJ, et al. Decreased plasma tryptophan levels in major depression. J Affect Disord. 1989;16:27.
7. Young SN. The use of tryptophan in combination with other antidepressant treatments: A review. J Psychiatry Neurosci. 1991;16:241.
8. Young SN. Some effects of dietary components (amino acids, carbohydrate, folic acid) on brain serotonin synthesis, mood and behavior. Can J Physiol Pharmacol. 1991;69:893.
9. Sandyk R. L-tryptophan in neuropsychiatrc disorders: A review. Int J Neurosci. 1992;67:127.
10. Hertzman PA, et al. The eosinophilia-myalgia syndrome: status of 205 patients and results of treatment 2 years after onset. Ann Intern Med. 1995;122:851.

Taurine

Taurine, like methionine and cysteine, contains a sulfur group. Taurine is unique in that, unlike all the other amino acids, it is not used to form structural proteins. It plays important functional roles and is the most abundant free amino acid in platelets, the nervous system, and muscle.[1] Body requirements for taurine are supplied by both dietary sources and synthesis within cells. However, humans can only synthesize small amounts of taurine, and diets low in taurine can cause body levels of taurine to fall.[2] Particularly in conditions when demand for taurine increases, dietary sources become important.

Functions

Growth and development. Taurine is important for growth and development of the brain and eye.[1]

Nerve metabolism. Taurine is a component of several small proteins and neurotransmitters important in regulation of nervous function.

Membrane stabilization. In conjunction with calcium, taurine has a stabilizing, inhibitory action on excitable membranes in the heart, nerves, and platelets.

Antioxidant actions. Taurine contains a sulfur group that allows it to function as an effective antioxidant.[1]

Detoxification. Taurine can bind to and help detoxify chemicals, drugs, and other xenobiotics in the liver.[1]

Bile acid metabolism. Bile acids secreted by the liver are bound to taurine (or glycine). Taurine is essential for proper bile acid function and fat absorption.[4]

Good Dietary Sources

Food	Serving size	mg
Clams, fresh	100 g	240
Tuna	100 g	70
Oysters	100 g	70
Pork loin	100 g	50
Lamb, filet	100 g	47
Beef, filet	100 g	36
Chicken, dark meat	100 g	34
Cod	100 g	31
Milk	1 dl	6

Usual dietary intake of taurine is in the range of 40–400 mg/day. Because taurine is virtually absent from plant foods, vegetarians have very low intakes.

Recommended Daily Intakes

Normal daily synthesis of taurine is estimated to be about 50–125 mg.[1] Supplemental taurine is usually given in the range of 0.5–4.0 g/day. Taurine can be synthesized in the liver from cysteine, so supplements of cysteine can enhance endogenous production and increase taurine stores. Because vitamin B6 is an essential cofactor in this synthesis, cysteine is most effective if taken with vitamin B6.

Preferred Form and Dosage Schedule

As a salt of taurine	Take in divided doses between meals

Use in Prevention and Therapy

Newborns. Infants have increased taurine requirements because of rapid growth, yet they cannot synthesize taurine efficiently. Breast milk is high in taurine, but many infant formulas are not. Therefore, newborns, particularly those fed formula, are at risk of taurine deficiency.[5]

Thrombotic disorders. Taurine supplementation reduces platelet aggregation, lowering the risk of heart attack, stroke, and venous thrombosis.[1] This effect is particularly marked in diabetes, where taurine supplements may reduce risk of eye and kidney disease.

Heart disease. Taurine has multiple beneficial actions on the heart.[6,7] It stabilizes the myocardium and reduces risk of dysrhythmias.[8] It also helps the heart pump stronger and more effectively. Taurine can be beneficial in coronary artery disease and congestive heart failure.

Hypertension. Taurine helps reduce high blood pressure[7] (Fig. 3.**23**) and is particularly effective when given with calcium supplements.

Epilepsy. Taurine, located in nerve membranes in a complex with zinc, stabilizes nerve membranes and can be effective in the treatment of epilepsy.[2]

Environmental hazards. Taurine protects the body from damage by toxic compounds in the environment and diet. Taurine binds to, detoxifies, and enhances excretion of chemicals, pesticides, and other toxins.[1] Taurine helps prevent liver damage from chronic, heavy alcohol consumption.

Cataract. Taurine is the most abundant free amino acid in the lens of the eye. Its antioxidant actions may help reduce risk of cataract.

Gallstones. Supplemental taurine can enhance bile acid function and reduce the likelihood of cholesterol-type gallstones.[1] Taurine can also enhance fat and fat-soluble vitamin absorption from the diet, particularly in people who have difficulty absorbing fats due to liver, gallbladder, or pancreatic diseases.[8]

Toxicity

Taurine supplements can occasionally cause stomach irritation and may cause drowsiness in children. Otherwise, there are no reports of taurine toxicity.

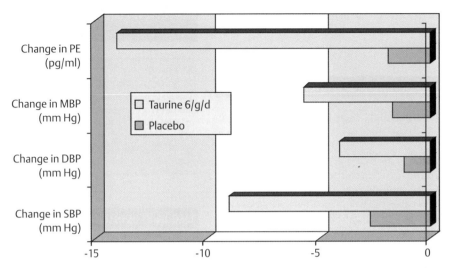

Fig. 3.**23**: **Reduction of blood pressure in hypertensive adults with taurine supplementation.** 19 hypertensives were given either 6 g/day taurine or placebo for 1 week. Treatment with taurine resulted in significant decreases in systolic blood pressure (SBP), diastolic blood pressure (DBP), mean blood pressure (MBP), and plasma epinephrine (PE), compared with placebo.
(From: Fujita T, et al. Circulation. 1987;75:525)

References

1. Hayes KC, Trautwein EA. Taurine. In: ME Shils, JA Olson, M Shike, eds. Modern Nutrition in Health and Disease. 8th ed. Philadelphia: Lea&Febiger; 1994.
2. Trautwein EA, et al. Taurine concentrations in plasma and whole blood during normal diets and during taurine supplementation and taurine deficiency. Z Ernährungswiss. 1995;34:137.
3. Takahashi R, Nakane Y. Clinical trial of taurine in epilepsy. In: Barbeau A, Huxtable RJ, eds. Taurine and Neurological Disorders. New York: Raven Press; 1978.
4. Kendler BS. Taurine: An overview of its role in preventive medicine. Prev Med. 1989;18:79.
5. Sturman JA, Chesney RW. Taurine in pediatric nutrition. Pediat Clin North Am. 1995;42:879.
6. Azuma J, et al. Therapeutic effect of taurin in congestive heart failure: A double-blind crossover trial. Clin Cardiol. 1985;8:276.
7. Fujita T, Sato Y. Hypotensive effect of taurine. J Clin Invest. 1988;82:993.
8. McCarty MF. Complementary vascular protective actions of magnesium and taurine: A rationale for magnesium taurate. Med Hypotheses. 1996;46:89.
8. Zamboni G, et al. Influence of dietary taurine on vitamin D resorption. Acta Pediatr. 1993;82:811.

Carnitine

Carnitine is an amino acid that plays a central role in the oxidation of fatty acids for energy. Over 95% of the body's carnitine is located in the heart and skeletal muscle, tissues where energy needs are high. Carnitine can be obtained from the diet or synthesized in our cells by joining methionine and lysine, a process that requires vitamins C, B6, and niacin. During periods of increased demand or increased loss, body synthesis of carnitine may be inadequate to supply needs, and carnitine from the diet becomes essential.[2]

Functions

Energy metabolism. Carnitine is the "shuttle" that carries fatty acids into the mitochondria so they can be oxidized for energy.[3] This is particularly important in the myocardium and in skeletal muscle when energy needs for physical activity are high.

Detoxification. Carnitine is also important for liver detoxification and excretion of chemicals and drugs.[3]

Increased Risk of Deficiency

● High fat diets increase carnitine requirements and reduce carnitine levels in blood.

● Inadequate amounts of the precursors for carnitine synthesis–the amino acids lysine and methionine and vitamins C, B6, and niacin–can impair carnitine synthesis and produce deficiency. For example, the profound muscle weakness of scurvy (the vitamin C deficiency disease) appears to be due to carnitine deficiency.

● Pregnant and lactating women have increased carnitine requirements; if dietery amounts are low, deficiency can occur (with symptoms of fatigue and weakness).[4]

Good Dietary Sources

Food	Serving size	mg
Beef, filet	100 g	3680
Ground beef	100 g	3615
Pork chop	100 g	1075
Cod	100 g	210
Chicken, breast	100 g	150
Milk	1, large glass	125
Hard cheese	30 g	48
Whole-wheat bread	100 g	14

Animal foods are rich in carnitine: vegetables, fruits, and cereals have negligible amounts. The average adult diet that includes meat, milk, and eggs provides about 100–300 mg/ day of carnitine.[1] Vegetarians are at increased risk for deficiency.

Recommended Daily Intakes

Supplemental carnitine is usually given in oral doses ranging from 1–3.5 g/day.

Preferred Form and Dosage Schedule

As a salt of L-carnitine. Only pure L-carnitine should be used as a supplement; D-carnitine can interfere with the action of L-carnitine in the body and produce signs of deficiency	Take in divided doses between meals

Use in Prevention and Therapy

Heart disease. By enhancing energy use in heart muscle, carnitine is beneficial in coronary heart disease and angina pectoris.[5,6] Carnitine can reduce the number of anginal attacks and increase the ability to exercise and be active without symptoms. Cardiomyopathy and congestive heart failure are often associated with carnitine deficiency.

Peripheral vascular disease. In intermittent claudication, carnitine increases efficiency of muscle function and may reduce symptoms.

High blood fats. People with high levels of fats and cholesterol in the blood may benefit from carnitine supplementation. Carnitine can reduce blood levels of triglyceride and total cholesterol and raise HDL cholesterol.

Exercise. Carnitine may increase endurance in sports where fat is an important energy source, such as long-distance cycling, running, or swimming.[7,8]

Detoxification. If the liver has to detoxify large burdens of chemicals, drugs, or alcohol over long periods, carnitine stores in the liver can be depleted, producing a deficiency. Supplemental carnitine can maintain optimum stores for this important function.

Liver disease. Because the liver is the principal site for carnitine synthesis, liver disorders, such as cirrhosis and hepatitis, reduce carnitine synthesis.[9]

Infancy. Newborns are at risk of carnitine deficiency due to a high reliance on fatty acids for energy and a poorly developed ability to synthesize carnitine. Although breastmilk is rich in carnitine, infant formulas are often low. Infants fed with formula may need additional amounts of carnitine to avoid deficiency.[1]

AIDS. People with AIDS are at increased risk of carnitine deficiency and, if deficient, may benefit from supplementation by improved immune function.[10]

Toxicity

L-carnitine in doses up to 4 g/day has no side effects other than occasional and temporary diarrhea. There have been reports that DL-carnitine (containing the potentially toxic D-isomer) can produce muscle weakness. Only L-carnitine should be used as a supplement.

References

1. ReBouche CJ. Carnitine In. Modern Nutrition in Health and Disease. Shils ME, Olson JA, Shike M, Ross AC, eds. Baltimore: Williams & Wilkins; 1999.
2. Pons R, DeVivo DC. Primary and secondary carnitine deficiency syndromes. J Child Neurol. 1995;10(S2):8.
3. Carter AL, et al. Biosynthesis and metabolism of carnitine. J Child Neurol. 1995;10(S2):3.
4. Rebouche CJ. Carnitine function and requirements during the life cycle. FASEB J. 1992;6:3379.
5. Goa KL, Brogden RN. Carnitine: A preliminary review of its pharmacokinetics and its therapeutic use in ischemic heart disease and primary and secondary carnitine deficiencies in relationship to its role in fatty acid metabolism. Drugs. 1987;34:1.
6. Chierchia SL, Fragasso G. Metabolic management of heart disease. Eur Heart J. 1993;14:2.
7. Starling RD, et al. Relationships between muscle carnitine, age and oxidative status. Eur J Appl Physiol. 1995;71:143.
8. Brass EP, Hiatt WR. Carnitine metabolism during exercise. Life Sci. 1994;54:1383.
9. Krahenbuhl S. Carnitine metabolism in chronic liver disease. Life Sci. 1996;59:1579.
10. Mintz M. Carnitine in HIV-1 infection/AIDS. J Child Neurol. 1995;10:S40.

Antioxidants and Free Radicals

Free Radicals

Free radicals are incomplete molecules, unstable because they have an unpaired, "free" electron. The presence of the unpaired electron makes a free radical a strong oxidant and highly reactive. Free radicals can damage cell membranes, fatty acids, cholesterol, proteins, and DNA and play a role in the pathogenesis of many chronic degenerative diseases.[1] Oxidation of cell proteins and membranes can produce tissue damage in rheumatoid arthritis, inflammatory bowel diseases, and Parkinson's disease.[2] Oxidation of LDL cholesterol increases risk of atherosclerosis.[3] Oxidative damage to DNA may contribute to development of cancer.[1,4]

Sources

● The respiratory chain in mitochondria produces a number of reactive oxygen species (e.g., the hydroxyl radical OH and superoxide radical O_2-) as by-products. Exercise, stress, and illness increase oxidative metabolism and thereby increase formation of free radicals.

● The immune system produces free radicals (including the superoxide radical O_2-) to destroy phagocytized bacteria and viruses.[2] Also, the inflammatory response to allergens and other foreign substances greatly increases production of free radicals. During chronic infection and inflammation, controlling the flood of free radicals is vital to protect nearby cells.

● Free radicals also come from the environment. Cigarette smoking sharply increases oxidative stress.[5] Exposure to industrial chemicals, radiation, and air pollution increases production of free radicals.[2] Potential environmental sources of free radicals are shown in the following table.

- Air pollution
- Cigarette smoke
- Radiation
- Excessive exposure to sunlight
- Industrial chemicals and solvents
- Medicines and drugs
- Herbicides and pesticides in foods
- Food additives: preservatives, colorings

● Disorders associated with free radical damage[1,3,4,9–12]

- Cancer
- Cardiovascular disease (Fig. 3.**25**)
- Adverse drug reactions
- Alcohol-induced liver damage
- Cataracts and macular degeneration
- Allergy and hypersensitivity
- Osteoarthritis and rheumatoid arthritis
- Inflammatory bowel disease (ulcerative colitis, Crohn's disease)
- Neurologic degeneration (multiple sclerosis, Parkinson's disease)
- Ischemia/reperfusion injury after heart attack or stroke
- The catabolic response associated with operation, injury, or chronic infection
- Complications of diabetes mellitus
- Oxidative damage to muscles during intense exercise

Antioxidants

Our bodies have evolved several lines of antioxidant defense against free radicals. Antioxidants are able to interact with and reduce free radicals. By donating electrons, antioxidants convert the radicals to stable, nontoxic metabolites.[3]

Both individual antioxidants and antioxidant enzyme systems are important in free-radical scavenging. Four of the major antioxidants are essential micronutrients (vitamins C, E, beta-carotene, cysteine), while two can be synthesized in limited amounts by the body (glutathione and coenzyme Q10). Riboflavin and the trace elements selenium, copper, zinc, manganese, and iron are essential components of the major antioxidant enzymes.

The major antioxidants

- Vitamin E
- Vitamin C
- Beta-carotene
- Glutathione
- Coenzyme Q10
- Cysteine

Major antioxidant enzymes and their vitamin and trace-element components

Antioxidant enzymes	Trace element
Glutathione peroxidases	Selenium
Catalase	Iron
Superoxide dismutases	Zinc, manganese, and copper
Glutathione reductase	Riboflavin

Most antioxidants scavenge free radicals by donating an electron. In the process the antioxidant is oxidized. For this reason the body's antioxidant reserves must be continually replenished. Antioxidants work in concert and their actions are synergistic.[6–8] Vitamin E and selenium both enhance the antioxidant actions of the other.[7] Vitamin C, coenzyme Q10, and glutathione peroxidase regenerate tocopherol that is oxidized, thereby recycling vitamin E for reuse by tissues. Vitamin C or selenium deficiencies therefore sharply increase requirements for vitamin E and increase risk of vitamin E deficiency.[8] A complete and balanced supply of all the major antioxidants is important.

Good Dietary Sources

A diet rich in fresh fruits and vegetables, whole grains, nuts, and seeds provides a balanced intake of antioxidants.[13] In addition, many foods contain non-nutritive antioxidants that may be important in protection from oxidative stress.[14,15] However, it is very difficult to obtain the recommended amounts of many of the antioxidants using only food sources. For example, to obtain 200 mg of vitamin E one would need to eat 2 kg of peanuts or 300 g of sunflower seed oil. To obtain 500 mg of vitamin C in a day, one would need to eat more than 0.5 kg of oranges or broccoli. Supplementation with a complete antioxidant formula is an efficient way to maintain antioxidant levels in the body.

Non-nutritive antioxidants in the diet

Source	Antioxidants
Soybeans	Isoflavones, phenolic acids
Tea	Polyphenols, catechins
Red wine	Phenols
Rosemary, sage, and other spices	Carnosic acid, rosmaric acid
Citrus and other fruits	Bioflavonoids, chalcones
Onions	Bioflavonoids, kaempferol
Olives	Polyphenols

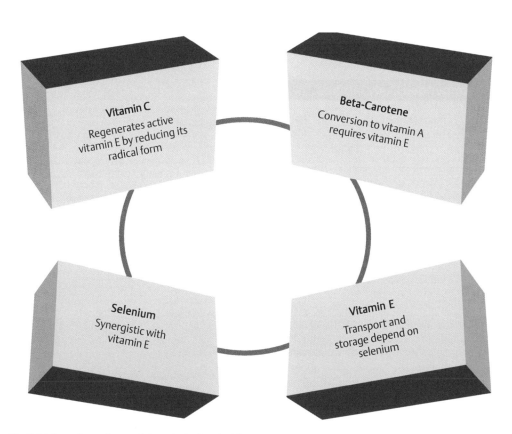

Fig. 3.**24**: Interdependence of the principal antioxidants.

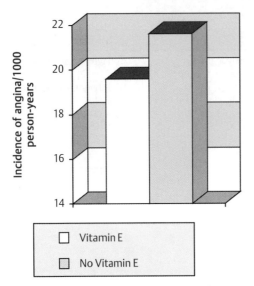

Fig. 3.**25**: **Vitamin E supplementation and angina pectoris.** In 20 000 male smokers, supplementation with 50 mg/day vitamin E significantly reduced the incidence of angina pectoris. Those not receiving vitamin E had a 10% greater risk of developing angina. (From: Rapola JM, et al. JAMA. 1996;275:693)

Recommended Daily Intakes

To maintain optimum antioxidant levels in the body, the following daily ranges of intake are recommended for healthy adults:

Vitamin C	250–500 mg
Vitamin E	100–200 mg
Beta-carotene	10–15 mg
L-Cysteine	0.5–1.0 g
Coenzyme Q10	30–100 mg
Selenium	50–100 µg
Zinc	15 mg
Manganese	5.0–7.5 mg

Because glutathione supplements are expensive and their absorption is uncertain, cysteine supplements are usually recommended. Cysteine is used by the body to build glutathione, and supplemental cysteine enhances endogenous synthesis of glutathione (see pp. 105).

For further details on the functions and recommended dosages of the antioxidants, see the separate discussions of the individual antioxidants.

References

1. Ames BN, et al. Oxidants, antioxidants and the degenerative diseases of aging. Proc Natl Acad Sci U S A. 1993;90:7915.
2. Halliwell B. Antioxidants. In: Ziegler EE, Filer LJ, eds. Present Knowledge in Nutrition. Washington D.C.: ILSI Press; 1996:596.
3. Diaz MN, et al. Antioxidants and atherosclerotic heart disease. N Engl J Med. 1997;337:408.
4. Borek C. Antioxidants and cancer. Sci Am Sci Med. 1997;6:52.
5. Marangon K et al. Diet, antioxidant status and smoking habits in French men. Am J Clin Nutr. 1998;67:231.
6. Rock CL. Update on the biological characteristics of the antioxidant micronutrients: vitamin C, vitamin E and the carotenoids. J Am Diet Assoc. 1996;96:693.
7. Baker H et al. Human plasma patterns during 14 days of ingestion of vitamin E, beta-carotene, ascorbic acid and their various combinations. J Am Coll Nutr. 1996;15:159.
8. Kubena KS, McMurray DN. Nutrition and the immune system: A review of nutrient-nutrient interactions. J Am Diet Assoc. 1996;96:1156.
9. Fahn S. An open trial of high-dosage antioxidants in early Parkinson's disease. Am J Clin Nutr. 1991;53:S380.
10. Kushi LH et al. Dietary antioxidant vitamins and death from coronary heart disease in postmenopausal women. N Engl J Med. 1996;334:1156.
11. Manson JE, Stampfer MJ, Willett WC, et al: Antioxidant vitamin consumption and incidence of stroke in women. Circulation. 1993;87:678.
12. McAlindon TE, Jacques P, Zhang Y, et al. Do antioxidant nutrients protect against development and progression of knee osteoarthritis? Arthritis Rheum. 1996;39:648.
13. Block G, Patterson B, Subar A. Fruit, vegetables and cancer prevention: A review of the epidemiological evidence. Nutr Cancer. 1992;18:1.
14. Hertog MGL, et al. Dietary antioxidant flavonoids and risk of coronary heart disease. Lancet. 1993;342:1007.
15. Serafini M, et al. In vivo antioxidant effect of green and black tea in man. Eur J Clin Nutr. 1996;50:28.

Coenzyme Q10

Coenzyme Q10 is an essential component of the respiratory chain in mitochondria. It is found in large amounts in the heart, muscles, kidney, and liver where energy production is high.[1] Coenzyme Q10 can be obtained in small amounts from the diet or may be synthesized in our cells. During periods of increased demand or increased loss, body synthesis may be inadequate to supply needs, and coenzyme Q10 from the diet becomes essential.[1]

Functions

Energy production. The activity of the respiratory chain in mitochondria is strongly dependent on optimum levels of coenzyme Q10.

Antioxidant actions. Coenzyme Q10 is an important lipid-soluble antioxidant.[2] It helps protect lipids thoughout the body from peroxidative damage from free radicals. Coenzyme Q10 works in concert with other antioxidant defenses–for example, it can regenerate oxidized vitamin E.

Good Dietary Sources

Coenzyme Q10 is widely distributed in foods, but only in small amounts. Soybeans, walnuts, and almonds (and their oils), meats, certain fish (particularly abundant in mackerel and sardines), nuts, wheat germ, and some vegetables (e.g., green beans, spinach, cabbage, and garlic) are the best sources. Sardines are particularly rich in coenzyme Q10. However, it is necessary to eat 1.6 kg of sardines to obtain 100 mg of coenzyme Q10. Therefore, in times of increased need, supplements of coenzyme Q10 may be the most efficient way to maintain body levels.

Recommended Daily Intakes

Usual supplementation with coenzyme Q10 is in the range of 30–120 mg/day.[1] In most people, increasing dietary intake by supplementing with 60–100 mg will double plasma levels of coenzyme Q10.[3] Supplemental doses do not impair endogenous synthesis.

Preferred Form and Dosage schedule

Coenzyme Q10	Take with meals

Use in Prevention and Therapy

Coronary heart disease and congestive heart failure (CHF). Coenzyme Q10 has been used to treat heart disease in Japan for over 20 years. Coenzyme Q10 may improve cardiac output and reduce the symptoms of CHF.[4,5] Coenzyme Q10 levels in the myocardium of patients with CHF are often low, and supplementation helps maintain normal levels.[5] Coenzyme Q10 helps protect LDL cholesterol from oxidation.[6] It can reduce the frequency and intensity of angina.[7] Supplements may also reduce risk of arrhythmias in coronary artery disease.

High blood pressure. Supplemental coenzyme Q10 may lower blood pressure in hypertension.[8]

Cancer. Supplemental coenzyme Q10 can reduce the toxic side effects of certain types of chemotherapy.[1]

Athletics and exercise. Endurance events sharply increase the demand for coenzyme Q10, and repeated training can lower body stores. Coenzyme Q10 can help reduce muscle damage from oxidation during strenuous exercise and reduce muscle soreness.

Muscular disorders. In certain forms of muscular dystrophy the ability of mitochondria to use oxygen for energy production is impaired. Supplemental coenzyme Q10 may be effective in increasing muscle cell function and level of activity.[9]

Toxicity

Even very large oral doses of coenzyme Q10 (600 mg/day) for prolonged periods do not appear to produce significant adverse side effects.[1] Some people may experience mild nausea or gastrointestinal discomfort when taking coenzyme Q10.

References

1. Biomedical and Clinical Aspects of Coenzyme Q10. Volumes 1–7. 1977–1993, Elsevier, Amsterdam.
2. Kontush A et al. Antioxidative activity of ubiquinol-10 at physiological concentrations in human low density lipoprotein. Biochim Biophys Acta 1995; 1258:177
3. Chopra RK et al. Relative bioavailabilty of coenzyme Q10formulations in human subjects. Internat J Vit Nutr Res 1998;68:109.
4. Greenberg S, Frishman WH.Coenzyme Q10: A new drug for cardiovascular disease. J Clin Pharmacol 1990;30:596.
5. Langsjoen PH, Folkers K. Long-term efficacy and safety of coenzyme Q10 therapy for idiopathic dilated cardiomyopathy. Am J Cardiol 1990;65:521.
6. Mohr D et al. Dietary supplementation with coenzyme Q10 results in increased levels of ubiquinol-10 within the circulating lipoproteins and increased resistance of human LDL to the initiation of lipid peroxidation. Biochem Biophys Acta 1992; 1126:247.
7. Kamikawa T et al. Effects of coenzyme Q10 on exercise tolerance in chronic stable angina pectoris. Am J Cardiol 1985;56:247.
8. Digiesi V et al. Effect of coenzyme Q10 on essential arterial hypertension. Curr Ther Res 1990;47:841.
9. Folkers K, Simonsen R. Two successful double-blind trials with coenzyme Q10 on muscular dystrophies and neurogenic atrophies. Biochim Biophys Acta. 1995;1271:281.

4 Micronutrition through the Life Cycle

Planning a Pregnancy

One of the best ways to achieve a healthy pregnancy outcome is to actively plan for pregnancy and enter pregnancy in good nutritional health. A critical time for nutrition is the periconceptional period: the 2 months just before and the 2–3 months after conception. Fetal development occurs rapidly after conception and most organs are formed in the first 8–10 weeks of pregnancy, before many women realize they are pregnant. During this period the tiny embryo is particularly vulnerable to alcohol, environmental toxins, drugs, maternal medications, and nutritional deficiencies. Deficiencies of thiamine, riboflavin, vitamin B12, vitamin A, zinc, and folic acid may increase risk of abnormal fetal development, miscarriage, and birth defects.[1]

During the child-bearing years, many women chronically diet to lose weight or maintain a

Recommended micronutrient intakes in preparation for pregnancy

Nutrient	Recommended daily intake (combined intake from food and supplement sources)
Vitamins:	
Vitamin A (preferably as beta-carotene)	800 μg
Vitamin D	10–15 μg
Vitamin E	15–20 mg
Vitamin K	75–150 μg
Thiamine (Vitamin B1)	1.5–2.0 mg
Riboflavin (Vitamin B2)	1.6–2.2 mg
Niacin	20 mg
Vitamin B6	2.5–5.0 mg
Pantothenic acid	5–10 mg
Biotin	75–150 μg
Folic acid	0.8 mg
Vitamin B12	3–5 μg
Vitamin C	100 mg
Minerals:	
Calcium	600–800 mg
Magnesium	300–400 mg
Iron	10–20 mg
Zinc	15 mg
Copper	2 mg
Manganese	2–5 mg
Fluoride	1–3 mg*
Iodine	200 μg
Selenium	100–150 μg
Chromium	100–200 μg
Molybdenum	100–250 μg

* If water or salt supply is not fluoridated

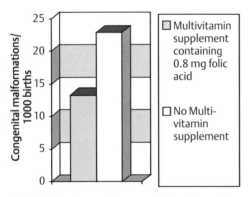

Fig. 4.1: **Vitamin supplements during the periconceptional period and birth defects.** 4150 women planning a pregnancy received either a multivitamin containing 0.8 mg folic acid or a control for at least 1 month before conception and until the date of the second missed menstrual period or later. Congenital malformations were significantly more frequent in the group not receiving the multivitamin than in the vitamin-supplement group (23/1000 vs. 13/1000). There were six cases of NTDs in the group not receiving the vitamins and none in the vitamin-supplemented group.
(Adapted from: Czeizel AE, et al. N Engl J Med. 1992;327:1832)

slim figure. Most low-calorie diets, whether self-selected or from published dieting programs, are nutritionally inadequate. They often lack the nutrients that young women need most, such as folic acid, iron, calcium, and zinc.[2] Chronic dieting that depletes nutrient stores may have adverse effects if a women becomes pregnant.

Nutrition and Birth Defects

Folic acid is a nutrient of vital importance in early pregnancy. Low body stores of folic acid during the periconceptional period sharply increase risk of birth defects. Folic acid is important in the early development of the central nervous system, and deficiency during this period can cause a neural tube defect (NTD).[3] The most common NTD is spina bifida, a condition in which the spine does not completely develop and close around the spinal cord. Babies born with spina bifida often have a permanently damaged spinal cord. When severe, NTDs result in miscarriages and stillbirths. Nearly half a million infants worldwide are born with NTDs each year and in the USA, NTDs affect 1–2% of pregnancies.[4]

All women of childbearing age should consume at least 0.4 mg/day of folic acid to reduce risk of birth defects in case of pregnancy. However, in the USA and Western Europe only one in 10 women have intakes near 0.4 mg/day. [6] Although folic acid intake can be increased by a diet high in whole grains, veg-etables, and fruits, the best way to ensure adequate intake during this crucial period is to supplement with folate (see Fig. 4.2).[7] Folate supplementation (0.4–0.8 mg/day) during the months just before and after conception can reduce risk of NTDs by more than 50% (see Fig. 4.1).[4] It can also reduce risk of other birth defects, such as cleft lip, cleft palate, and heart defects.[5]

Prepregnancy Weight

Women who are planning a pregnancy should strive to maintain a normal body weight. Maternal weight before pregnancy has a major influence on fetal growth and pregnancy outcome.[8]

Underweight

Women who are lighter than ideal body weight before pregnancy tend to deliver infants that are smaller than those of heavier women, even if they gain adequate weight during pregnancy. Women who enter preg-

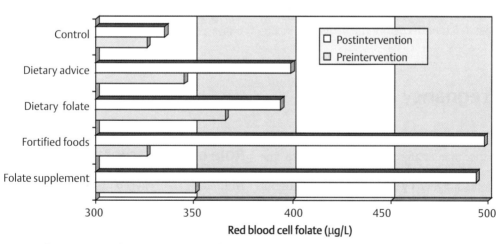

Fig. 4.2: **Changes in supplemental and dietary folic acid and the effect on red cell folate levels.** Sixty healthy women were randomly assigned to one of five groups receiving: 1) a 0.4-mg folate supplement; 2) folic-acid-fortified foods (an additional 0.4 mg folate); 3) folate-containing foods (an additional 0.4 mg folate); 4) dietary advice to increase folate intake; or 5) control. Although in groups 1–4 dietary folate intake increased significantly, only the folate supplement and the folate-fortified foods produced significant increases in tissue levels of folate. Eating folate-fortified foods or taking a folate supplement is the most effective way to improve folate status. (Adapted from Cuskelly GJ, et al. Lancet. 1996; 347:657)

nancy underweight have a higher risk of delivering a premature or low-birth-weight infant. In addition, anemia is more common in women who are underweight before conception.

Overweight

Women who are overweight are also at higher risk for a poor pregnancy outcome. In women weighing more than 130% of their ideal body weight serious complications, such as diabetes and hypertension during pregnancy, are more common. Weight loss during pregnancy, even in very obese women, is dangerous for the fetus, thus overweight women should try to lose weight before becoming pregnant. However, "crash" diets for rapid weight loss should be avoided because they are low in important micronutrients, such as folic acid, zinc, and iron.

Oral Contraception before Pregnancy

Oral contraceptive pills interfere with metabolism of folic acid and vitamin C, vitamin B6, and vitamin B12. When planning a pregnancy, oral contraception should be discontinued at least 3–6 months before the planned conception and substituted with another form of birth control. During this period a supplement containing ample amounts of the B vitamins and additional vitamin C (100–200 mg/day) should be taken to replenish body stores.

References

1. Keen CL, et al.(eds.) Maternal nutrition and pregnancy outcome. Ann NY Acad Sci. 1993;678.
2. Block G, et al. Vitamin and mineral status of women of childbearing potential. Ann NY Acad Med. 1993;678:245.
3. Botto LD, et al. Neural tube defects. N Engl J Med. 1999;341:1509.
4. Centers for Disease Control and Prevention. Recommendations for the use of folic acid to reduce the number of cases of spina bifida and other neural tube defects. MMWR Morb Mortal Wkly Rep. 1992;41:14.
5. Shaw GM, et al. Risk of orofacial clefts in children born to women using multivitamins containing folic acid periconceptionally. Lancet. 1995;345:393.
6. Life Sciences Research Office, FASEB. Nutrition monitoring in the U.S.: an update report. DHHS Publ., Hyattsville, MD. 1989;89:1255.
7. Elkin AC, et al. Folic acid supplements are more effective than increased dietary folate intake in elevating serum folate levels. Br J Obstet Gynecol. 2000;107:285.
8. Cnattingius S, et al. Prepregnancy weight and the risk of adverse pregnancy outcomes. N Engl J Med. 1998;338:147.

Pregnancy

The nutrient needs of a pregnant woman are higher than at any other time in her life. The developing fetus is formed entirely out of nutrients supplied by the mother's diet, thus optimum nutrition is vital for healthy fetal growth. Maternal lifestyle choices take on extra importance during pregnancy – the fetus is highly vulnerable to environmental chemicals, heavy metals, drugs, alcohol, and cigarette smoke.

Role of the Placenta

Nutrients and oxygen coming from the mother's bloodstream are moved to the fetus across the placenta. The placenta is a dynamic organ that actively pulls nutrients from the maternal blood and transfers them to the fetus. Many vitamins are present in higher concentrations in fetal than in maternal blood; for example, fetal blood levels of vitamin C are 50% higher than those of the mother. The placenta also carefully regulates the concentration of minerals crossing to the fetus. Nutrient transfer by the placenta accelerates during the last weeks of pregnancy, building up fetal stores in preparation for birth. During the final month, over 300 mg of calcium are moved across to the fetus each day. However, the placenta is not an effective barrier keeping harmful substances from the fetus. Many drugs, industrial chemicals, alcohol, substances in cigarette smoke, and other toxins readily cross the placenta and can harm the fetus.

Fetal Growth

In the first 2 months after conception – the period of embryogenesis – the fetus develops very rapidly. By 9 to 10 weeks after conception, although the fetus weighs only about 6 g, all of the major organ systems are present, the heart begins to beat, and the fetus begins to move. Optimum, balanced nutrition is very important during this period – the embryo is extremely vulnerable to changes in nutrient supply and adverse effects from environmental toxins. Absence of micronutrients (e.g., folate and zinc) during this critical period may impair development and produce a birth defect or cause miscarriage.[1] During this stage the pregnant woman should be very careful to avoid environmental hazards (e.g., alcohol and cigarette smoke) and to eat a micronutrient-dense, high-quality diet.[2]

During the remainder of pregnancy the fetal-organ systems mature and acquire their basic adult characteristics. The weight of the developing fetus increases from 6 g to over 3000 g during the second and third trimesters – a remarkable 500-fold increase. Fetal growth draws heavily on the nutrient resources of the mother in the second half of pregnancy. During this time, both quantity and quality of the diet are important.

A major goal of pregnancy is to obtain an infant birth weight greater than 2500 g. Babies weighing less than 2500 g at birth are termed low birth weight (LBW) infants. Compared with normal weight infants, LBW infants have much higher rates of illness[2] and are 40 times more likely to die in the first few weeks of life.

Many LBW infants do not "catch up" after birth; even with adequate nutrition after birth, most will be shorter than average for the rest of their lives, and many show long-term impairments in intellect and mental development. In addition, LBW infants tend to have more chronic health problems in later life. Thus, poor nutrition in utero may have profound effects that cannot be reversed after birth. A multivitamin/mineral supplement taken during pregnancy may decrease risk of delivering a LBW infant.[3]

Nutritional Needs during Pregnancy

Weight Gain

Normal, steady weight gain is a characteristic of a pregnancy that is progressing well. On average, a woman should gain approximately 0.45 kg/week during the middle months of pregnancy, and about 0.4 kg/week during the final 3 months. In well-nourished women, average total weight gain during pregnancy is about 10.5–12.5 kg.[4]

In the USA and Western Europe many mothers gain too much weight during pregnancy. This can harm both the baby and the mother. Excess weight gain increases the chance of having a larger baby, which can prolong labor and may reduce oxygen supply to the baby during delivery. In the mother, too much weight gain increases risk of developing high blood pressure during pregnancy and makes returning to the prepregnancy weight more difficult, increasing risk of later obesity.[4]

Energy, Protein, and Fat

Although a pregnant women is "eating for two," there is no need to double food intake. The average pregnant woman needs only an additional 300 kcal/day during the last 6 months of pregnancy.[4] As an example, an additional two cups of whole milk together with an extra apple or banana each day would provide the extra 300 kcal. For most pregnant women, diet quality is more important than quantity. Weight gain within the recom-

Components of weight gain in a typical pregnancy	
Infant	3 kg
Placenta	0.5 kg
Amniotic fuid	1 kg
Uterus	1 kg
Increased breast size	1.5 kg
New maternal blood	2 kg
Protein accumulation	1 kg
Maternal fat stores	1.5 kg

mended ranges is the best sign that energy intake is appropriate. Weight gain of more than 0.5 kg/week for several weeks may mean energy intake is too high.

In the second half of pregnancy, protein needs almost double – the average woman requiring 40–50 g/day before pregnancy now requires 70–90 g/day.[4] The choice of dietary fat is important. A pregnant woman's diet should be rich in the omega-3 fatty acids, eicosapentanoic acid (EPA), and docosahexanoic acid (DHA). These fatty acids are important components of the developing baby's central nervous system and eyes. Because most of the cells in the central nervous system are formed during pregnancy and the first year after birth, ample intakes of EPA and DHA are vital during this period.[5] Although adults are able to synthesize some EPA and DHA from linolenic acid (see pp. 89), the fetus cannot because the necessary metabolic pathways have not fully developed. These fatty acids need to be supplied to the fetus by the mother.

Vitamins

Fat-soluble vitamins. Daily vitamin D requirements more than double during pregnancy. Besides eating more vitamin D-rich foods, pregnant women should obtain regular sunlight exposure to increase vitamin D production in the skin. Vitamin E requirements also increase, particularly during the last 8–10 weeks of pregnancy. The baby accumulates important stores of fat during this period, and vitamin E is needed to protect fetal fat stores from oxidation. Most well-nourished mothers have ample vitamin A stores to provide for the growing fetus. If total fetal needs for vitamin A

during pregnancy were drawn from maternal stores, only about 10% of those stores would be used during pregnancy.[4] Therefore, no significant increase in vitamin A intake is necessary during pregnancy. Although newborn babies have low vitamin K stores and most require supplemental vitamin K at birth, transport of vitamin K in utero is minimal. Therefore, supplementing maternal diets with the vitamin does not significantly affect fetal levels, and no additional vitamin K is recommended during pregnancy.[4]

Water-soluble vitamins. Pregnancy sharply increases requirements for the water-soluble vitamins. Thiamin, riboflavin, niacin, and vitamin B12 requirements increase by about 50%, and vitamins C and B6 requirements double. If these requirements are not met, maternal stores will be depleted. For example, the fetus is dependent on a steady supply of vitamin B6, and levels of B6 in fetal blood are two to five times higher than in maternal blood. This fetal "drain" causes vitamin B6 stores to fall sharply during the second and third trimester in most pregnant women, many of whom develop signs of vitamin B6 deficiency.[6] Similarly, increased demands for folate are often not met by the maternal diet, and impaired folate status is a common cause of anemia in pregnancy. To maintain maternal stores and support fetal growth, pregnant women need more than twice the amount of folate than nonpregnant women.

Minerals and Water

Calcium. A total of 30–40 g of calcium are transferred to the fetus during pregnancy, most of it during the third trimester. The efficiency of maternal calcium absorption doubles during pregnancy. Even so, many maternal diets will not cover increased calcium needs in late pregnancy, and calcium must be withdrawn from maternal bone and transferred to the fetus. However, if calcium intake is maintained at 1000–1200 mg/day throughout pregnancy, bone loss is minimized. At this intake, calcium stores built up early in pregnancy before fetal needs become significant can be transferred to the fetus in the third trimester. Thus, a steady, high supply of calcium is important, and needs during pregnancy are double those before pregnancy.[4]

Iron. Iron requirements increase dramatically during pregnancy as the mother produces millions of new red blood cells. In response, maternal intestinal absorption of iron increases. Compared with nonpregnant women, pregnant women are about three to five times more efficient at absorbing iron from foods.[7] However, in most women dietary iron cannot cover the demands of pregnancy, and maternal stores of iron are depleted. By the third trimester, iron stores are low or absent in most women. During pregnancy, the iron status of the fetus is maintained near normal even if depletion of iron stores and anemia occur in the mother.

Requirements for absorbed iron during pregnancy more than double and are estimated to be as high as 30 mg/day.[4] This amount of iron is very difficult to obtain, even from carefully chosen diets, and the iron intake of most pregnant women falls far short. Iron deficiency during pregnancy produces anemia, fatigue, and irritability in the mother and may impair growth of the fetus. Because of this, iron supplementation (preferably as part of a multivitamin/mineral), is indicated for most pregnant women. [4] Iron supplements should be taken with foods that enhance iron absorption (meat, fish, and fruits and vegetables rich in vitamin C).

Magnesium. During pregnancy, magnesium intake should be 400 mg/day. Many pregnant women do not obtain this amount and become deficient, particularly during the second half of pregnancy. Magnesium deficiency during pregnancy can cause fatigue and muscle cramps, and increase risk of premature birth and maternal hypertension.

Zinc. Low zinc intake during pregnancy increases risk of delivering a low birth weight baby and may increase risk of birth defects.[8] Zinc requirements are about 50% higher during pregnancy, and many women's diets do not cover these increased needs. In most pregnant women, zinc levels in hair and blood decline during the later half of pregnancy, indicating depletion of body stores.

Micronutrient Deficiency and Its Effect On Pregnancy

The rapidly growing fetus is very sensitive to an inadequate supply of micronutrients. The potential adverse effects of micronutrient deficiency during pregnancy, both for the mother and the baby, are shown in the following table.

Effects of micronutrient deficiencies during pregnancy[1]		
Nutrient	Effects on mother	Effects on fetus/infant
Vitamin D	Reduced bone density; may increase risk of osteoporosis	Impaired skeletal and tooth development, hypocalcemia, rickets
Vitamin A	Anemia	Low birth weight, premature birth
Vitamin E		Birth defects, spontaneous abortion
Folate	Anemia	Low birthweight, birth defects, miscarriage
Thiamin		Infant beri beri (severe thiamin deficiency producing heart failure)
Iodine	Hypothyroidism	Severely impaired mental and motor development
Calcium	Increased risk of hypertension and eclampsia, reduced bone density, may increase risk of osteoporosis	Impaired skeletal and tooth development, rickets
Magnesium	Increased risk of hypertension and eclampsia	Premature birth
Zinc		Birth defects, premature birth, low birth weight
Iron	Anemia	Low birth weight, premature birth, increased infant mortality

Dietary and Environmental Hazards during Pregnancy

Alcohol

Regular alcohol consumption during pregnancy has potentially devastating effects on the infant. Alcohol causes a group of birth defects, termed the fetal alcohol syndrome (FAS).[9] FAS is characterized by abnormal facial structure (small eyes and a poorly developed nose, upper jaw, and lip) and impairments in growth and intellectual development. FAS is the leading cause of mental retardation in children in the industrialized countries of the world. Both alcohol and its toxic breakdown product acetaldehyde readily cross the placenta into the fetus. Since the fetus does not have enzyme systems to break down alcohol and acetaldehyde, they circulate in the baby before they pass back through the placenta to the mother for metabolism. Thus, the fetus is exposed to prolonged high concentrations of alcohol.

Although severe FAS usually occurs in babies of heavy, chronic users (more than six drinks per day), smaller amounts of alcohol may also have detrimental effects. Mothers who consume more than three drinks per day double the risk of mental retardation in their children. Even one to two drinks per day may increase risk of growth impairment. No absolutely safe level of alcohol consumption has yet been established, thus every effort should be made to limit or eliminate alcohol intake during pregnancy.[9] (A "drink" is any alcoholic beverage containing approximately 15 g of ethanol, equivalent to about 360 ml of beer, 120 ml of wine, or 30 ml of hard liquor).

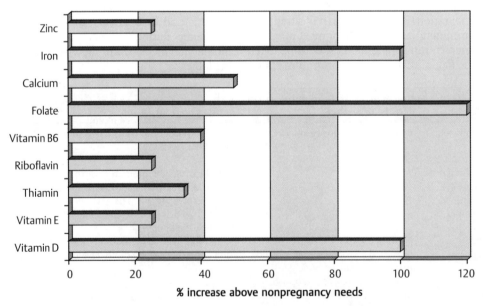

Fig. 4.3: Increased micronutrient requirements during pregnancy: selected vitamins, minerals and trace elements. (Source: National Research Council. RDAs. 10th ed. Washington DC: NAP; 1989. For folic acid: CDC. MMWR Morbid Mortal Wkly Rep. 1992;41:RR-14.

Caffeine

Pregnant women should limit their intake of caffeine. Metabolism of caffeine is slowed during pregnancy – caffeine takes two to three times longer to be metabolized and excreted – so levels in the maternal blood are elevated for longer periods. Caffeine readily passes through the placenta to the fetus. Ingestion of more than 300 mg caffeine/day (more than three cups of coffee) during pregnancy may be harmful to the fetus – impairing growth and development and increasing risk of miscarriage.[10] Even at lower levels of intake (about two cups of coffee), caffeine constricts the blood vessels in the placenta. This can restrict blood flow through the placenta and reduce the supply of oxygen and nutrients to the fetus.[10] Pregnant women should limit or eliminate their caffeine intake by avoiding coffee, black tea, chocolate, and colas.

Food Additives

The non-nutritive sweeteners saccharin, cyclamate, and aspartame should be avoided by pregnant women. Saccharin crosses the placenta and may be carcinogenic, particularly when exposure begins in utero and continues into adult life. Although aspartame does not cross the placenta, it is broken down into aspartate, phenylalanine, and small amounts of methanol, all of which can pass into the fetus. The health effects of methanol (a toxic alcohol) on the fetus are uncertain.

Heavy Metals

The developing fetus is very vulnerable to the toxic effects of mercury, lead, cadmium, and nickel, as well as industrial and agricultural chemicals. Small amounts of lead ingested by the mother in food and water can easily cross the placenta. Lead exposure of the fetus increases risk of premature birth. Moreover, the adverse effects of low-level lead exposure in utero can last long after birth – irreversibly impairing intellectual and motor development throughout childhood and lowering IQ.[1]. Exposure to mercury or polychlorinated biphenyls (widely used industrial chemicals) can retard fetal growth and cause birth defects.

High Doses of Vitamin A

High doses of vitamin A during pregnancy are teratogenic. Chronic intake of more than 25000 IU during pregnancy has been linked to birth defects, including malformations of the skull, heart, and central nervous system.[12] Pregnant women should be careful to maintain vitamin A intake (from food and supplements) at levels near 2500 IU. Choline and vitamin E deficiencies enhance the toxicity of high doses of vitamin A during pregnancy.

Tobacco

About one-third of pregnant women in the USA and Western Europe are smokers, and mothers who smoke are at increased risk for premature delivery and miscarriage. Children of mothers who smoked during pregnancy may have long-term impairments in physical growth and intellectual performance. These adverse effects are dose-dependent – the greater the number of cigarettes smoked during pregnancy, the greater the likelihood of harm. Smoking may reduce blood flow through the placenta and restrict oxygen and nutrient flow to the fetus. Smoking can deplete maternal stores of zinc, vitamin C, vitamin B6, folate, and vitamin B12. Levels of vit-

Effects of maternal smoking on the antioxidant status of the mother and newborn		
Nutrient	Smokers	Nonsmokers
Vitamin C in umbilical-cord blood (mg/dl)	0.61	1.68
Placental vitamin C (mg/100 g)	10.1	20.9*
Maternal plasma vitamin E (mg/dl)	0.4	0.8*
Vitamin E in umbilical-cord blood (mg/dl)	0.2	0.3*
Maternal plasma beta-carotene (g/dl)	19	44*
Beta-carotene in um-bilical-cord blood (g/dl)	7	20*

Values are means. * $P < 0.05$
(Source: Bendich A. Ann NY Acad Sci. 1993;678)

amins C and E in the fetus and placenta are markedly lower in women who smoke during pregnancy, compared to those who do not.

Maternal Health Problems during Pregnancy

Heartburn, Nausea, and Constipation

During pregnancy, high progesterone levels relax muscular tone and slow down peristalsis in the digestive tract.[14] This can be beneficial in that slower food transit times allow for increased nutrient absorption from foods. Absorption efficiency of iron, calcium, and vitamin B12 increases during pregnancy. However, reduced muscle tone can also cause problems. In the lower esophagus, it allows gastric reflux, causing irritation and discomfort ("heartburn"). Reflux can be minimized by eating multiple small meals. Meals should not be eaten immediately prior to physical activity or exercise. Also, because reflux is usually worse when lying down, elevating the head of the bed and not eating or drinking within 3 hours of bedtime can be helpful.[14]

Nausea is common in pregnant women, particularly in the first half of pregnancy. It is usually worse early in the day ("morning sickness"). Simple changes in diet may help diminish the symptoms. Eating smaller, frequent meals can help. Reducing meal volumes by drinking liquids between, and not with, meals may be of benefit.[14] Eating dry toast or crackers may help settle the stomach. Nausea often responds well to supplemental vitamin B6 (25–75 mg/day) and magnesium (200–500 mg/day) (see Fig. 4.4).[15]

Because movement of food through the intestines is slower, more water is absorbed from the stool and constipation is a problem for many pregnant women. Ample fluid and fiber intake can help (fiber intake should be gradually increased to more than 25–30 g/day through intake of fresh fruits and vegetables and whole grains).[14] Extra vitamin C (100–500 mg/day) and regular moderate exercise may also be helpful. Hemorrhoids, another common complaint during pregnancy, can also be reduced by including ample fiber, fluid, and vitamin C in the diet.

Hypoglycemia

Because the placenta pulls glucose from the mother's blood for use by the fetus, pregnant women more easily develop hypoglycemia, particularly in the morning before breakfast or if meals are skipped during the day. Hypoglycemia can produce lightheadedness, faintness, or headache. Also, skipping meals may increase levels of ketone bodies in the blood that can cross the placenta and adversely affect fetal development. Women should consume regular meals and snacks and avoid long periods of fasting while pregnant.

Diabetes

Pregnancy reduces the ability of insulin to control blood sugar. Most pregnant women secrete more insulin to balance this effect, and glucose control remains normal. However, about 5% of pregnant women develop glucose intolerance or diabetes.[16] Diabetes during pregnancy can harm both the mother and fetus and increase risk for complications during delivery. Because diabetes can develop without visible symptoms, all women should be screened midway through pregnancy. Nutrition and moderate exercise are the cornerstones of the prevention and treatment of diabetes during pregnancy. Eating small, frequent meals high in complex carbohydrate and fiber can help control blood sugar. Moderate exercise can enhance the action of insulin, along with supplemental zinc and chromium.[16] In over 95% of women, diabetes during pregnancy disappears after delivery.

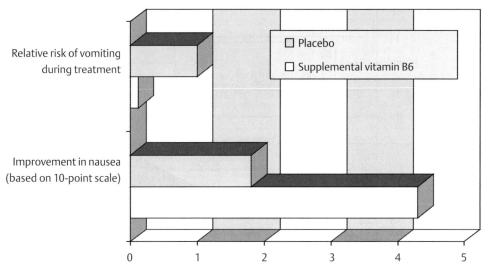

Fig. 4.**4**: **Vitamin B6 for nausea and vomiting in pregnancy.** In a trial of vitamin B6 (75 mg/day) in 59 pregnant women with nausea, supplementation was effective in reducing severity of nausea and vomiting. Using a "difference in nausea" score before and after treatment, women who received vitamin B6 had significant improvement and risk of vomiting was reduced 89% in the treated group. (Adapted from Sahakian V, et al. Obstet Gynecol. 1991;78:33.

Hypertension and Toxemia of Pregnancy

Toxemia is characterized by extreme hypertension, protein loss in the urine, and fluid retention and can be fatal for the mother and/or the fetus.[17] Fortunately, optimal nutrition can help prevent this disorder. Both too much and too little weight gain increase risk of hypertension during pregnancy. Inadequate salt intake may also increase the risk, so women should not attempt to restrict salt intake during pregnancy. Low calcium and/or zinc intake sharply increases risk of toxemia. Calcium supplementation (2 g/day) during pregnancy may reduce risk of toxemia by a third (see Fig. 4.**5**).[17] Supplemental vitamin B6 (25–50 mg/day) and evening primrose oil (containing GLA) (see pp. 89) may also be helpful in preventing and/or treating this disorder.

Vitamin and Mineral Supplementation during Pregnancy

Nutritional supplementation during pregnancy should not aim to replace a healthy, balanced diet. On the other hand, a balanced diet does not guarantee nutritional adequacy for every individual. How well do pregnant women meet the increased need for micronutrients during pregnancy? In the USA and Western Europe, many pregnant women do not obtain adequate vitamin B6, vitamin D, vitamin E, folate, iron, calcium, zinc, and magnesium in their diets.[4] For example, in most pregnant women iron intake is only about 10 mg/day, far below daily needs of 30 mg. It is not surprising that over two-thirds of pregnant women show signs of one or more nutrient deficiencies. Careful attention to diet is essential – while energy intake during pregnany should increase by only 15–20%, requirements for many micronutrients increase by 50–200%. A balanced multivitamin/mineral helps reduce risk of birth defects such as

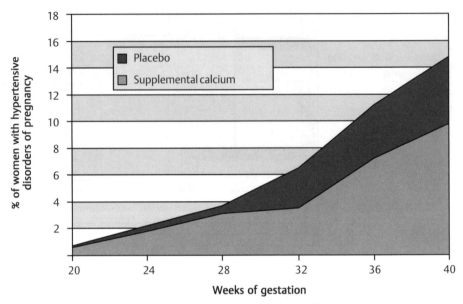

Fig. 4.**5**: **Calcium supplements and hypertensive disorders of pregnancy**. 1200 pregnant women with normal blood pressure began taking 2 g/day calcium or placebo at week 20 of gestation. There was a significant reduction in hypertensive disorders of pregnancy in the supplemented group: the overall rates of hypertensive disorders of pregnancy were 14.8% in the control group vs. 9.8% in the supplemented group. (From Belizan, et al. N Engl J Med. 1991;325:1399)

neural-tube defects and cleft palate.[18,19] It also helps prevent maternal problems, such as anemia, diabetes, and hypertension. A broad-spectrum, balanced nutritional supplement is a sensible part of any healthy pregnancy.[20]

The key to nutritional supplementation during pregnancy is balance. Many pregnant women are given a supplement containing high doses of iron and folic acid, but insufficient zinc. Both folic acid and iron reduce zinc absorption – and zinc deficiency can increase risk of problems during pregnancy. Mineral intake should be balanced, with optimum ratios of zinc to copper, as well as calcium to phosphorus and magnesium.

Summary

● Eat a well-balanced and nutrient-dense diet, including fruits, vegetables, whole grains, milk products, and protein foods (e.g., meat, eggs, legumes, nuts, and tofu). Emphasize foods that supply ample iron, calcium, vitamin D, zinc, fiber, and folate. Limit consumption of refined carbohydrates, fats, and other "micronutrient-empty" foods.

● Total weight gain for most women should be in the range of 10–12 kg, or about 0.4–0.5 kg/week during the second and third trimesters. Weight gain for women underweight before pregnancy should be at the upper end of this range, and for those overweight before pregnancy at the lower end.

● To obtain adequate calcium and vitamin D, eat milk products (milk, yogurt, cheese) at least three times daily.

● To absorb more iron, eat foods containing heme iron (meat, poultry, fish) regularly. To maximize iron absorption, include vitamin C-rich foods (e.g., orange juice, broccoli, strawberries) with meals.

Recommended nutrient intakes for pregnant women

Nutrient	Recommended daily intake (combined intake from food and supplement sources)
Macronutrients:	
Energy	2400–2600 kcal (for 60 kg female of average activity)
Protein	70–90 g
EFAs (linoleic plus linolenic acids)	25–30 g
Omega-3 fatty acids (EPA and DHA)	4–6 g
Fiber	25–30 g
Vitamins:	
Vitamin A (preferably as beta-carotene)	800 µg
Vitamin D	10–20 µg
Vitamin E	20 mg
Vitamin K	100 µg
Thiamin (Vitamin B1)	2 mg
Riboflavin (Vitamin B2)	2 mg
Niacin	20 mg
Vitamin B6	5 mg
Pantothenic acid	5–10 mg
Biotin	100–150 µg
Folic acid	0.8 mg
Vitamin B12	3 µg
Vitamin C	100 mg
Minerals:	
Calcium	1.5–2 g
Magnesium	400–600 mg
Iron	30 mg
Zinc	20–30 mg
Copper	2–3 mg
Manganese	2–4 mg
Fluoride*	2 mg
Iodine	200 µg
Selenium	100–150 µg
Chromium	200 µg
Molybdenum	200–250 µg

* only if water or salt supply is not fluoridated

● Food can be salted moderately to taste. For healthy women there is no need to restrict salt intake during pregnancy.

● Avoid foods with additives, and wash and/or peel fresh produce to remove agricultural chemicals (if not obtained from organic sources).

● Avoid supplementing with megadoses of micronutrients. This is no time to experiment with excessive levels of nutrients, since optimum nutrition is a question of balance. Both too much and too little can cause harm.

● Miniminze consumption of coffee or other caffeinated beverages, particularly near mealtime (coffee reduces iron and zinc absorption).

● The only sure way to avoid the possible harmful effects of alcohol on the fetus is to avoid drinking alcoholic beverages entirely.

References

1. Keen CL, et al. (eds.) Maternal Nutrition and Pregnancy Outcome. Ann NY Acad Sci. 1993;678.
2. Bendich A: Lifestyle and environmental factors that can adversely affect maternal nutritional status and pregnancy outcomes. Ann NY Acad Sci. 1993;678:255.
3. Taren DL, et al. The association of prenatal nutrition and educational services with low birthweight rates in a Florida program. Pub Health Rep. 1991;106:426.
4. Institute of Medicine. Nutrition during Pregnancy. Washington DC: National Academy Press; 1990.
5. Crawford MA. The role of essential fatty acids in neural development: implications for perinatal nutrition. Am J Clin Nutr. 1993;57:S703.
6. Schuster K, et al. Effect of maternal pyrodoxine supplementation on the vitamin B6 status of the infant and mother and on pregnancy outcome. J Nutr. 1984;977:114.
7. Rosso P. Nutrition and Metabolism in Pregnancy. Oxford University Press: New York; 1990.
8. King JC. Determinants of maternal zinc status during pregnancy. Am J Clin Nutr. 2000;71:1334S.
9. Beattie JO. Alcohol exposure and the fetus. Eur J Clin Nutr. 1992;46:S7.
10. Hinds TS, et al. The effect of caffeine on pregnancy outcome variables. Nutr Rev. 1996;54:203.
11. Andrews KW, et al. Prenatal lead exposure in relation to gestational age and birthweight: a review. Am J Indust Med. 1994;26:13.
12. Azais-Braesco V, Pascal G. Vitamin A in pregnancy: requirements and safety limits. Am J Clin Nutr. 2000;71:1325S.
13. Floyd RL, et al. A review of smoking in pregnancy: Effects on pregnancy outcomes and cessation efforts. Annu Rev Pub Health. 1993;14:379.
14. Baron TH, et al. Gastrointestinal motility disorders during pregnancy. Ann Int Med. 1993;118:366.
15. Sahakian V, et al. Vitamin B6 is effective therapy for

nausea and vomiting of pregnancy: A randomized double-blind placebo-controlled study. Obstet Gynecol. 1991;78:33.

16. Jovanovic-Peterson L, Peterson CM. Vitamin and mineral deficiencies which may predispose to glucose intolerance of pregnancy. J Am Coll Nutr. 1996;15:14.

17. Ritchie LD, King JC. Dietary calcium and pregnancy-induced hypertension: Is there a relation? Am J Clin Nutr. 2000;71:1371S.

18. Centers for Disease Control. Recommendations for the use of folic acid to reduce the number of cases of spina bifida and other neural tube defects. MMWR Morbid Mortal Wkly Rep. 1992;41:RR-14.

19. Shaw GM, et al. Risk of orofacial clefts in children born to women using multivitamins containing folic acid periconceptionally. Lancet. 1995;345:393.

20. Keen CL, Zidenberg-Cherr S. Should vitamin-mineral supplements be recommended for all women of childbearing potential? Am J Clin Nutr. 1994;59:S532.

Breastfeeding and Infancy

The breast is much more than a passive reservoir of milk. The mammary glands in the breast extract water, amino acids, fats, vitamins, minerals, and other substances from the maternal blood. They package these substrates, synthesize many new nutrients, and secrete a unique fluid specifically tailored to the needs of the infant. The glands balance milk production with infant demand, so that the volume of milk produced during lactation is determined by infant need. Milk production in the first 6 months averages about 750 ml/day,[1] but breastfeeding mothers have the potential to produce far more milk. Mothers who breastfeed twins can produce over 2000 ml/day.

Composition of Breast Milk

Breast milk is a remarkably complex substance, with over 200 recognized components. Breast milk contains:

● all the nutrients (energy, protein, EFAs, vitamins, and minerals) needed by the newborn to grow and develop

● enzymes to help the newborn digest and absorb nutrients

● immune factors to protect the infant from infection

● hormones and growth factors that influence infant growth

Although the basic components of breast milk are the same in all women, concentration of the individual components may vary considerably, depending on the mother's nutritional status.

An immature milk, called colostrum, is produced during the first week after birth. It is thicker than mature milk, and slightly yellow. The yellow tint is due to high concentration of beta-carotene. The carotene content of colostrum is about 10 times higher than in mature milk. High levels of carotenes and vitamin E in colostrum provide antioxidant protection during the vulnerable newborn period.[2] Colostrum is also rich in immunoglobulins and other immune proteins which help protect the newborn from infections in the digestive tract. This protective effect provides a temporary defense while the infant's own immune system is maturing.

Nutritional Needs during Breastfeeding

Eating a healthy diet while breastfeeding is important. A healthy infant doubles its weight in the first 4 to 6 months after birth, and, for a mother who is exclusively breastfeeding, breastmilk must provide all the energy, pro-

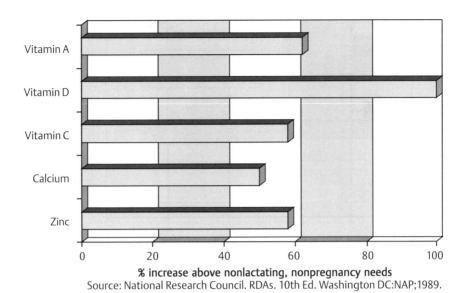

% increase above nonlactating, nonpregnancy needs
Source: National Research Council. RDAs. 10th Ed. Washington DC:NAP;1989.

Fig. 4.**6**: Increased micronutrient needs during lactation: selected vitamins, minerals and trace elements.

tein, and micronutrients to support this rapid growth. Moreover, the diet also needs to support maternal health – allowing the breastfeeding mother to lose weight gained during pregnancy, replenishing nutrient stores depleted by the demands of pregnancy, and maintaining nutrient stores to support milk production.

Breastfeeding women need significantly more energy, protein, and micronutrients during lactation to support milk formation. For women exclusively breastfeeding, synthesis and secretion of breast milk requires an additional 750 kcal/day and an extra 15–20 g of high-quality protein.[1] Requirements for most vitamins and minerals are 50–100% higher, compared with before pregnancy. Figure 4.**6** compares the nutritional needs of lactating versus nonlactating women for several important micronutrients.

Food choice can substantially influence the quality of the breast milk. For example, the type of fat eaten while breastfeeding influences the fat composition of the breast milk.[3] About one-third of the fatty acids present in the milk are derived directly from the maternal diet. Vegetarians produce milk with greater amounts of the fatty acids present in plant foods. Because EFAs (particularly linolenic acid and the omega-3 fatty acids EPA and DHA) (see pp. 89) are vital for the developing nervous system of the newborn,[4] nursing mothers should consume generous amounts.

Poor intake of vitamins or trace minerals can reduce the nutritional quality of the mother's breastmilk and produce a deficiency in her infant. For example, women who are deficient in vitamin D (from little sunlight exposure and poor dietary intake) have very low levels of vitamin D in their breast milk. Infants fed breast milk low in vitamin D may develop skeletal abnormalities and rickets.[5] On the other hand, a high maternal intake of vitamin D can substantially increase amounts secreted in the breast milk (see Fig. 4.**7**). Similarly, levels of the B vitamins, vitamin C, and vitamin E in human milk are very sensitive to the mother's intake. Even a small supplement of vitamin B6 (at a level of 2.5 mg/day) can more than double levels of vitamin B6 in breastmilk.[6] For the trace minerals – particularly

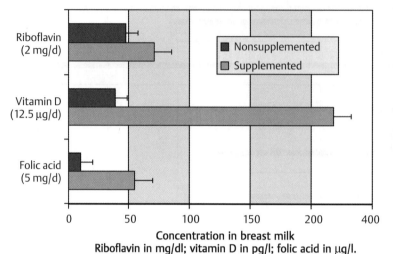

Fig. 4.7: Increase in vitamin concentration in breast milk in response to maternal supplementation. (From Nail PA, et al. Am J Clin Nutr. 1980;33: 198. Lönnerdal J. J Nutr. 1986;116:499. Cooperman. Am J Clin Nutr. 1982;36:576)

Concentration in breast milk
Riboflavin in mg/dl; vitamin D in pg/l; folic acid in μg/l.

zinc, selenium, and iodine – maternal dietary intake also influences concentrations in milk. For example, zinc supplementation during lactation (15–25 mg/day) can produce a significant rise in milk zinc levels.[7]

In contrast, major minerals like calcium and magnesium continue to be secreted into milk even if maternal intake is poor, with maternal stores making up the difference. If the maternal diet is chronically low in calcium, body stores can be significantly depleted. The skeleton of an average adult woman contains 1 kg of calcium. Daily secretion of calcium into breastmilk is about 10 g per month. If extra calcium is not consumed to cover losses into the milk, during 8 months of breastfeeding about 7% of calcium in the bones will be removed and used for milk production.[1] Large losses of calcium during lactation may increase risk of developing osteoporosis later in life. Calcium supplementation (along with vitamin D) during lactation and during the weaning period is important to maintain calcium balance and maternal skeletal health (see Fig. 4.8).[8]

Recommended daily intake for selected micronutrients during breastfeeding	
Vitamin A	1200 μg
Vitamin D	10 μg
Vitamin E	50 mg
Vitamin C	200 mg
Vitamin B6	5–10 mg
Folate	0.4 mg
Calcium	1500 mg
Magnesium	400 mg
Zinc	30 mg
Omega-3 fatty acids	1.0–1.5 g

Postpartum Depression

Some mothers become depressed in the first few months after their baby is born. Pregnancy and lactation may drain maternal nutrient stores, producing deficiencies that can contribute to postpartum depression. A lack of B vitamins may be the cause, along with deficiencies of calcium, magnesium, and iron. A supplement containing ample amounts of the B-vitamin complex (emphasizing thiamin and vitamin B6) along with an iron-containing mineral supplement may help provide energy and an emotional lift. Also helpful are a carefully chosen, well-balanced diet, adequate rest, and emotional support.

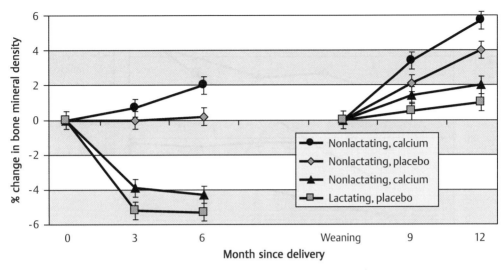

Fig. 4.**8**: **Calcium supplementation increases bone density during lactation and weaning.** Effects of calcium supplementation and lactation in 389 women on the % change in bone mineral density of the lumbar spine during the first 6 months postpartum and postweaning. Significant differences were found between the calcium and placebo groups in the nonlactating women during the first 6 months, and for the calcium and placebo groups in both the lactating and nonlactating women after weaning.
(Adapted from Kalkwarf HJ, et al. N Engl J Med. 1997; 337:523)

Dietary Hazards: Caffeine and Alcohol

About 1% of a maternal dose of caffeine (whether from coffee, tea, soft drinks, chocolate, or medicines) is transported into the breastmilk. Infants metabolize caffeine more slowly than adults, and caffeine in breast milk may cause irritability and wakefulness. High intake of alcohol can inhibit milk production. Moreover, infant exposure to alcohol during breast-feeding may have serious adverse effects on development. Ethanol itself readily passes into the milk at concentrations approaching those in maternal blood and can produce lethargy and drowsiness in the breast-feeding infant. Heavy alcohol consumption (more than 4–5 "drinks"/day) by nursing mothers may impair psychomotor development in their infants.[10] The effects of occasional light drinking are unknown.

Breastfeeding and Infant Health

Human milk is a superior source of nutrition for infants. No manufactured formula can duplicate the unique, biologically specific physical structure and nutrient composition of human milk. Human milk has several advantages over formula[9]:

● Nutrient bioavailability from breast milk is superior. For example, the absorption of minerals such as calcium, zinc, and iron from breast milk is five to 10 times higher than from formula.

● The nutrient content of human milk is uniquely suited to the newborn's needs A good example is vitamin D. Vitamin D from foods must first be converted in the liver to the 25-OH form before it can be stored. However, during early infancy the liver is immature and it cannot readily convert dietary forms of vitamin D to 25-OH vitamin D. Fortunately, unlike other foods and formula, most

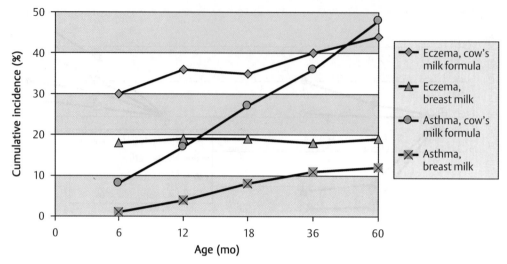

Fig. 4.**9**: **Infant feeding and incidence of childhood eczema and asthma.** The incidence of eczema and asthma up to the age of 5 years in children is significantly lower in those who were breast-fed during infancy, compared with those given cow's milk formula.
(Adapted from Chandra RK. J Ped Gastroenterol Nutr. 1997;24:380)

of the vitamin D in human milk is present as 25-OH vitamin D.

● A variety of digestive enzymes are present in human milk. They are important in that they help the immature gastrointestinal tract of the newborn digest and absorb nutrients in the milk.

● Breast-feeding protects the infant against infection. Human milk contains anti-infective substances and cells, including white blood cells and antibodies, not found in infant formula. The frequency of gastrointestinal infections is much lower in breast-fed infants than in formula-fed infants. Breast-fed infants also mount a more vigorous immune response to certain respiratory viruses – respiratory illnesses tend to be milder and shorter than those in formula-fed infants.

● Breast-feeding helps protect against food allergies and asthma (see Fig. 4.**9**).

● Human milk contains a variety of factors that hasten the maturation of the newborn's immune system. Breast-feeding helps protect against several diseases with immunologic causes that occur later in life, including juvenile-type diabetes, childhood lymphoma, and Crohn's disease.

● Breastfeeding costs less, is more convenient to prepare and clean-up, and is guaranteed to be clean and hygienic.

Nutrients of Special Importance For Infants

Physical growth during the first few months after birth is explosive. By age 4 months, the birth weight of most healthy infants has doubled, and by the end of the first year has tripled. Per unit body weight, an infant's nutritional needs are markedly higher than at any other time in life. Optimum nutrition can strongly influence the infant's growth, development, and disease resistance.

Protein and Amino Acids

Protein needs are high during infancy. Large amounts of amino acids are needed for the formation of new muscle, connective tissue, and bone, and for synthesis of a large number of enzymes and hormones. The nine amino acids that are essential for adults are also essential for infants. However, several additional amino acids – cysteine, arginine, carnitine, and taurine – are essential in infancy. In older children and adults, these amino acids can be synthesized by the body, but in the newborn the synthetic pathways are not fully developed. Requirements must be at least partially met by dietary sources.

Essential Fatty Acids

Ample intake of the EFAs (see pp. 89) is vital during infancy. Because infants absorb fat poorly and have low fat stores, they are particularly sensitive to EFA deficiency and quickly develop signs of deficiency if fat intake is low. Infants fed formulas deficient in linoleic acid for just a few days may develop a dry, eczema-like, flaky skin rash, diarrhea, hair loss, and impaired wound healing. Deficiency also impairs platelet function and lowers resistance to infection. Regular intake of EFAs is therefore critical during infancy, and although breast milk is rich in EFAs, not all infant formulas have adequate amounts.

Vitamins

In northern climates during the winter months when maternal and infant sunlight exposure is minimal, the level of vitamin D in breast milk may not be sufficient to maintain optimum skeletal growth. Infants from such regions fed only breast milk without supplemental vitamin D have lower bone mineral content, compared with those given a 10-µg daily supplement of the vitamin.[5] Therefore, most experts recommend that breast-fed infants who do not get regular sunlight exposure should receive a supplement. Vitamin D supplementation should be at the level of 5–10 µg/day. Toxicity can occur if infants are given higher doses of vitamin D.

Newborn infants have low body stores of vitamin E and needs for the vitamin are high. The requirement for vitamin E increases as dietary intake of polyunsaturated fatty acids (PUFAs) increases, and human milk is rich in PUFAs. Also, because of reduced absorption of fat-soluble compounds, it is difficult for many infants to absorb sufficient vitamin E. During the 1960s and 1970s, infants were often fed formulas high in PUFAs, but with low vitamin E : PUFA ratios. These formulas caused vitamin E deficiency and anemia. Current formulas have been modified and now contain less PUFAs and more vitamin E. To compensate for poor intestinal absorption, infants may benefit from daily supplementation with 5–10 mg of vitamin E.

Vitamin K is important during the newborn period for normal blood clotting. However, the infant requirement for vitamin K cannot be met by usual levels in breast milk. Poor vitamin K status can lead to hemorrhagic disease of the newborn. Therefore, to prevent bleeding problems and provide adequate body stores, newborns often receive a single dose of 0.5–1 mg of vitamin K soon after birth.

Ample vitamin B6 is important for infant growth. Infants with low vitamin B6 intakes (less than 0.1 mg/day) may show signs of deficiency – irritability, digestive problems, and, if deficiency is severe, seizures.

Body stores of folate at birth are small and can be quickly depleted by the high requirements of growth. Although human milk contains ample folate, cow's milk has little. Moreover, if the cow's milk is boiled, folate levels will fall even further. Therefore, infants receiving boiled cow's milk or boiled evaporated milk need supplemental folate.

Because vitamin B12 is only found in animal foods, infants of vegetarians (vegans) who are exclusively breast-fed may develop anemia and neurological problems due to vitamin B12 deficiency.[11] Lactating women who are vegetarians should consider taking a vitamin-B12 supplement – the vitamin will then be passed to their infant in their milk.

Minerals

It is important that infants receive foods rich in calcium and other minerals as they wean from the breast. Rickets can develop in infants who are fed weaning foods low in calcium and vitamin D. However, cow's milk, although rich in calcium, is not an ideal weaning food. Cow's milk has a much higher amount of phosphorus than human milk – the ratio of calcium to phosphorus is only about 1 : 1 in cow's milk, while it is over 2 :1 in human milk. Newborns who are fed only cow's milk may develop hypocalcemia and seizures. This occurs because the excess phosphorus in cow's milk deposits into the skeleton, pulling calcium with it and lowering blood levels of calcium. In general, infants should not be fed large amounts of cow's milk or milk products until after the first year. [12]

The rapidly growing infant requires large amounts of iron for synthesis of new red blood cells and muscle. There are only small amounts of iron in human milk, and although the bioavailability of the iron is high, the amount absorbed is usually not able to meet the infant's needs. In the later half of the first year, breast-fed infants are at much higher risk for iron-deficiency and anemia compared with infants receiving supplemental iron (see Fig. 4.**10**).[13] By 9 months, about one-quarter of exclusively breast-fed infants will develop iron-deficiency anemia. Iron-deficiency can seriously harm a growing infant. Infants deficient in iron are more likely to suffer from infections, grow more slowly than their healthy counterparts, and may have impaired mental development and lower IQs.[14] Thus iron supplementation is important for full-term, breast-fed infants beginning between 4 and 6 months. When weaning begins, foods rich in iron, such as iron-fortified infant cereals, pureed green leafy vegetables, and strained meats should be given.

Flouride is incorporated into the teeth as they slowly mineralize inside the jaws during infant development. Deposition of fluoride into the enamel sharply reduces later susceptibility to dental caries. Both the unerupted primary and permanent teeth mineralize in early infancy. Because only trace amounts of fluoride are found in breast milk, fluoride supplements should be given to breast-fed infants (and infants receiving formula without fluoride) beginning at about 4–6 months. A daily supplement of 0.25 mg of fluoride should be provided until the infant begins to consume fluoridated water or salt. Fluoride intakes from all sources during infancy should not exceed 2.5 mg/day to avoid mottling of tooth enamel.

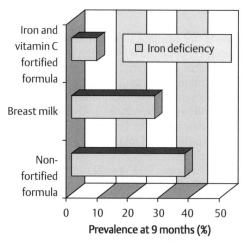

Fig. 4.**10**: **Iron status with different feeding regimens during infancy.** Prevalence of iron deficiency at 9 months among infants fed exclusively nonfortified cow's milk formula, breast milk, or an iron and vitamin C fortified formula (15 mg iron and 100 mg ascorbic acid/100g). Iron supplements (with vitamin C) may be beneficial in infants fed nonfortified formula and infants who are exclusively breast-fed, especially after 4–6 months.
(Adapted from Pizarro F, et al. J Pediatr. 1991;118:687)

Nutrient supplements during infancy	
Nutrient	**Recommended daily intake**
Omega-3 fatty acids	500 mg
Vitamin D	5 µg*
Vitamin E	5 mg
Iron	10 mg**
Fluoride	0.2 mg***

* Particularly important for breast-fed infants during winter months
** Particularly important during breastfeeding, before iron-rich supplemental foods become a major part of the infant's diet[15]
*** Only until the infant begins to consume fluoridated water

References

1. Institute of Medicine. Nutrition during Lactation. Washington DC: National Academy Press; 1991.
2. Patton S, et al. Carotenoids in human colostrum. Lipids. 1990;25:159.
3. Jensen CL, et al. Effect of docosahexanoic acid supplementation of lactating women on the fatty acid composition of breast milk lipids and maternal and infant plasma phospholipids. Am J Clin Nutr. 2000;71:292S-99S.
4. Crawford MA. The role of essential fatty acids in neural development: Implications for perinatal nutrition. Am J Clin Nutr. 1993;57:S703.
5. Greer FR, Marshall S. Bone mineral content, serum vitamin D metabolite concentrations, and ultraviolet B light exposure in infants fed human milk with and without vitamin D2 supplements. J Pediatr. 1989;114:204.
6. Sneed SM, et al. The effects of ascorbic acid, vitamin B6, vitamin B12 and folic acid supplementation on the breast milk and maternal nutritional status of low socioeconomic lactating women. Am J Clin Nutr. 1981;34:1338.
7. Walravens PA, et al. Zinc supplements in breastfed infants. Lancet. 1992;340:683.
8. Kalwarf HJ, et al. The effect of calcium supplementation on bone density during lactation and weaning. N Engl J Med. 1997;337:523.
9. Newman J. How breast milk protects newborns. Sci Am Dec. 1995;12:58.
10. Little RE, et al. Maternal alcohol use during breastfeeding and infant mental and motor development at one year. N Engl J Med. 1989;321:425.
11. Dagniele PC, et al. Increased risk of vitamin B12 and folate deficiency in infants on macrobiotic diets. Am J Clin Nutr. 1989;50:818.
12. Wharton BA. Milk for babies and children; No ordinary cow's milk before 1 year. BMJ. 1990;301:775.
13. Fomon SJ. Nutrition of Normal Infants. St. Louis: Mosby-Year Book Inc.; 1993.
14. Sheard NF. Iron deficiency and infant development. Nutr Rev. 1994;52:137.
15. Lönnerdal B. Regulation of mineral and trace elements in human milk: Exogenous and endogenous factors. 2000;58:223–9.

Childhood and Adolescence

Optimum nutrition is important during childhood and adolescence for three major reasons:

● It allows a child to grow and develop and reach his or her genetic potential for physical size and intelligence.

● Childhood offers an important opportunity to establish healthy eating patterns and food preferences. Diet habits learned during this period often become lifelong habits.

● A poor quality diet during childhood and adolescence can increase risk of chronic diseases, such as osteoporosis and heart disease, later in life.[1]

Nutritional Needs

Energy

Because of high levels of activity and rapid growth, children's energy needs are high. For example, on average a 7-year-old girl has nearly the same calorie requirement as her mother. An active 14-year-old male in the midst of his pubertal growth spurt may need over 4000 kcals/day, almost double the energy requirement of a middle-aged adult.[2]

Fats

Although children have small stomachs and appetites, making fats important as concentrated sources of calories for growth, fat intake during childhood should be kept moderate. High fat intakes increase risk of obesity and heart disease later in life.[1] However, strict restriction of fat intake may lead to inadequate energy consumption and poor growth.[3]

Calories from fat should provide about one-third of energy requirements. Saturated fat intake should be minimized by avoiding fatty meats and substituting reduced-fat milk products for whole-fat products. Regular consumption of cold-pressed plant oils (rich in the EFAs, linoleic acid and linolenic acid) is important.

Sugars

Many children have a preference for sweet, carbohydrate-rich foods. Overconsumption of foods high in sugar may increase risk of dental caries and obesity. However, rigorous elimination of sugar-containing foods from a child's diet without adequate energy substitution may lead to weight loss and poor growth. Again, moderation is the key. Decreasing refined-sugar intake during childhood can be difficult, as it is often added to processed foods popular with children.

Micronutrients

Although most children and adolescents obtain adequate amounts of energy and protein, their diets are often low in micronutrients (see Fig. 4.**11**). Micronutrient needs are very high – especially during the adolescent growth spurt – and micronutrient deficiencies are common among teenagers.[5] Many adolescent girls, concerned about their body shape and weight, regularly consume only 1600–1800 kcal/day. At this level of intake, unless foods are very carefully chosen, obtaining adequate amounts of the micronutrients is difficult. The nutrients most often lacking in the diets of children and adolescents are the minerals iron, zinc, and calcium, and the B vitamins (particularly vitamin B6 and folate) along with vitamin C.[4,5]

Vitamins. Requirements for thiamin, riboflavin, and niacin peak during the teenage years. This occurs because demand for these B-vitamins increases proportionately with increasing energy intake – and energy needs are highest during adolescence. Vitamin B6 plays a central role in protein synthesis and generous amounts of this vitamin are needed for building muscle, bone and other organs. The synthesis of new blood proteins and cells requires large amounts of folic acid, and vitamins B12 and B6. Because of its central role in the building of collagen (the major protein component of connective tissue and bone), ample vitamin C is needed for optimal devel-

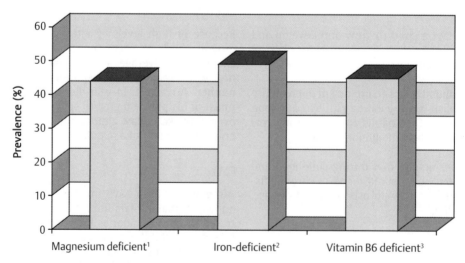

Fig. 4.**11**: **Micronutrient deficiencies in adolescence.** Between 40 and 50% of adolescents have biochemical signs of magnesium, iron, and vitamin B6 deficiency.
(From: 1. Am J Clin Nutr. 1997;66:1172;2. AJDC. 11992;46:803;3. J Am Diet Assoc. 1987;87:307)

opment of cartilage, bone, and the connective tissue in skin and blood vessels. In children with erratic diets who eat few vegetables and fruits, a balanced supplement containing the B-vitamin complex with vitamin C ensures regular intake of these important micronutrients.

Calcium and magnesium. Formation of the skeleton during childhood and adolescence requires high amounts of calcium, phosphorus, and magnesium. A 2-year-old child needs 800 mg of calcium each day.[2] For children and adolescents with poor appetites, a calcium supplement may be beneficial. Although many children do not consume enough calcium,[4,5] their diets tend to be too high in phosphorus. Processed foods, soft drinks, and meats are very rich in phosphorus, and milk has twice as much phosphorus as calcium. Imbalanced intake of too much phosphorus can interfere with normal growth of the skeleton. A healthy ratio of calcium, phosphorus, and magnesium in the diet is approximately 2:2:1. Balanced sources of these minerals include sesame seeds (50 g contain 400 mg of calcium and 300 mg of phosphorus) and dark green leafy vegetables like spinach.

Iron. Children and adolescents have very high iron needs – a rapidly growing boy needs more iron each day than his father.[2] Iron is required to build hemoglobin in red blood cells and myoglobin in muscle, yet the diets of many children do not supply adequate amounts. Milk is a major source of calories at this age and is very low in iron. Iron deficiency is the most common nutritional deficiency in children – about one-quarter of children and adolescents are iron deficient in Western Europe and the USA.[5,6] The symptoms of iron deficiency are easy to recognize when they become severe – children appear listless and develop pallor, easy fatigue, and anemia. But anemia is only one manifestation of iron deficiency. Children who are deficient in iron have poor appetites, are more likely to develop infections, and grow more slowly than their healthy counterparts. They are often irritable, inattentive, and perform more poorly on tests of motor and mental development (see Fig. 4.**13**). Even adolescents who are mildly iron deficient (without signs of anemia) have impaired learning and memory and may benefit from iron supplementation (see Fig. 4.**14**).[7] Iron deficiency is more common among adolescent athletes than nonathletes and can decrease exercise capacity and endurance.

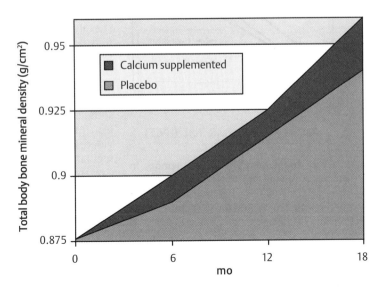

Fig. 4.**12**: **Increased bone density in adolescent girls by calcium supplementation.** In 94 teenage girls, supplemental calcium (500 mg/d) produced significant increases in total body bone mineral density (1.3%), spine bone mineral density (2.9%), and content (4.7%). (From Lloyd TL, et al. JAMA. 1993;270:841)

Total body bone mineral density (g/cm²)

■ Calcium supplemented
□ Placebo

0.95
0.925
0.9
0.875

0   6   12   18

mo

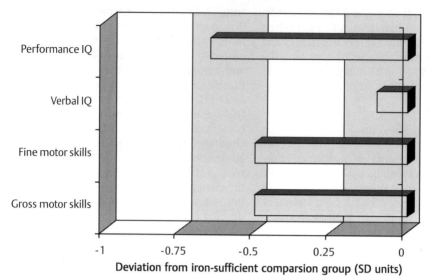

Deviation from iron-sufficient comparsion group (SD units)

Fig. 4.**13: Iron deficiency and mental and motor development during childhood.** The graph shows the differences in the results of developmental tests (the Bruininks-Oseretsky Test of Motor Proficiency and the Wechsler Preschool and Primary Scale of Intelligence) at 5 years between children who had iron-deficiency anemia in infancy and an iron-sufficient control group. Children who are iron-deficient during infancy are at risk of long-lasting developmental impairment.
(Adapted from Lozoff B, et al. N Engl J Med. 1991; 325:687)

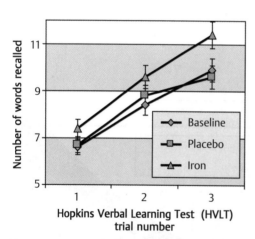

Hopkins Verbal Learning Test (HVLT)
trial number

Fig. 4.**14: Iron supplements improve memory in nonanemic, iron-deficient adolescents.** Iron supplementation (260 mg/d) for 8 weeks in nonanemic, iron-deficient adolescent girls improved tests of verbal learning and memory.
(Bruner AB, et al. Lancet. 1996;348:992)

What can be done to ensure ample dietary iron during childhood and adolescence? The choice of beverage with meals is important. Orange juice doubles the absorption of iron from a meal (vitamin C is a potent enhancer of iron absorption), whereas milk or iced tea sharply decreases it.[8] When the principal protein of a meal is meat, fish, or chicken, iron absorption is about four times higher than when the prinicipal protein is dairy products or eggs. In order to prevent iron-deficiency anemia in children and adolescents, regular sources of iron, such as green leafy vegetables, lean meat, poultry, and fish should be provided. In children and adolescents who do not regularly eat these foods, a daily-supplement containing 5–10 mg of iron is recommended.

Zinc. Many children do not get adequate zinc because of low dietary intake of whole grains, meat, and fish.[5] Severe zinc deficiency can stunt growth permanently and delay sexual development. Even mild zinc deficiency during childhood and adolescence may impair growth. In children with marginal zinc intakes (5–6 mg/day), adding a daily zinc supplement (10–15 mg) can significantly improve growth and development (see Fig. 4.**15**).[9,10]

Nutrition and Child Health

Dental Decay

Formation of healthy teeth is supported by proper diet during childhood – ample protein, calcium, phosphate, and vitamins C and D are particularly important. Diet is also important in the prevention of dental caries. Repeated exposure of the teeth to sugar by frequent snacking on sugary foods and drinks will substantially increase risk of dental caries. Resistance to dental caries is increased if the diet contains optimum amounts of fluoride. Fluoride is incorporated into the crystals that form the tooth enamel, making them more resistant to acid. In many areas, fluoridation of the water or salt supply provides children with ample fluoride. In areas where the flu-

oride content of the water is low or absent (less than 0.3 parts per million) and the salt is not fluoridated, supplemental fluoride should be given to children.[2] The best time to give fluoride supplements (1–2 mg, in the form of drops) is at bedtime, after brushing the teeth.

Behavior Problems

Most children have periods when they become unruly, excitable, or inattentive. These can be due to a lack of sleep or physical activity, emotional state, desire for attention, anxiety, and many other factors. Nutritional factors can also strongly influence childhood behavior. Timing of meals and snacks can affect behavior and performance at school. Children who skip breakfast or other meals are less able to concentrate at school and may have shorter attention spans.[11] A malnourished child is more likely to be a poor student and have behavioral problems. Children become sluggish and inattentive if they have deficiencies of iron, zinc, vitamin C, or the B vitamins.[12] A balanced vitamin/mineral supplement may help children improve their performance at school.[13]

Lead Toxicity

Millions of children in Europe and North America have body lead levels high enough to impair intellectual development and produce other adverse health effects.[14] Lead is distributed throughout the environment and makes its way into food through contaminated soil and water. Mainly due to the elimination of lead solder on food cans and the reduction in lead from automobile exhaust, levels of lead in foods today are 90% lower than 20 years ago. However, tainted food and drink continue to be sources of lead. Dishware is a potential source: small amounts of lead can leach from the glazes and decorative paints on ceramic ware, lead crystal, pewter, and silverplated holloware. Acidic liquids such as coffee, fruit juices, and tomato soup have a greater tendency to cause leaching of lead. A common source of lead exposure is lead-based paint. Most house paints used in the past were very high in lead – those used before 1940 contain up to 50% lead. Children may ingest lead by

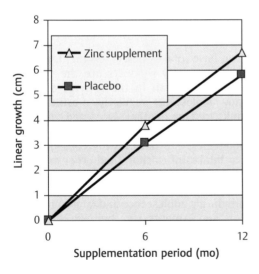

Fig. 4.**15**: **Mild zinc deficiency is growth-limiting in children.** In 40 low-income, mildly zinc-deficient children aged 2–6 years, a zinc supplement (10 mg/d) significantly increased growth.
(Adapted from Walravens PA, et al. Am J Clin Nutr. 1983;38:195)

eating paint chips (which are often colorful and sweet-tasting) or by ingestion of lead-contaminated dust and dirt around the house.

Children absorb lead more efficiently and are more sensitive to its effects than adults. They can absorb up to 50% of ingested lead, whereas adults absorb only about 10%. Deficiencies of iron and calcium enhance absorption of lead and may increase its toxic effects in children.[15] Compared with adults, children are more sensitive to lead toxicity because less can be deposited into their smaller skeleton, leaving a higher percentage of the lead in soft tissues and blood where it is more toxic. Lead affects almost every organ system – the kidney, bone marrow, and brain are particularly sensitive. It can slow growth, damage hearing, and impair coordination and balance. A child with chronic lead intoxication may be listless and irritable, and even low levels of lead exposure in childhood can impair neuropsychological development and classroom performance (see Fig. 4.**16**).[16] All children should be checked for body burden of lead at about 1 year of age and periodically thereafter.[17] This can be done by measuring lead levels in blood or hair. For children who live in areas with a high risk of environmental lead, a supplement containing calcium and zinc (at levels of 500 mg and 15 mg, respectively) can help block absorption of lead[16] and gradually reduce elevated body burdens.

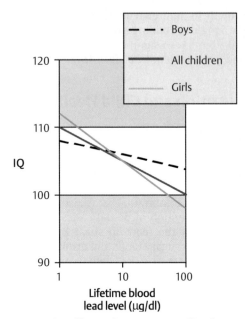

Fig. 4.**16**: **The effects of environmental lead exposure on children's intelligence.** Low-level exposure to lead during childhood has adverse effects on neuropsychological development and IQ. For an increase in blood lead level from 10 g/dl to 30 g/dl over the first 4 years of life, the estimated reduction in IQ is 4–5%. (Adapted from Baghurst PA, et al. N Engl J Med. 1992;327:1279)

Calcium, Minerals, and Skeleton Health

Ample calcium and mineral intake is particularly important for teenage females. Bone growth is rapid during adolescence, when about half of the total skeleton is formed. The amount of bone mineral that has accumulated in the skeleton during this period is a major determinant of risk of osteoporosis in later life. More calcium deposited into the skeleton during childhood and adolescence means a greater "calcium bank" to draw from during aging.

Although teenagers need about 1200–1500 mg/day of calcium,[18] the average calcium intake of adolescent females in the USA is only about 750 mg/day and only about one in seven have intakes near 1200 mg/day.[4] Milk and other dairy products are the primary source of calcium in the teenage diet, yet many adolescents regularly substitute soft drinks, iced tea, or other sweetened beverages for milk. Insufficient dietary calcium during adolescence can have lasting consequences. Poor intakes of calcium (and other minerals, such as zinc[19]) can compromise bone health and may increase incidence of bony fractures both during adolescence and later in life. Calcium supplements can help children and teenagers reach adequate calcium intake and can stimulate stronger, denser bone growth (see Fig. 4.**12**).[20]

Micronutrient supplements for children > 4 years and adolescents	
Nutrient	Recommended daily intake
Vitamins:	
Vitamin A	700 µg
Vitamin D	10 µg
Vitamin E	20–50 mg
Vitamin C	100 mg
Thiamin	2–5 mg
Riboflavin	2–5 mg
Niacin	25–50 mg
Vitamin B6	10–15 mg
Folic acid	0.4 mg
Vitamin B12	2–5 µg
Biotin	50–100 µg
Pantothenic acid	5–10 mg
Minerals:	
Calcium	600 mg
Magnesium	300 mg
Iron	10–20 mg
Zinc	10–20 mg
Copper	2–3 mg
Selenium	100 µg
Iodine	150 µg
Manganese	2–5 mg
Fluoride*	1–2 mg
Chromium	100–200 µg
Molybdenum	150–250 µg

* only it water or salt supply is not fluoridated

Summary

The diets of most children and adolescents are erratic and unpredictable, and it is often a problem getting them to eat healthy foods. Poor dietary intake combined with very high nutritional needs sharply increases risk of micronutrient deficiencies. For many children, taking a well-balanced vitamin/ mineral supplement to ensure adequate micronutrient intake is important. Appropriate levels for a supplement are shown in the table above.

Of course, multivitamin/mineral supplements cannot replace healthy foods and good dietary habits. Diets should be high in fruits, vegetables, whole grains, and legumes. Dairy products, lean meats, poultry, and fish are also important. Processed and refined foods should be avoided. Many contain additives, colorings, and flavorings, as well as high amounts of added sugar, salt, and hydrogenated fats. Healthy snacks, such as milk, yogurt, fruit, nuts, and whole-grain baked goods, should be available throughout the day.

References

1. McGill HC, et al. Origin of atherosclerosis in childhood and adolescence. Am J Clin Nutr. 2000; 72:1307S.
2. U.S. National Research Council. Recommended Dietary Allowances. 10th ed. Washington; National Academy Press: 1989.
3. Kaplan RM, Toshima MT. Does a reduced fat diet cause retardation in child growth? Prev Med. 1992;21:33.
4. Life Sciences Research Office, FASEB. Nutrition monitoring in the U.S.: an update report. DHHS Publ. 89 1255, Hyattsville, MD, Sept. 1989.
5. Roberts SB, Heyman MB. Micronutrient shortfalls in young children's diets: Common and owing to inadequate intakes both at home and at child care centers. Nutr Rev. 2000;58:27.
6. Samuelson G, et al. Dietary iron intake and iron status in adolescents. Acta Paediatr. 1996;85:1033.
7. Bruner AB, et al. Randomised study of cognitive effects of iron supplementation in non-anemic, iron deficient adolescent girls. Lancet. 1996;348:992.
8. Hurrell RF. Bioavailability of iron. Eur J Clin Nutr. 1997;51:S4.
9. Castillo Duran C, et al. Zinc supplementation increases growth velocity of male children and adolescents with short stature. Acta Paediatr. 1994;83:833.
10. Walravens PA, et al. Linear growth of low-income preschool children receiving a zinc supplement. Am J Clin Nutr. 1983;38:195.
11. Simeon DT, Grantham-McGregor S. Effects of missing breakfast on the cognitive functions of school children of differing nutritional status. Am J Clin Nutr. 1989;49:646.
12. Louwman MWJ, et al. Signs of impaired cognitive function in adolescents with marginal cobalamin status. Am J Clin Nutr. 2000;72:762.
13. Benton D. Vitamin-mineral supplements and intelligence. Proc Nutr Soc. 1992;51:295.
14. Tong S, et al. Environmental lead exposure: A public health problem of global dimensions. Bull World Health Organization. 2000;78:1068.
15. Sargent JD, et al. Randomized trial of calcium glycerophosphate-supplemented infant formula to prevent lead absorption. Am J Clin Nutr. 1999;69:122.
16. Baghurst PA, et al. Environmental exposure to lead

and children's intelligence at age of seven years. N Engl J Med. 1992;327:1279.

17. Schaffer SJ, et al. The new CDC and AAP lead poisoning prevention recommendations. Ped Annals. 1994;23:592.

18. Teegarden D, Weaver CM. Calcium supplementation increases bone density in adolescent girls. Nutr Rev. 1994;52:171.

19. King J. Does poor zinc nutriture retard skeletal growth and mineralization in adolescents? Am J Clin Nutr. 1996;64:375.

20. Caulfield LE, et al. Nutritional supplementation during early childhood and bone mineralization during adolescence. J Nutr. 1995;125:1104S.

Aging and Longevity

The average human life span in the industrialized countries has increased from 40–45 years to nearly 75 years over the past century.[1] This is due to improved living standards, including better nutrition, medical care, and sanitation. The maximum human life span is thought to be 120 years. Although our genetic potential should allow most people to live to 100 and beyond, few survive to 100 and not many make it to 90. Moreover, living longer does not necessarily mean living better. Degenerative disease – arthritis, heart disease, osteoporosis, cataracts – plague the elderly. There is little sense in striving to extend maximum life span until ways can be found to live out our present-day life span in reasonably good health, with physical and mental vitality. A goal of preventive nutrition is to find ways to compress illness and the degenerative process of aging into a short period preceding death. Rather than dreaming about living to 200, the aim should be to live past 100 and do so in generally good health up until the end. That is the goal of the guidelines in this section.

Aging

Aging is a gradual decline in the function of body organs and systems that, in general, follows a predictable path. However, the speed, timing, and chronology of aging varies dramatically between individuals. For example, as most people age the heart beats less efficiently and the functional capacity of the cardiovascular system declines. But some 70 and 80 year-olds maintain healthier cardiovascu-

lar systems than many 30 year-olds. This implies that a declining heart is not an inevitable, programmed sign of aging.

Similarly, scientists have traditionally believed that relentless and irreversible changes occur in the brain as we age, including loss of neurons, atrophy, and gradual functional decline. However, these changes are not as inevitable as previously believed. Many healthy older people (even in their late 90s) maintain memory and reasoning capabilities equivalent to much younger individuals, and their cerebral blood flow and oxygen uptake is similar to that of individuals 50 years younger. So much of what has been traditionally attributed to aging may actually be due to accumulated insults and stresses – in the form of poor nutrition, smoking, and a sedentary lifestyle. Many of the changes of aging are more the result of how one lives than how long one lives. A lifetime of poor nutritional choices can have a major impact on health and aging. Proper nutrition can delay or slow down the aging process and help one reach a maximum life span.

Nutrition, Lifestyle, and Longevity

Gerontologists now view the declines in physiologic function associated with advancing age as a combination of genetically programmed change accelerated by damage from free-radical reactions, disuse, and degenerative disease.[2]

Free Radicals and Antioxidants

Over the past two decades, a persuasive theory of why cells gradually lose function has evolved – the free radical theory of aging. A free radical is a highly reactive molecule whose structure contains an unpaired, unstable electron. Free radicals in the body react with and oxidize nearby molecules and damage cell membranes, fatty acids, proteins, and DNA. Many free radicals are toxic derivatives of oxygen, produced by cell metabolism (as byproducts of energy-producing reactions) or environmental toxins (chemicals, radiation). To help protect themselves against free radicals, our cells evolved a complex array of free-radical defenses, or "antioxidants." These antioxidants can neutralize free radicals and protect the cell. (For a detailed discussion of free radicals and antioxidants, see pp. 115).

These mechanisms are not perfect, however. Low-level free-radical damage does occur in cells, gradually reducing cell function and the ability of the cell to divide and replace itself. Free radical reactions produce a steady accumulation of breakdown products. A visible example are the brown "age spots" found on older skin. They are breakdown products of fats resulting from prolonged exposure to sunlight and other environmental factors.

Within the nuclei of cells, free-radical damage causes small errors to accumulate in genetic code of DNA. Eventually, the DNA can no longer serve as a template for synthesis of vital proteins needed for metabolism. This impairment of cell function leads to degenerative disease and premature aging.[3]

What is particularly intriguing about the free radical theory is that it suggests a practical means of modifying the effects of aging. Boosting levels of natural antioxidant compounds in cells – using micronutrient supplementation together with an optimum diet – may help protect cells from the damage of free radicals.[4,5] The major antioxidant nutrients are the carotenoids, the vitamins C and E, the minerals zinc, manganese, and selenium, the amino acid cysteine, and coenzyme Q10 (see pp. 116).

Exercise

Regular exercise can prolong life. People who expend at least 2000 kcal/week exercising during adulthood (equal to about 30 mins of jogging per day) live longer than those who are sedentary.[6] Mortality rates from most chronic diseases in the sixth, seventh, and eighth decades are roughly a third lower in men who exercise regularly. Regular physical activity also maximizes function during later life. Exercise can improve balance and mobility and maintain cardiovascular function. Exercise burns calories for energy, increases appetite, and allows older adults to eat more without becoming overweight. Exercise is also of significant benefit in many diseases common among the elderly, such as hypertension, heart disease, and diabetes.

The Major Degenerative Diseases

Good health late in life depends largely on avoiding the major degenerative diseases associated with getting old. These common disorders greatly accelerate the aging process – preventing these conditions would allow many to live a healthy life well past the age of 100. (A detailed discussion of the nutritional prevention and treatment of each of these important disorders can be found in later sections.

● **Cancer.** The chances of getting cancer double every 10 years after the age of 50. The accumulated effects of poor nutrition and exposure to cancer-causing substances in the environment weaken the immune system and impair DNA repair mechanisms – making cancer more likely in later years. It is estimated that about 30–50% of all cancers are due to dietary factors.[7] Proper eating habits, antioxidant supplementation, and a healthy lifestyle can dramatically reduce risk of cancer.

● **Cardiovascular disease.** The risk of heart attack and stroke rises steadily with age and become much more common after age 60. The major contributing factors – nutritional deficiencies, too much dietary fat and alcohol, smoking, lack of exercise – can all be avoided.

● **Type 2 diabetes.** After age 40, the chances of developing diabetes double every 10 years. Most cases occur in individuals who are overweight, do not exercise regularly, and eat too much fat. Proper nutrition, exercise, and maintaining a normal weight can cut the risk substantially.

● **Obesity.** Obesity increases the risk of many of the chronic diseases that affect older adults. Overweight adults are three times more likely than normal-weight people to be hypertensive. Overweight people are more often hyperlipidemic and have more heart attacks and strokes at younger ages, compared with normal-weight people. Obese people have three to four times the risk of developing type 2 diabetes and osteoarthritis.[8]

● **Immune weakness.** Susceptibility to infections and cancer steadily increases with age. The immune system is dependent on many micronutrients, particularly zinc, selenium, vitamin E, and the B vitamins. Optimizing body levels of these nutrients can help maintain immune function into older age.[9]

● **Dementia.** Many older people are disabled by a gradual loss of brain functions, a condition referred to as dementia. About 5% of people over the age of 65 have dementia and the incidence increases sharply with age – over 30% of those older than 85 are affected. Dietary factors, including nutritional deficiencies and overconsumption of fats and alcohol – contribute to one-third to half of all cases.[10]

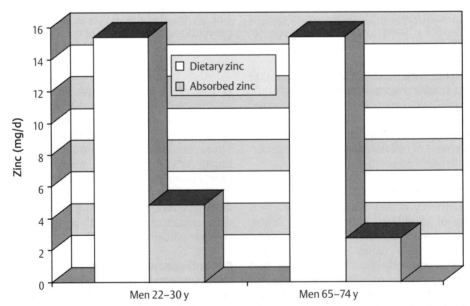

Fig. 4.**17**: **Reduced zinc absorption in older adults.** A study of the effect of aging on zinc metabolism showed a significant difference in zinc absorption between younger and older men. While younger men absorbed 31% of the zinc from the test meal, older men absorbed only 17%.
(Adapted from Turnlund JR, et al. J Nutr. 1986; 116:1239)

Physical Changes of Aging and Their Impact on Nutritional Health

Digestive System

Thinning and gradual loss of function of the secretory mucosa of the stomach (termed atrophic gastritis) affects one of four adults in their 60s and nearly 40% of those over 80 years. This common condition sharply increases risk of micronutrient deficiency. As secretion of gastric acid falls, the absorption of iron, calcium, and the vitamins B6, B12, and folate is reduced.[11] Decreased secretion of intrinsic factor, the protein required for vitamin B12 absorption, further decreases absorption of vitamin B12. As a result, deficiencies of vitamin B12 are common among the elderly. Mild deficiency causes fatigue, weakness, and impaired concentration. If severe, vitamin B12 deficiency leads to anemia, neurologic damage, and dementia[12]. Vitamin B12 supplementation (if necessary, by intramuscular injection) may benefit older people with these symptoms.

Liver function also declines in older adults, decreasing clearance of many drugs and increasing the potential for adverse drug-nutrient interactions (see appendix I). Constipation is a common complaint in older adults. Immobility, dehydration, and foods low in fiber contribute to this problem. Increasing physical activity, consuming more dietary fiber – eating whole-grain products, legumes, fruits, and vegetables – and drinking from six to eight glasses of water per day is beneficial. Additional vitamin C (0.5 g–1.0 g) per day may also help soften and ease passage of the stool.

Skeleton

Risk of developing osteoporosis increases steadily with age. More than half of all women and about one-third of all men will experience osteoporotic fractures during their lives, almost all occuring after age 55.[13] Often the first sign of the disease is a fracture of the spine or the hip from a minor fall. Vitamin D deficiency is found in 20–25% of older people and increases risk of osteoporosis.[14] Over 50% of older adults consume inadequate vitamin D. With age, the kidney is less able to convert dietary vitamin D to the active form, 1,25 (OH) vitamin D.[15] The aging intestine is also less responsive to the signal from vitamin D to increase absorption of calcium. In younger people, significant amounts of vitamin D can be synthesized in sun-exposed skin, but aging skin is less able to synthesize the vitamin. Compounding this, many older adults, particularly those with disabilities, obtain little sunlight exposure. In older adults, particularly during the winter months in northern climates, vitamin D supplementation helps maintain bone density and prevent fractures.[16]

Calcium intakes of many older women and men are substantially below optimum levels. The average calcium intake of men and women above age 65 in Western Europe is only 700 and 550 mg/day, respectively. Calcium intake in this age group should be at least 1200 mg/day, and older women at high risk for osteoporosis need even higher amounts – up to 1500 mg/day. Compounding the problem of low intake, intestinal calcium absorption decreases with age. While younger adults respond to low calcium diets by increasing the efficiency of calcium absorption, older people are less able to adapt to low calcium diets by increasing absorption.[17] Older people who take daily supplements of vitamin D (10–15 µg) and calcium (1–2 g) lose less bone and have fewer osteoporotic fractures.[16] Other minerals and trace elements also play a role in osteoporosis (see pp. 192).

Immune System

Immune strength often diminishes with age. Production of antibodies falls, B and T cells react weakly to antigens, and phagocytes destroy bacteria less efficiently. These changes make many older people more vulnerable to infection. However, not all older adults show these changes – some have immune systems that function as well as those of younger adults. Differences in diet and micronutrient status are critical determinants of immune competence in old age. Nutrients often lack-

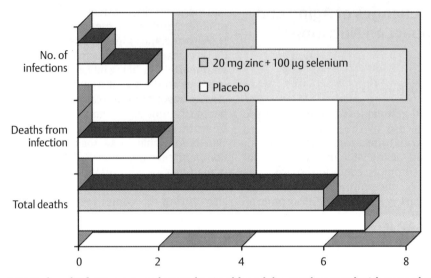

Fig. 4.**18**: **Reduced infection rate and mortality in older adults supplemented with trace elements.** In 81 older people (mean age 84 ± 8 years), a supplement containing 20 mg zinc and 100 µg selenium given daily for 2 years reduced mortality from infections and significantly reduced the mean number of infections. Compared with the placebo group, the trace-element group had two to four times fewer infections during the study. (Adapted from Girodon F, et al. Ann Nutr Metab. 1997;41:98)

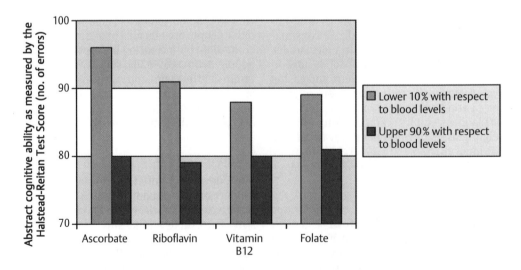

Fig. 4.**19**: **"Subclinical" malnutrition and impairment of cognitive function in older adults.** In 260 free-living, ambulatory people (aged 60–94 years), low blood levels of vitamin C, vitamin B12, riboflavin, and folate were associated with significant reductions in cognitive ability. Values are means (SE). (Adapted from Goodwin JS, et al. JAMA. 1983; 249:2917)

Micronutrient supplements for older adults	
Nutrient	Recommended daily intake
Compensating for reduced nutrient absorption:	
Vitamin D	10 µg
Vitamin B6	20–25 mg
Vitamin B12	5 µg (may need injectable form if malabsorption is severe)
Folic acid	0.4–0.8 mg
Calcium	1–2 g
Magnesium	500 mg
Zinc	10–20 mg
Antioxidant protection:	
Vitamin C	1 g
Vitamin E	200–400 mg
Beta-carotene	15 mg
L-Cysteine	500–1500 mg
Coenzyme Q10	100 mg
Selenium	200 µg
Zinc	20 mg
Manganese	10 mg
Immune-system support:	
Vitamin B6	10–25 mg
Vitamin E	200–400 mg
Vitamin C	0.5–1 g
Zinc	10–15 mg
Selenium	50–100 µg
plus a balanced vitamin/ mineral supplement	
Maintaining bone health:	
Vitamin D	10 µg
Calcium	1–2 g
Magnesium	400–600 mg
plus a balanced multi- mineral supplement	

were not deficient in any micronutrients at the beginning of the study. Supplementation with individual micronutrients can also benefit older adults. In healthy older adults, additional zinc, vitamin B6, or vitamin E improves immune function.[18,19] Older adults absorb vitamin B6 less efficiently, and inadequate reserves of vitamin B6 contribute to decreased immune function in older people.

Brain and Mental Function

Many older adults suffer a gradual loss of brain functions, and memory and concentration often diminish with age. About one-third of people above age 80 have significant mental impairment. However, many healthy older people (including some in their late 90s) maintain mental powers equal to younger individuals. "Exercising" the brain by reading, playing games, crossword puzzles, and lively conversation can help preserve mental ability as we age. In addition, optimum nutrition plays an important role. Brain function, memory, and alertness are significantly better in older adults who have sufficient body reserves of thiamin, riboflavin, and iron, compared with those with marginal status.[20] Subclinical deficiencies of vitamin B12 and folate can cause fatigue, weakness, impaired concentration, and depression, even in the absence of anemia (see Fig. 4.**19**).[12] Supplemental niacin and vitamins E and C may help maintain blood flow through the small blood vessels in the brain.

Drugs and Nutritional Health

Older adults (above age 65) consume one-quarter to one-third of all medicinal drugs. Most common prescription and over-the-counter drugs have significant nutrient interactions, and the elderly are particularly vulnerable to their side effects.[21] For example, thousands of older people are hospitalized each year in the USA and Western Europe because of diuretic depletion of potassium and magnesium stores. The liver and kidneys of older people metabolize and excrete drugs slower than younger adults. Many elderly people have marginal underlying nutritional

ing in older people's diets –zinc and vitamins C, E, and B6 – are vital to proper functioning of the immune system (see Fig. 4.**18**).[18]

In a recent study, 100 healthy older adults were divided into two groups: one group was given a multivitamin/mineral supplement, the other group received a placebo. After 1 year the supplemented group had better immune function and fewer infections than the placebo group.[19] Many of the participants had micronutrient deficiencies that were corrected by the supplement, but improvements occurred even in supplemented people who

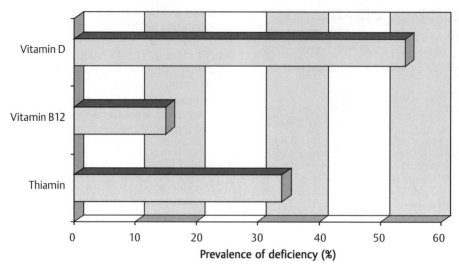

Fig. 4.**20**: **Vitamin deficiencies among older adults.** Three recent large surveys of free-living, ambulatory elderly people in the USA have documented widespread deficiencies of vitamin D, vitamin B12, and thiamin. (Sources: Gloth FM, et al. JAMA. 1995;274:1683. Lindenbaum J, et al. Am J Clin Nutr. 1994;60:2. Wilkinson TJ, et al. Am J Clin Nutr. 1997;66:925)

status, and so are more susceptible to drug-nutrient interactions (see appendix I). The micronutrient status of older adults taking multiple medications should be periodically reassessed.

Micronutrient Supplementation for Older Adults

Micronutrient supplementation is particularly beneficial in older age groups because many older people eat less and are less able to absorb micronutrients from foods.[22] Moreover, in older adults even mild micronutrient deficiencies can weaken the immune system and impair memory and concentration. Together with eating a well-balanced diet, maintaining a lean body shape, and keeping physically active, micronutrient supplementation can be a powerful tool to maintain function in later years.

References

1. Kinsella K. Changes in life expectancy 1900–1990. Am J Clin Nutr. 1992;55:S1196.
2. Miller RA. The biology of aging and longevity. In: Hazard WR, ed. Principles of Geriatric Medicine and Gerontology. New York: McGraw-Hill; 1994.
3. Ames BN, Shigenaga MK, Hagan TM. Oxidants, antioxidants and the degenerative diseases of aging. Proc Natl Acad Sci. 1993;90:7915.
4. Monget AL, et al. Effect of 6 month supplementation with different combinations of an association of antioxidant nutrients on biochemical parameters and markers of the antioxidant defence system in the elderly. Eur J Clin Nutr. 1996;50:443.
5. Stähelin HB. The impact of antioxidants on chronic disease in aging and in old age. Int J Vit Nutr Res. 1999;69:146.
6. Paffenbarger RE, et al. Physical activity, all-cause mortality and longevity of college alumni. N Engl J Med. 1985;314:605.
7. Doll R. The lessons of life. Keynote address to the nutrition and cancer conference. Cancer Res. 1992;52:S2024.
8. Pi-Sunyer PX. Health implications of obesity. Am J Clin Nutr. 1991;53:1595S-603S.
9. Bell RA, et al. Alterations of immune defense mechanisms in the elderly: The role of nutrition. Infect Med. 1997;14:415.

10. Gray GE: Nutrition and dementia. J Am Diet Assoc. 1989;89:1795.

11. Russell RM. Changes in the gastrointestinal tract attributed to aging. Am J Clin Nutr. 1992;55:S1203.

12. Lindenbaum J, Healton EB, Savage DG, et al. Neuropsychiatric disorders caused by cobalamin deficiency in the absence of anemia or macrocytosis. N Engl J Med. 1988;318:1720.

13. Ross PD. Osteoporosis: Frequency, consequences and risk factors. Arch Intern Med. 1996;156:1399.

14. Russell RM, Suter PM. Vitamin requirements of elderly people: An update. Am J Clin Nutr. 1993;58:4.

15. Gloth FM, et al. Vitamin D deficiency in homebound elderly persons. JAMA. 1995;274:1683.

16. Dawson-Hughes B, et al. Effect of calcium and vitamin D supplementation on bone density in men and women 65 years of age or older. N Engl J Med. 1997;337:670.

17. Wood RJ, et al. Mineral requirements of elderly people. Am J Clin Nutr. 1995;62:493.

18. Chandra RK. Nutrition and immunity in the elderly. Nutr Rev. 1992;50:367.

19. Chandra RK. Effect of vitamin and trace-element supplementation on immune responses and infections in elderly subjects. Lancet. 1992;340:1124.

20. Goodwin JS, et al. Association between nutritional status and cognitive function in a healthy elderly population. JAMA. 1983;249:2917.

21. Schümann K. Interactions between drugs and vitamins at advanced age. Int J Vit Nutr Res. 1999;69:173.

22. Tucker K. Micronutrient status and aging. Nutr Rev. 1995;53:S9.

5 Micronutrients as Prevention and Therapy

Skin Care

Introduction: Healthy Skin

The skin is the largest organ of the body. It is a dense web of nerves, blood vessels, and glands: a section the size of a postage stamp contains nearly a meter of blood vessels, 3 meters of nerves, and over 100 sweat and oil-secreting glands. Healthy, intact skin is an extremely effective barrier against harmful bacteria, viruses, and chemicals. It also synthesizes vitamin D and helps regulate body temperature. Therefore, caring for skin is much more than just a cosmetic concern. Skin cells are among the most rapidly dividing cells in our bodies. Older cells are constantly shed and replaced by younger ones produced deeper in the skin, and a steady supply of micronutrients is essential to support this rapid growth. For this reason the skin is particularly susceptible to nutritional imbalances or deficiencies.[1]

Skin, hair, and nails are built mainly of protein. Several micronutrients that are important for synthesis of body protein, including zinc and vitamins C and B6, are important for skin health. Folic acid and vitamins A and B12 are needed in high amounts to support rapid cell turnover in skin.

The skin's moisture and integrity depend on a constant synthesis and secretion of oils – keeping the skin smooth and intact and preventing excess water loss by evaporation. Because these natural skin oils are synthesized by means of precursors provided by the diet, the form and quality of dietary fatty acids strongly influences skin health.[2] Generous intake of the essential polyunsaturated fatty acids (linoleic and linolenic acid) in vegetables, nuts and seeds, and fish are important.

Metabolites of linoleic and linolenic acid are central components of our natural skin oils.[2]

Particularly important is gamma-linoleic acid (GLA), a fatty acid that can be synthesized in small amounts from dietary linoleic acid. GLA is also found in high amounts in a few plant oils, including borage oil and evening primrose oil. Without adequate GLA and its products, skin will dry out, wrinkle, and age prematurely. Because the skin cannot easily synthesize adequate GLA during times of increased need – exposure to cold, dry air, allergens, aging, eczema, stress – supplementation with evening primrose oil rich in GLA can be beneficial.[3] To protect and maintain the natural skin oils, ample vitamin E and beta-carotene are essential. (For a more detailed discussion of these important polyunsaturated fats, including GLA, see pp. 89).

Dry Skin

Skin needs moisture to stay flexible. If too much water is lost through evaporation, skin becomes stiff, dry, and brittle. The most important skin moisturizers are the natural skin oils – they hold water in the skin and maintain a barrier that prevents excess water loss and keeps skin moist.

Diet · Dry Skin

Eating too much saturated fat (from meat, milk, and eggs) and too little polyunsaturated fat (in plants, fish, nuts, and seeds) creates an imbalance that interferes with the synthesis of skin oils (see pp. 89). To maintain skin moisture, high-quality, cold-pressed plant oils (sesame, corn, sunflower, or safflower oil) and fish should be a regular part of the diet. The diet should also emphasize foods rich in vitamins A, E, C and zinc.

Micronutrients · Dry Skin

Nutrient	Suggested daily dose	Comments
Vitamin E	100 mg	Protects skin oils from oxidative damage
Vitamin A	1000 µg	Supports cell turnover and healthy skin growth
GLA	As 1–2 g evening primrose oil	Helps maintain skin's natural moisture barrier

Aging Skin: Wrinkles and Age Spots

With age the skin becomes thinner, drier, and loses its elasticity. This is particularly evident on the face and hands where wrinkles, loss of tone, and pigmented age spots appear. These changes are mainly the result of gradual, accumulated damage from sun overexposure, strong soaps, chemicals in the air and water, and poor nutrition.

Diet · Aging Skin

The degenerative changes in skin due to overexposure to sun and wind are caused mainly by free radical oxidation and damage (see discussion of antioxidants and free radicals on pp. 115). For example, age spots on the skin are accumulations of oxidized, pigmented lipids. Generous intake of the antioxidant nutrients – particularly vitamin C, beta-carotene, and vitamin E, and the minerals zinc and selenium – can help maintain antioxidant defenses and protect skin from sun damage.[4,5] To support the constant renewal of skin cells and to maintain elasticity and tone, foods rich in protein, zinc, and vitamins C and B6 should be eaten regularly. Consumption of two to three tablespoons of high-quality, plant-derived oils each day supports skin production of the natural skin oils. Vitamin A plays a central role in regulating division and growth of skin cells, and optimum intake of vitamin A (or its precursor beta-carotene) is important for skin health.

Micronutrients · Aging Skin

Nutrient	Suggested daily dose	Comments
Antioxidant formula (containing beta-carotene, vitamins C and E, zinc and selenium, cysteine)	See pp. 115 for discussion of recommended antioxidant doses	Protects skin from oxidative damage that can cause wrinkling and age spots[4,5]
Vitamin A[6]	1200 µg	Can be taken in the form of beta-carotene
Vitamin B complex (balanced and complete)	Should contain at least 10 mg of vitamins B1, B2, and B6	Important for normal skin cell development and healthy skin tone
GLA	As 1–2 g evening primrose oil	Maintains natural skin oils

Acne

Acne is caused by inflammation and infection of the sebaceous glands of the skin. More than three-quarters of adolescents and young adults have chronic acne. In severe cases, acne can cause scarring of the skin. Acne is common among young adults because sebum production in the sebaceous glands is stimulated by the hormonal changes of puberty and adolescence. Heredity, hormones (particularly androgens), oral contraceptives, contact and food allergies, excessively oily skin, stress, and dietary factors can all play a role in triggering acne.

Diet · Acne

Excess consumption of saturated fats (fatty meat, whole milk, and chocolate) and hydrogenated fats (margarines and processed foods) can aggravate acne by increasing sebum production. Foods high in refined carbohydrates (particularly sucrose) and low in fiber can also stimulate sebum production. Food sensitivities (especially to nuts and colas) can trigger acne in susceptible individuals. Acne can be caused by preparations containing iodine, such as kelp products and certain medicines.

To help reduce the frequency and severity of acne	
Reduce or eliminate:	**Eat more of:**
• Foods high in saturated fat: fatty meats, whole milk, cheese, butter, chocolate	Raw vegetables and whole-grain products
• Foods high in hydrogenated fat: margarine, processed baked products (pastries, cookies)	Fresh fruit and fruit juice
• Salty, fatty foods: potato chips, french fries	Fresh fish and other seafood
• Nuts, particularly salted almonds and peanuts	
• White flour and sugar, cola drinks	

Psoriasis

Psoriasis appears as red skin patches with silvery scales, most commonly on the elbows and knees. In severe cases it also affects the ears, scalp, and back. The patches are caused by rapid growth and proliferation of cells in the outer skin layers. Psoriasis is a chronic condition that waxes and wanes. Exacerbations can be triggered by many factors, including stress, illness, surgery, skin damage from abrasions or cuts, poison ivy, sunburn, food sensitivities, and certain drugs such as beta-blockers and lithium.

Diet · Psoriasis

In psoriasis, metabolism of essential fatty acids (EFAs) in the skin is abnormal. Production of EPA and DHA, the omega-3 fatty acids derived from dietary linolenic acid (see pp. 89) is impaired (see Fig. 5.1).[12] Skin synthesis of GLA from linoleic acid is also abnormal. To provide ample polyunsaturated fatty acids, regular consumption of high-quality, cold-pressed nut and seed oils is important. The diet should also be low in saturated fat and hydrogenated fat.[13] Vegetarian diets can sometimes dramatically improve psoriasis. They tend to be low in protein, which can aggravate the condition, and high in EFAs. Food sensitivities should be determined as they may promote psoriasis – in some cases careful food-elimination diets can lead to dramatic improvement of the condition (see pp. 205). Alcohol consumption can aggravate psoriasis in certain individuals.

Micronutrients · Acne

Nutrient	Suggested daily dose	Comments
Vitamin A	2000–10,000 µg	Can be effective in reducing severity and inflammation. High doses of vitamin A should only be taken with the advice of a physician
Vitamin E plus selenium	200–400 mg vitamin E, 200 µg selenium	Especially effective in treating pustules (whiteheads)[7]
Zinc	50–80 mg	Reduces inflammation and severity of acne[8–10]
GLA	As 1–2 g evening primrose oil	Reduces inflammation in the sebaceous glands. Take with 100 mg vitamin E
Vitamin B complex	Complete formula containing 25–50 mg pantothenic acid[11] and 50 mg vitamin B6	May be effective for premenstrual acne flare-ups. Take for 1 week prior to and during menstrual periods

Micronutrients · Psoriasis

Nutrient	Suggested daily dose	Comments
Omega-3 fatty acids	As fish-oil capsules, 1.0–1.5 g EPA plus DHA	Can reduce proliferation and inflammation.[12] Skin salves containing EPA can also be applied to patches. Take with at least 100 mg vitamin E
GLA	As 1–4 g evening primrose oil	Can reduce skin cell proliferation and inflammation. Take with at least 100 mg vitamin E
Selenium plus zinc	200 µg selenium, 50 mg zinc	Psoriasis is often linked with low blood levels of selenium. Zinc and selenium supplements can reduce skin inflammation, itching, and redness. These nutrients can also be effective when used topically as selenium-sulfide or zinc-oxide salves.
Vitamins A and D[14–16]	8000 µg vitamin A plus 20 µg vitamin D	Vitamins A and D play a central role in regulation and control of skin cell growth, and supplementation can help clear psoriasis. Calcitriol, the active form of vitamin D3, is effective in both oral and topical treatments. Skin salves containing vitamins A and D can be applied directly to psoriatic plaques. High doses of vitamin A should only be taken with the advice of a physician

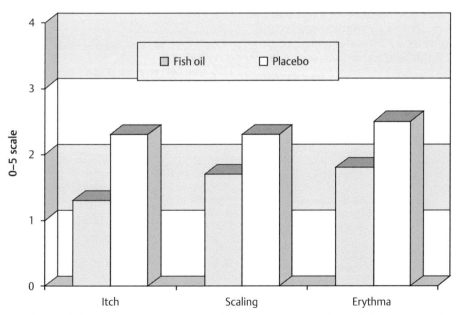

Fig. 5.**1**: **Omega-3 fatty acids and psoriasis.** 28 subjects with stable chronic psoriasis were given 1.8 g omega-3 fatty acids or placebo for 12 weeks. In the treatment group, itching, scaling, and erythema were all significantly reduced at 8 and 12 weeks compared with placebo. The percentage of surface area affected was also decreased by treatment with omega-3 fats (7% vs. 12%, treatment vs. control) (Adapted from Bittiner SB, et al. Lancet. 1988;1:378)

Eczema

Eczema is a dermatitis that usually begins as patchy redness. If untreated, small breaks develop in the skin patches and can progress to scaling, thickening, and cracking. It most often occurs on the hands, but can appear anywhere on the skin. Although there are many triggers of eczema, one of the most common causes is food sensitivity. Eczema can also be caused by exposure to environmental agents such as chemicals, soaps, and detergents. Metal compounds in earrings, watches, or other jewelry (particularly metal alloys containing nickel) can trigger eczema.

Diet · Eczema

A careful elimination diet (see pp. 205) can identify food sensitivities that trigger eczema.[17] The most common offending foods are milk, eggs, fish, cheese, nuts, and food additives. Cold-pressed nut and seed oils are high in beneficial EFAs important for skin health and should be consumed regularly. Disturbances in fatty acid metabolism in the skin can produce or aggravate eczema; impaired production of omega-3 fatty acids and GLA can increase inflammation in the skin (see pp. 89).[18]

Micronutrients · Eczema

Nutrient	Suggested daily dose	Comments
GLA[19]	As 1–2 g evening primrose oil	Can reduce inflammation and accelerate healing. Take with at least 100 mg vitamin E
Omega-3 fatty acids[18,20]	1.0–1.5 g EPA from fish-oil capsules	Skin salves containing EPA can also be applied to patches; take with at least 100 mg vitamin E
Zinc[21]	50 mg	Zinc-containing ointments can also be beneficial
Vitamin E[22]	100–200 mg	Can help regulate skin proliferation and reduce symptoms

References

1. Sherertz EF, Goldsmith LA. Nutritional influences on the skin. In: Goldsmith LA, ed. Physiology, Biochemistry and Molecular Biology of the Skin. Oxford: Oxford University Press; 1991.
2. Ziboh VA. The significance of polyunsaturated fatty acids in cutaneous biology. Lipids. 1996;31:S249.
3. Oliwiecki S, Burton JL. Evening primrose oil and marine oil in the treatment of psoriasis. Clin Exp Dermatol. 1994;19:127.
4. Biesalski HK, et al. The effect of supplementation with beta carotene on sun damaged skin. Ernähr Umschau. 1994;41:91.
5. Stahl W, et al. Carotenoids and carotenoids plus vitamin E protect against ultraviolet light-induced erythema in humans. Am J Clin Nutr. 2000;71:795.
6. Saurat JH. Retinoids and ageing. Horm Res. 1995;43:89.
7. Michaelsson G, Edqvist LE. Erythrocyte glutathione peroxidase activity in acne vulgaris, the effects of selenium and vitamim E treatment. Acta Derm Venereol. 1984;64:9.
8. Verm KC, et al. Oral zinc sulfate therapy in acne vulgaris: A double-blind trial. Acta Dermatovener. 1980;60:337.
9. Pohit J, et al. Zinc status of acne vulgaris patients. J Appl Nutr. 1985;37:18.
10. Dreno B, et al. Low doses of zinc gluconate for inflammatory acne. Acta Derm Venereol Stockh. 1989;69:541.
11. Leung LH. Pantothenic acid deficiency as the pathogenesis of acne vulgaris. Med Hypotheses. 1995;44:490.
12. Bittiner SB, et al. A double-blind, randomised, placebo-controlled trial of fish oil in psoriasis. Lancet. 1988;1:378.
13. Naldi L. Dietary factors and the risk of psoriasis. Br J Dermatol. 1996;134:101.
14. Lowe KE. Vitamin D and psoriasis. Nutr Rev. 1992;50:138.
15. Stewart DG; Lewis HM. Vitamin D analogues and psoriasis. J Clin Pharm Ther. 1996;21:143.
16. Majewski S, et al. Decreased levels of vitamin A in serum of patients with psoriasis. Arch Dermatol Res. 1989;280:499.
17. Mabin DC, et al. Nutritional content of few foods diet in atopic dermatitis. Arch Dis Child. 1995;73:208.
18. Bjorneboe A, et al. Effect of dietary supplementation with eicosapentaeonoic acid in the treatment of atopic dermatitis. Br J Dermatol. 1987;117:463.
19. Horrobin DF, Morse PF. Evening primrose oil and atopic eczema. Lancet. 1995;345:260.
20. Soyland E, et al. Dietary supplementation with very long-chain n-3 fatty acids in patients with atopic dermatitis. A double-blind, multicentre study. Br J Dermatol. 1994;130:757.

21. Endre L, et al. Incidence of food allergy and zinc deficiency in children treated for atopic dermatitis. Orv Hetail. 1989;130:2465.

22. Olson PE, et al. Oral vitamin E for refractory hand dermatitis. Lancet. 1994;343:672.

Eye and Ear Care

Healthy Eyes

Diet · Healthy Eyes

To maintain good eyesight foods rich in vitamins A, C, E, riboflavin, selenium, and zinc should be consumed. All these nutrients are important for vision and are supplied by a balanced diet with generous amounts of fruits and vegetables, such as carrots, cantaloupe, oranges, and broccoli. Generous intake of antioxidant nutrients (see pp. 115) over a lifetime may help prevent cataract, the most common cause of impaired vision in older adults.[1] Age-related macular degeneration (AMD) is a common cause of vision impairment in older people, and the risk of AMD can be reduced by a diet high in antioxidants, carotenoids, and zinc.[2,3] Nutrient supplementation may help correct minor eye troubles such as dry, burning, itchy eyes and eyestrain.

Micronutrients · Healthy Eyes

Nutrient	Suggested daily dose	Comments
Vitamin A	1000 µg	Maintains health and function of the retina and cornea[4]
Vitamin C	500 mg	Maintains clarity of the lens[1] and health of the retina[2,3]
Zinc	20 mg	Together with vitamin A, zinc supports optimum function of the retina[3]

Conjunctivitis and Styes

Red, itchy, inflamed eyes (conjunctivitis) can be due to irritation of the conjunctiva by dry air, smoke, air pollution, contact-lens solutions, or eye make-up. Infection by viruses or bacteria can also produce conjunctivitis. A stye (a tender, raised red papule on the eyelid) is an infection within the oil glands in the eyelid.

Diet · Conjunctivitis

Foods such as carrots, cantaloupe, liver, oranges, strawberries, and broccoli, which are rich sources of vitamins A and C, should be consumed. Additionally, hot, damp compresses on an eyelid with a stye can relieve discomfort and help a stye open and drain.

Micronutrients · Conjunctivitis

Nutrient	Suggested daily dose	Comments
Vitamin A	5000 µg	Supports healing of the conjunctiva. Itchy, red eyes can be an early sign of vitamin A deficiency[4]
Vitamin C	0.5 g-1.0 g	Enhances immune response to infection. Take until redness clears
Zinc	60 mg	Supports healing and enhances immune response. Take until redness clears

Cataracts

A cataract is a clouding and loss of transparency in the lens that intereferes with the ability to see clearly. Cataracts are very common – half of all people over 75 years are affected. Most cataracts develop slowly over many years. Once established, surgery is usually needed to remove the damaged lens. The risk of cataract can be strongly influenced by diet and nutrient intake.[1]

Diet · Cataracts

Most cataracts are caused by oxidative damage from lifetime exposure of the lens to light and radiation entering the eye. The antioxidant vitamins A, C, and E are a major defense against oxidative damage, and eating foods rich in these nutrients each day can reduce the risk of cataract (see Fig. 5.2).[1] Regular consumption of galactose, found in the milk sugar lactose, may cause cataracts in people with inherited defects in galactose metabolism. In cases of an inability to metabolize galactose, milk and dairy product consumption should be sharply restricted. Hyperlipidemia, diabetes, and obesity also increase the risk of cataract. All these conditions are modifiable by dietary changes and nutritional supplementation.

Micronutrients · Cataracts

Nutrient	Suggested daily dose	Comments
Vitamin C	1–2 g	May reduce further clouding of the lens[5]
Vitamin E[6]	100–400 mg	Plays a crucial role in maintaining clarity of the lens
For prevention of cataract:		
Antioxidant formula[1,5,6]	Generous amounts of vitamins A, C, and E, riboflavin and zinc (see pp. 115)	Long-term supplementation helps prevent cataract development

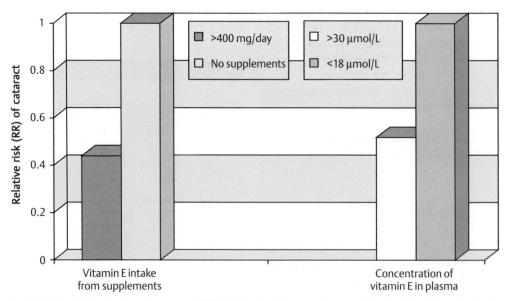

Fig. 5.**2**: **Vitamin E and cataracts.** Among 300 individuals taking supplemental vitamin E (> 400 mg/day), the prevalence of cataract was 56% lower than in those not consuming supplements. Another study found the prevalence of nuclear cataract in 671 adults to be 48% less among individuals with higher plasma concentrations of vitamin E.
(Adapted from Robertson JM, et al. Ann NY Acad Sci. 1989;570:372 and Vitale S, et al. Epidemiol. 1994, 4:195)

Glaucoma

In glaucoma, impaired fluid circulation in the eye produces high pressure in the posterior chamber that damages the optic nerve. Glaucoma is the second leading cause of blindness (after diabetes) in the developed countries of the world. Glaucoma usually develops slowly over months to years. The warning signs are halos appearing around lights, blurred vision, watering in the eyes, headache, and, when advanced, constriction of the visual field. Those with a family history of glaucoma, who are nearsighted, or who are taking antihypertensive drugs or steroids have a greater risk of glaucoma.

Diet · Glaucoma

Food sensitivities may increase intraocular pressure in people with glaucoma. Caffeine ingestion increases pressure in the eye, and people with glaucoma should avoid caffeine[7]. Excess dietary protein and trans-fatty acids (in hydrogenated fats) are associated with increased risk of glaucoma.

Micronutrients · Glaucoma

Nutrient	Suggested daily dose	Comments
Vitamin C with bioflavonoids[8]	1–2 g vitamin C with 200 mg rutin	Vitamin C, particularly together with rutin bioflavonoids may help reduce eye pressure in glaucoma
Thiamin	25 mg	Thiamin deficiency may contribute to development of glaucoma
Multimineral supplement	Should contain zinc (10–20 mg) and chromium (200 μg)	Reduced zinc and chromium intake is associated with higher eye pressure, and deficiencies may aggravate glaucoma

Middle Ear Infection (Otitis Media)

Infections of the middle ear are very common in childhood; up to 95% of children have had an ear infection by age 6. Persistent ear infections can damage the ear and cause hearing loss. During childhood growth, the developing structure of the ear increases susceptibility to infection. However, a weakened immune system caused by poor nutrition, and food and environmental allergies may sharply increase susceptibilty.

Diet · Otitis

In infants and children with frequent ear infections, food or environmental allergies should be investigated. Allergy to cow's milk can cause inflammation and swelling of the nasopharynx, which may increase risk of infection. Eliminating the offending food can prevent reinfection. Optimum nutrition can support the immune system and reduce the chance of recurrent infections and the need for antibiotics.

Micronutrients · Otitis

(To reduce or prevent inner ear infections in children aged 1–6 years: older children and adults may need higher doses)

Nutrient	Suggested daily dose	Comments
Multivitamin supplement for children	Should contain 400 μg vitamin A[9], and 10 mg vitamin E	Maintains optimum functioning of the immune system
Vitamin C	250 mg	Supports the immune system and helps fight infection[10]

References

1. Seddon JM, et al. Dietary carotenoids, vitamins A,C, and E and advanced age-related macular degeneration. JAMA. 1994;272:1413.
2. Hung S, Seddon JM. The relationship between nutritional factors and age-related macular degeneration. In: Bendich A, Deckelbaum RJ, eds. Preventive Nutrition. Totowa, New Jersey: Humana; 1997:245–66.
3. Jacques PF, Taylor A. Antioxidant status and risk for cataract. In: Bendich A, Deckelbaum RJ, eds. Preventive Nutrition. Totowa, New Jersey: Humana; 1997:267–84.
4. Sommer A. Vitamin A: Its effect on childhood sight and life. Nutr Rev. 1994;52:60.
5. Jacques PF, et al. Long-term vitamin C supplement use and prevalence of early age-related lens opacities. Am J Clin Nutr. 1997;66:911–6.
6. Lyle BJ, et al. Serum carotenoids and tocopherols and incidence of age-related nuclear cataract. Am J Clin Nutr. 1999;69:272–7.
7. Higginbotham EJ, et al. The effect of caffeine on intraocular pressure in glaucoma patients. Ophthalmology. 1989;96:624.
8. Virno M, et al. Oral treatment of glaucoma with vitamin C. Eye Ear Nose Throat Month. 1967;46:1502.
9. Bates CJ. Vitamin A. Lancet. 1995;345:31.
10. Bendich A, Langseth L. The health effects of vitamin C supplementation: A review. J Am Coll Nutr. 1995;14:124.

Oral Health

Gingivitis and Periodontal Disease

The periodontal tissues consist of three components: the gums, the bone in which the teeth are set, and the periodontal ligament, a thin layer of connective tissue that attaches the roots of teeth to the bone. Gingivitis (redness and inflammation of the gums) is caused by a nearly invisible sticky film of bacteria and other debris along the gum line, called dental plaque. An early sign of gingivitis is easy bleeding when brushing or flossing the teeth. Dental plaque contains harmful bacteria that can damage both the teeth and periodontal tissues. Early gingivitis is reversible. But untreated it progresses over months to years to periodontal disease. Periodontal disease is marked by permanent damage to the underlying bone and tissue, causing swollen and receding gums, and, ultimately, loose, unstable teeth.

Diet · Gingivitis

A diet high in refined carbohydrates (especially sucrose) promotes periodontal disease.[1] Frequent consumption of sugar increases plaque build-up and risk of gingivitis. Sugars also promote periodontal disease by reducing the ability of the white blood cells in the gums to destroy the pathogenic plaque bacteria. Sucrose is particularly destructive in sticky form (like candy and baked goods) because it clings longer to the teeth. Regular intake of foods rich in vitamin C[2], high-quality protein, and zinc can help maintain the integrity of the periodontal tissues.

Micronutrients · Gingivitis

Nutrient	Suggested daily dose	Comments
Vitamin C	0.5–1.0 g (best if taken together with a bioflavonoid complex)	Vitamin C may help heal inflamed gums and reduce bleeding. It also helps maintain the immune system to fight periodontal infection[2–4]
Folic acid	500 µg–1 mg (can also be taken as a 0.1 % solution of folate mouthwash, rinsing with 1 tablespoon twice daily)	Can be an effective treatment for periodontal disease[5]; diseased gums may contain only low levels of folate
Vitamin D and calcium	5–10 µg vitamin D and 600 mg calcium	Can help maintain the bones surrounding and supporting the teeth[6,7]

Dental Caries

Although dental caries (tooth decay) is one of the most common childhood diseases, with proper nutrition and tooth care it is entirely preventable. Tooth decay occurs when bacteria on the teeth ferment sugar and other carbohydrates to produce acid, which dissolves the tooth enamel.[8] This leads to cavity formation and infection of the dental pulp.

Diet · Caries

Sucrose is extremely cariogenic, whereas lactose (milk sugar) and fructose are less likely to cause caries. Unlike sugars, fats and protein cannot be used by bacteria to produce acid. Moreover, fats can coat the teeth and form a protective layer, whereas proteins increase the buffering capacity of the saliva. Milk products or cheese rather than sugary foods at the end of meals can reduce acid formation and help prevent tooth decay.

Optimum nutrition during childhood can encourage formation of thick, acid-resistant enamel. The teeth gradually form and calcify from birth through the teen years, and a generous dietary supply of protein, calcium, fluoride, and vitamins C and D are important. Fluoride, incorporated into the enamel structure, sharply increases resistance of enamel to acid (see Fig. 5.**3**). Insufficient fluoride leaves teeth vulnerable to tooth decay. Low-level fluoride supplementation has great benefits; adding trace amounts of fluoride to the water or salt supply can reduce risk of caries in children by more than two-thirds.[9] However, too much can actually impair enamel formation and cause weakened, discolored teeth. In areas where water is fluoridated, supplementation with fluoride mouthwashes or tablets is unnecessary. However, in areas where the fluoride content of the water is very low or nonexistant, supplements are beneficial. The best time to give a fluoride supplement is at bedtime, after cleaning the teeth. [10]

Micronutrients · Caries

Nutrient	Suggested daily dose	Comments
Fluoride	0.25 mg as drops during infancy; then 0.5–1 mg during childhood and adult years (see pp. 87)	Only indicated if fluoride levels in drinking water are <0.7 ppm. Can substantially toughen enamel against acid attack[9,10]
Multivitamin supplement for children	Should contain 10 µg vitamin D and 20–50 mg vitamin C	Vitamin D and C are important for tooth formation

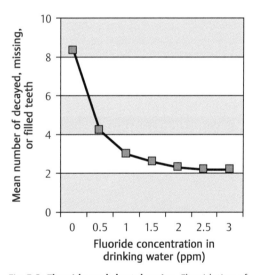

Fig. 5.**3**: **Fluoride and dental caries.** Fluoridation of the water supplyat the level of about 1–1.5 parts per million (ppm) sharply reduces prevalence of dental caries.
(Adapted from Rugg-Gunn AJ, Hackett AF. Nutrition and Dental Health. Oxford: Oxford University Press; 1993)

Canker Sores (Oral Aphthae)

Oral aphthae, commonly called canker sores, are small painful ulcers that occur on the oral mucosa. They can be triggered by multiple factors. Certain forms of streptococci can produce aphthae, particularly after minor trauma (from the toothbrush, accidentally biting the cheek) produces a break in the tissue.[11]

Diet · Aphthae

In certain individuals aphthae may be caused by food sensitivity.[12] An elimination diet can identify the offending foods (see pp. 205), which can then be avoided. Highly acidic foods – tomatoes, citrus fruits – can produce aphthae in susceptible individuals. Stress can also be a trigger. Because they compete with and reduce the number of oral streptococci, *Lactobacillus* in yogurt and other fermented milk products can reduce the frequency and severity of aphthae. People who have frequent aphthae may benefit from daily consumption of *Lactobacillus*-containing foods.

Micronutrients · Aphthae

Nutrient	Suggested daily dose	Comments
Zinc	30–60 mg	Can help prevent aphthae, particularly in individuals with marginal zinc status[13,14]
Vitamin B complex	Balanced supplement containing all the B vitamins; ample folic acid and vitamin B12 are particularly important	B vitamins promote health and strength of the oral mucosa[15]
Vitamin A	2000 µg	Helps maintain health and integrity of oral tissues

References

1. Sewon LA, Makinen KK. Dietary shifts may explain the incidence of periodontitis in industrialized countries. Med Hypotheses. 1996;46:269.
2. Fontana M. Vitamin C (ascorbic acid): Clinical implications for oral health–A literature review. Compendium. 1994;15:916.
3. Vogel RI, et al. The effects of megadoses of ascorbic acid on PMN chemotaxis and experimental gingivitis. J Periodontol. 1986;57:472.
4. Leggott PJ, et al. The effect of controlled ascorbic acid depletion and supplementation on periodontal health. J Periodontol. 1986;57:480.
5. Pack ARC. Folate mouthwash: Effects on established gingivitis in periodontal patients. J Clin Periodontol. 1984;11:619.
6. Whalen JP, Krook L Periodontal disease as the early manifestation of osteoporosis. Nutrition. 1996;12: 53–4.
7. Wical KE, Brussee P. Effects of a calcium and vitamin D supplement on alveolar ridge resorption in immediate denture patients. J Prosthet Dent. 1979;41:4.
8. Mandel ID. Caries prevention: Current strategies, new directions. J Am Dent Assoc. 1996;127:1477.
9. Richmond VL. Thirty years of fluoridation: A review. Am J Clin Nutr. 1985;41:129.
10. Horowitz HS. Commentary on and recommendations for the proper uses of fluoride. J Public Health. 1995;55:57.
11. Wray D. Aphthous stomatitis is linked to mechanical injuries, iron and vitamin deficiencies and certain HLA types. JAMA. 1982;247:774.
12. Wray D, Vlagopoulos TP, Siraganian RP. Food allergens and basophil histamine release in recurrent aphthous stomatitis, Oral Surg Oral Med Oral Pathol. 1982;54:388.
13. Endre L. Successful treatment of recurrent ulcerative stomatitis, associated with cellular immune defect and hypozincaemia, by oral administration of zinc sulfate. Orv Hetil. 1990;131:475.
14. Wang SW, et al. The trace element zinc and aphthosis. The determination of plasma zinc and the treatment of aphthosis with zinc. Rev Stomatol Chir Maxillofac. 1986;87:339.
15. Wray D, Ferguson MM, Mason DK, et al. Recurrent aphthae; Treatment with vitamin B12, folic acid and iron. BMJ. 1975;5:490.

Digestive Disorders

Constipation and Diverticulitis

Constipation is a disorder characterized by the need to strain to pass hard stools and decreased frequency of stools (two to three times a week). Chronic constipation can lead to diverticulosis, in which multiple small sacs of the colonic mucosa are pushed out through the muscular wall of the colon. Diverticulosis occurs because chronic straining to pass feces produces increased pressure inside the colon. Inflammation often develops within the small sacs (diverticula) producing diverticulitis, with abdominal pain and bleeding. Constipation and diverticulitis are so-called "diseases of civilization." They occur in near epidemic proportions in the industrialized countries, where one-fifth of the adult population suffers from chronic constipation and diverticulosis occurs in about one-third of people older than 65 years.

Diet · Constipation

The primary cause of both constipation and diverticulosis are highly refined and processed diets that are low in dietary fiber. Dietary fiber passes into the colon intact and absorbs water – increasing the bulk of the stool and softening it.[1] This stimulates peristalsis in the colon, pushing the stool forward more rapidly. Dietary fiber is found in large amounts in whole grains, corn, vegetables, fruits (dried prunes, apples, raisins, and figs), seeds, and legumes. Increasing intake of these foods will soften the stool, and often eliminate constipation. Supplements of fiber, such as corn or wheat bran and psyllium-seed preparations, can also be beneficial. However, because large amounts of fiber can produce gas and abdominal discomfort, fiber intake should be increased gradually as tolerated over a period of several weeks. Ample fluid intake (8–10 large glasses per day) should accompany increases in dietary fiber.[2]

Micronutrients · Constipation

Nutrient	Suggested daily dose	Comments
Vitamin C	250 mg-2 g	Pulls water into the colon and softens stools. Start with 250 mg and increase gradually until constipation improves. Take as single dose on arising in the morning
Folic acid	0.4–0.8 mg	Deficiency can aggravate constipation

High-dose calcium supplements (more than 2 g/day) may worsen constipation. Chronic use of laxatives should be avoided. Most interfere with normal colonic function and reduce absorption of nutrients. They can also precipitate development of irritable bowel syndrome.

Gastroesophageal Reflux (Heartburn)

Heartburn is sour, substernal burning pain often occurring after large meals, particularly when lying down. It is caused by gastric reflux of acid back into the lower esophagus, causing inflammation and pain.

Diet · Reflux

Meals containing large amounts of fat slow stomach emptying and can aggravate heartburn. Large meals distend the stomach and may trigger symptoms, so multiple small meals throughout the day are often beneficial. In certain individuals spicy foods may precipitate symptoms. If heartburn occurs at night, sleeping slightly propped up on pillows can reduce symptoms. Obesity aggravates heartburn by increasing intrabdominal pressure, which may cause gastric reflux.

Foods that Most Often Cause Heartburn

- Alcohol

- Citrus fruits and pineapple

- Tomatoes

- Coffee, black tea

- Chocolate

- Spicy foods (peppers, onions)

- Fatty meals

- Peppermint and spearmint

Cigarette smoking and certain drugs, including oral contraceptives and antihistamines, can worsen heartburn.

Micronutrients · Reflux

Follow recommendations for peptic ulcer.

Peptic Ulcer

Peptic ulcers are small erosions in the wall of the stomach or duodenum. These areas are normally protected from gastric acid by mucosal secretions that form a protective barrier. When this barrier breaks down, damage occurs and an ulcer forms. Symptoms are pain, nausea, and bleeding. Ulcers are common, occurring in about one in 15 adults. The causes are multiple: stress, poor diet, food sensitivities, and infection of the stomach by *Helicobacter pylori* can all contribute. Optimum nutrition can maintain the health of the protective lining of the stomach and duodenum. It can also support the immune system to increase resistance to chronic *Helicobacter* infection.

Diet · Ulcer

Dietary factors play a central role in ulcer frequency and severity.[3,4] High intakes of sugar and refined carbohydrate can contribute to ulcers.[5] Milk, traditionally recommended to reduce acidity, actually produces only a transient rise in pH. This is often followed by a large rebound increase in acid secretion, which can worsen ulcers. Heavy alcohol consumption can cause erosions and ulceration of the stomach lining. Both decaffeinated and regular coffee can aggravate heartburn and ulcers. Food sensitivities (such as allergy to cow's milk) may contribute to ulcer formation; identifying and avoiding the offending foods often improves healing and may prevent recurrence.[6] Raw cabbage juice contains large amounts of S-methylmethionine and glutamine, two amino acids that can accelerate healing of ulcers.

Micronutrients · Ulcer

Nutrient	Suggested daily dose	Comments
Vitamin A	8000–10 000 µg	Supports the gastric mucosa, may protect against ulceration and promote healing (see Fig. 5.4).[7] High doses of vitamin A should only be taken with the advice of a physician
Vitamin E	400 mg	Helps protect against ulcer development and may aid healing of ulcers both in the stomach and duodenum[8]
Zinc	30–60 mg	Speeds healing of ulcers[9]
L-Glutamine	1.0–1.5 g	Glutamine promotes healing of the gastric and duodenal mucosa

Blood tests are available to detect the presence of *Helicobacter* infection. If tests are positive, along with antibiotic therapy, the nutritional regimen suggested to support the immune system should be followed (see pp. 195). Taking drugs that can irritate the stomach lining, such as aspirin, other nonsteroidal anti-inflammatory drugs (NSAIDS), and steroids, should be avoided. Smoking should be reduced or stopped, as smokers have sharply increased risk for ulcers.

Gallstones

The gallbladder stores bile produced in the liver until mealtimes when it is secreted into the intestine and aids in fat emulsification and digestion. Most gallstones are composed mainly of cholesterol from the bile that precipitates into small stones. Gallstones can irritate the lining of the gallbladder, causing in-flammation and pain. They are found in about 10% of adults in the industrialized countries.

Diet · Gallstones

Diet can have a major influence on the development of gallstones. High-fat diets, particularly saturated fat, and overconsumption of refined carbohydrates can stimulate gallstone development. Ample dietary fiber and moderate intake of alcohol decrease the risk. Being overweight sharply increases risk of gallstones, whereas weight loss in obese persons can cause chronic stones to dissolve and clear.[10] In individuals with gallstones, consumption of fatty foods or coffee can bring on painful gallbladder spasms. Food sensitivities are often an unrecognized trigger of gallbladder symptoms – eggs, pork, and onions are the most commonly implicated.

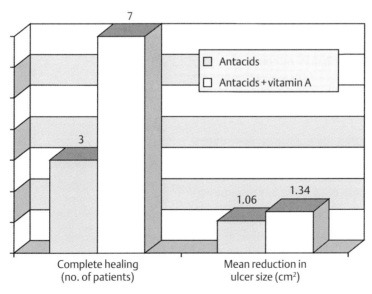

Fig. 5.**4**: **Vitamin A as adjunctive therapy in gastric ulcer.** 56 men with chronic gastric ulcers were given standard antacid therapy (in doses necessary to reduce stomach pain) or antacid therapy plus 150 000 IU/day vitamin A for 4 weeks. Ulcer sizes, which did not differ between groups at the beginning of treatment, were reduced in both groups, but healing was significantly greater in the vitamin A group. Complete healing of ulcers occurred in 19% of men treated with antacids alone, compared with 39% from the antacids plus vitamin A group. (Adapted from Patty I, et al. Lancet. 1982;2:876)

Micronutrients · Gallstones

Nutrient	Suggested daily dose	Comments
Taurine	1 g	Taurine is a component of the bile and helps prevent cholesterol precipitating in the gallbladder.[11] Supplementation may reduce risk of stone formation
Vitamin C	250 mg	Deficiency increases risk of gallstones[12]

Inflammatory Bowel Disease: Ulcerative Colitis and Crohn's Disease

There are two major forms of chronic inflammatory bowel disease (IBD). Ulcerative colitis is an ulcerative disorder of the mucosa of the colon, whereas Crohn's disease is characterized by transmural inflammation, most often in the small intestine. Both produce abdominal pain and diarrhea, which can be bloody. IBD tends to wax and wane, with periods of intense active disease followed by long periods of remission. Although the cause is not clear, IBD appears to be an autoimmune reaction, in which "overzealous" immune cells attack the tissues of the intestinal wall.

Diet · IBD

Active IBD often leads to severe malnourishment due to loss of appetite and malabsorption of nutrients. Dietary deficiencies are common, and nutritional status must be carefully monitored. Body levels of minerals (calcium, magnesium, zinc, and iron) are often depleted. In severe cases, parenteral administration of nutrients is required to bypass the diseased intestine.[13] In Crohn's disease affecting the ileum vitamin B12 is poorly absorbed and B12 injections may be needed. Often a high-fiber, low-refined carbohydrate diet reduces the severity of and recurrences in IBD and, if followed long-term, reduces the need for hospital care and intestinal surgery. Food sensitivities may aggravate IBD, and identification and avoidance of offending foods may increase chances of remission.[14] During acute exacerbations of Crohn's disease, enteral nutrition with protein hydrolysate diets is effective and reduces need for steroid therapy.[15]

Micronutrients · IBD

Nutrient	Suggested daily dose	Comments
Omega-3 fatty acids	2.5–3.0 g EPA (as fish oil capsules)	May reduce extent and severity of inflammation and improve symptoms[16–18]
Vitamin E	400 mg	Can reduce bowel inflammation and aid healing
L-Glutamine	1.0–1.5 g	Glutamine promotes healing of intestinal mucosa
Zinc	30–60 mg	Can promote healing[19,20]
Multivitamin/mineral supplement	A balanced supplement containing at least 0.8 mg folate and 50 µg vitamin B12 as well as magnesium, zinc, and iron	Malabsorption is common during active IBD. Folic acid and vitamin B12 may help protect against development of colon cancer in chronic ulcerative colitis[21]

References

1. Cranston D, et al. Dietary fibre and gastrointestinal disease. Br J Surg. 1988;75:508.
2. Yang P, Banwell JG. Dietary fiber: Its role in the pathogenesis and treatment of constipation. Practical Gastroenterology. 1986;6:28.
3. Katschinski BD, et al. Duodenal ulcer and refined carbohydrate intake: a case-control study assessing dietary fibre and refined sugar intake. Gut. 1990;31:993.
4. Aldoori WH, et al. Prospective study of diet and the risk of duodenal ulcer in men. Am J Epidemiol. 1997;145:42.
5. Tovey F. Diet and duodenal ulcer. J Gastroenterol Hepatol. 1994;9:177.
6. Kaess H, et al. Food intolerance in duodenal ulcer patients, non ulcer dyspeptic patients and healthy sub-

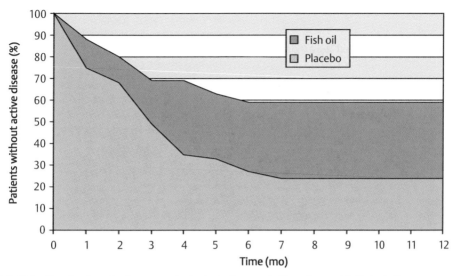

Fig. 5.**5**: **Fish oil and reduced relapse rate in Crohn's disease.** In 78 patients with Crohn's disease, treatment with 2.7 g/day of omega-3 fatty acids in an enteric-coated formula significantly reduced the rate of relapse over the course of 1 year.
(Adapted from Belluzzi A, et al. N Engl J Med. 1996; 334:1557)

jects. A prospective study. Klin Wochenschr. 1988;66:208.

7. Patty I, et al. Controlled trial of vitamin A therapy in gastric ulcer. Lancet. 1982;2:876.

8. Moutairy AR, Tariq M. Effect of vitamin E and selenium on hypothermic restraint stress and chemically-induced ulcers. Dig Dis Sci. 1996;41:1165.

9. Escolar G. Zinc compounds, a new treatment in peptic ulcer. Drugs Exp Clin Res. 1989;15:83.

10. Maclure KM, et al. Weight, diet, and the risk of symptomatic gallstones in middle-aged women. N Engl J Med. 1989;321:563.

11. Wang WY, Liaw KY. Effect of a taurine-supplemented diet on conjugated bile acids in biliary surgical patients. J Parenteral Enteral Nutr. 1991;15:294.

12. Simon JA, Hudes ES. Serum ascorbic acid and gallbladder disease prevalence among US adults: The Third National Health and Nutrition Examination Survey (NHANES III). Arch Intern Med. 2000;160:931.

13. Harries AD, Heatley RV. Nutritional disturbances in Crohn's disease. Postgrad Med J. 1983;50:690.

14. Heaton KW, et al. Treatment of Crohn's disease with an unrefined-carbohydrate, fibre-rich diet. BMJ. 1979;2:764.

15. Griffiths AM, et al. Meta-analysis of enteral nutrition as a primary treatment of active Crohn's disease. Gastroenterology. 1995;108:1056.

16. Belluzzi A, et al. Effect of an enteric coated fish oil preparation on relapses in Crohn's disease. N Engl J Med. 1996;334:1557.

17. Greenfield SM, et al. A randomized controlled study of evening primrose oil and fish oil in ulcerative colitis. Aliment Pharmacol Ther. 1993;7:159.

18. Belluzi A, et al. Polyunsaturated fatty acids and inflammatory bowel disease. Am J Clin Nutr. 2000;71:339S.

19. Dronfield MW, et al. Zinc in ulcerative colitis; A therapeutic trial and report on plasma levels. Gut. 1977;18:33.

20. Hendricks KM, Walker WA. Zinc deficiency in inflammatory bowel disease. Nutr Rev. 1988;46:401.

21. Lashner BA, et al. Effect of folate supplementation on the incidence of dysplasia and cancer in chronic ulcerative colitis: A case controlled study. Gastroenterology. 1989;97:255.

Obesity

Obesity is usually defined as a condition in which accumulation of body fat causes a person to weigh more than 20% of their ideal, healthy weight. Overweight is common in the industrialized countries, where about one-third of adults are obese. Obesity sharply increases risk of heart disease, stroke, cancer, high blood pressure, and diabetes.[1] Accumulation of body fat occurs when energy intake is greater than energy used for daily activities and basal metabolism.[2] The difference is mostly stored as fat. Obesity is often defined by body mass index (BMI). BMI is calculated as body weight in kilograms divided by height in meters squared (see Fig. 5.**6**).

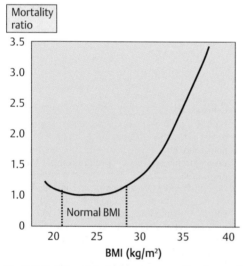

Fig. 5.**6**: **Relationship between mortality from all causes and body weight as defined by body mass index (BMI).** Very low or very high BMIs correlate with increased early mortality risk.

Diet · Obesity

Diets high in fat increase risk of weight gain. Protein and carbohydrate each contain 4 kcal of energy per gram, whereas fat has 9 kcal per gram. Moreover, dietary fat is efficiently stored as body fat, while protein and carbohy-

drate must first be converted to fat before storage, a more complex, less efficient process that requires energy. For the average person to lose about 0.5 kg of body fat per week, energy intake must be cut by about 500 kcal per day. Reducing caloric intake to between 1000 and 1500 kcal/day, particularly when combined with moderate exercise, produces a gradual but steady loss of body fat and weight.

Many popular weight-loss diets are unscientific and can be hazardous. Unbalanced diets that severely limit foods and are deficient in many important micronutrients[2] should be avoided. Although "high-protein" diets produce rapid initial weight loss, the loss is transient because water is lost, not fat. High-protein diets can also cause kidney damage and a life-threatening fall in blood potassium. Very low-calorie diets are those providing about 300–400 kcal per day. They should only be used in selected cases and must be carefully supervised by a doctor or dietitian. They often have harmful side effects (e.g., they may trigger gallstones) and are deficient in important micronutrients.

Weight-loss diets should contain generous amounts of dietary fiber.[3] Fiber adds nondigestible bulk, so that eating fiber-rich foods results in satiety with lower caloric intake, encouraging weight loss. Fruits, vegetables, whole grains, and legumes are fiber-rich foods that should be a part of diets for weight loss. Alcoholic drinks (beer, wine, and spirits) contain large amounts of calories; for example, a medium-sized glass of dry wine contains about 120 kcal.

The following plan provides a healthy way to trim body fat and will usually produce weight loss of about 0.5–1 kg of body fat per week:

● Diet
Should be low-fat (less than 20 g fat/day) and low-calorie (about 1000 cal/day). One-third of calories should be from high-quality protein (low-fat milk products, eggs, fish) Half of calories should be from carbohydrates (whole grains, fruits, vegetables, peas, and beans).

● Exercise
Combine diet with 30–45 minutes of aerobic exercise (walking, jogging, swimming) at least three to four times per week.

● Supplements
Take a complete, balanced multivitamin/mineral to supply micronutrient needs.

References

1. Pi-Sunyer, FX. Medical hazards of obesity. Ann Intern Med. 1993;119:655.
2. Rosenbaum M, et al. Obesity. N Engl J Med. 1997;337:396.
3. Rigaud D, et al. Overweight treated with energy restriction and a dietary fibre supplement: A 6-month randomized, double-blind, placebo-controlled trial. Int J Obes. 1990;14:763.
4. Krotkiewski M. Effect of guar gum on body weight, hunger ratings and metabolism in obese subjects. Br J Nutr. 1984;52:97.

Micronutrients · Obesity

Nutrient	Suggested daily dose	Comments
Fiber	Guar gum or other fiber supplement	Increases feeling of satiety and may help reduce caloric intake[4]
Multivitamin/mineral supplement	Containing balanced amounts of all the vitamins (including 100–250 mg vitamin C) and minerals	Ensures micronutrient balance during periods of low food intake

Cardiovascular Disease

Introduction: Atherosclerosis

Cardiovascular disease is the major cause of death in the industrialized countries of the world. Most cardiovascular disease is caused by atherosclerosis. Atherosclerosis is a disorder in which fatty plaques deposit within arteries, thickening the walls and reducing blood flow. Often the final event that abruptly closes off a narrowed vessel is the formation of a thrombus. About half of all deaths in Europe and North America are due to the two main forms of cardiovascular disease – myocardial infarction (heart attack) and stroke. These disorders kill nearly three times as many people each year as all types of cancer combined.

Several major physiologic risk factors for atherosclerosis can be influenced by diet and micronutrient intake. The major risk factors are:

● *Elevated blood levels of total and low-density lipoprotein (LDL) cholesterol.* Diets high in saturated fat, hydrogenated fat and cholesterol but low in polyunsaturated fatty acids (PUFAs), increase blood cholesterol levels.[1]

● *Low blood levels of high-density lipoprotein (HDL) cholesterol.* HDLs are the "protective" form of cholesterol, and higher levels lower the risk of cardiovascular disease. HDLs can be increased by exercise, weight loss if overweight, and moderate alcohol intake.

● *High levels of blood homocysteine.* Homocysteine, an amino acid that is a toxic byproduct of cell metabolism, can damage the lining of blood vessels and promote atherosclerosis. Vitamins B6 and B12 and folate are essential for metabolism and clearance of homocysteine (see Fig. 5.**7**). Poor intake of these B vitamins increases levels of homocysteine in the blood. An elevated blood homocysteine level increases risk of heart attack and stroke by two to five times.[2]

● *Low intake of essential PUFAs.* Essential fatty acids and their metabolites – the omega-6 and omega-3 fatty acids – protect against atherosclerosis and heart disease (see pp. 89). Omega-6 fatty acids (particularly GLA) and omega-3 fatty acids (eicosapentanioc acid [EPA] and docosahexanoic acid [DHA]) are precursors to important prostaglandins that tend to lower blood pressure and reduce platelet aggregation.[3] Lack of essential PUFAs in the diet, especially when combined with high intake of alcohol and saturated fat, lowers tissue levels of these protective prostaglandins. Deficiencies of the omega-6 and omega-3 fatty acids are aggravated by concurrent deficiencies of vitamin B6 and zinc.

● *High blood pressure.* High blood pressure damages arteries and accelerates development of atherosclerosis. Diets high in alcohol, sodium, and saturated fat and low in potassium, calcium, and PUFAs increase risk of high blood pressure. [4,5]

● *Low tissue levels of antioxidants* (see pp. 115), including vitamins E, C, and selenium. If levels of antioxidants in tissues and blood are low, LDL cholesterol and other blood lipids are susceptible to oxidation.[6] Oxidized cholesterol tends to deposit into the walls of arteries and is highly atherogenic.

The major cause of the epidemic of cardiovascular disease in Europe and North America is the typical affluent "Western" diet; it is high in saturated fat, hydrogenated fat, refined carbohydrates, processed foods, sodium, and alcohol and low in essential PUFAs, B vitamins, potassium, fiber, and antioxidant nutrients.

Coronary Heart Disease

Coronary heart disease (CHD) is caused by atherosclerosis in the coronary arteries. This limits the supply of oxygen to the heart and produces symptoms of angina (chest pain and shortness of breath) during exercise or stress

when oxygen demands increase. If a thrombus develops in a diseased artery and myocardial blood flow is blocked, heart tissue dies, producing a myocardial infarct (heart attack).

Diet · CHD

Dietary Fat

Eating saturated fat raises levels of LDL cholesterol. At the same time, it lowers HDL cholesterol and increases the tendency for platelet aggregation. Substituting polyunsaturated fats from nut and seed oils or monounsaturated fats from olive, peanut, and canola oil helps lower levels of LDL cholesterol.[1]

Hydrogenated Fat

Hydrogenation is a chemical process that alters fats to make them more solid. Hydrogenated oils are found in many processed baked goods and snacks, such as margarines and potato chips. They are as atherogenic as saturated fat, and intake should be minimized.[7]

Dietary Cholesterol

The amount of saturated fat in the diet influences blood cholesterol levels much more than intake of dietary cholesterol. If values of blood cholesterol are normal, dietary cholesterol has little effect on blood cholesterol levels. However, individuals who are hypercholesterolemic can benefit from a lower cholesterol intake.[1]

Fiber

Vegetables, fruits, beans, and whole grains are high in fiber. Fiber lowers blood cholesterol, and the soluble fiber found in fruits, oats, and vegetables is particularly beneficial.[8]

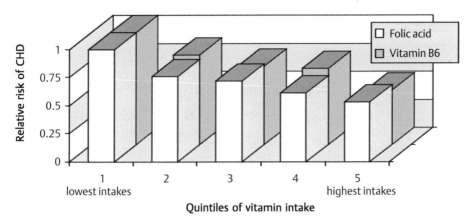

Fig. 5.**7**: **Folic acid and vitamin B6 intake and CHD.** Among 80,000 women, those with the highest intakes of folic acid and vitamin B6 had 30% lower risk of developing coronary heart disease (CHD). Women in the highest quintile for intake on average consumed 696 mg folate and 4.6 mg vitamin B6 daily. (Adapted from Rimm E, et al. JAMA. 1998;279:359)

Garlic, Ginger, Peppers, and Onions

These foods are rich in compounds that can help lower blood cholesterol and reduce platelet aggregation.[9]

Fish

Fish is rich in omega-3 fatty acids, which can lower blood cholesterol and triglycerides, lower blood pressure, and reduce platelet aggregation. Fish is also rich in protein and B vitamins and low in saturated fat. Eating fish two to three times a week as part of a healthy diet can reduce risk of heart disease by 50%.[10]

Coffee

High intake of regular or decaffeinated coffee (more than three cups per day) can raise blood cholesterol. Boiling methods of preparing coffee are particularly likely to raise cholesterol.

Dietary Antioxidants

Oxidative damage to blood lipids makes them much more atherogenic (see pp. 115). Antioxidants, both within lipopoteins (such as vitamin E) and circulating in the blood (beta-carotene and vitamin C) help protect against oxidation (see Fig. 5.**8**).[6] Regular, daily intake of citrus fruits and green and yellow vegetables supplies these vitamins as well as other important antioxidant food compounds.

Alcohol

Moderate alcohol consumption can raise HDL cholesterol and help protect against heart disease. People who consume one to two "drinks" per day (a drink is a medium-sized glass of beer or wine or 45 ml of spirits, all containing about 10 g of ethanol) have less risk of heart disease than those who abstain.[11] Red wine may also be beneficial because it contains natural antioxidants that can protect against oxidation of blood fats.

Micronutrients · CHD

Nutrient	Suggested daily dose	Comments
To reduce elevated blood homocysteine		
Folic acid plus vitamin B12	0.5–1.0 mg folic acid; 10–20 µg vitamin B12	Reduces blood homocysteine levels[12]
Vitamin B6	50 mg	Reduces blood homocysteine levels; lowers risk of platelet aggregation[12]
To reduce elevated blood cholesterol		
Niacin (in form of nicotinic acid)	Begin with 100 mg and gradually increase over several weeks to 1–3 g. Take with meals	Lowers LDL cholesterol and raises HDLs, thereby reducing risk of heart attack.[13] Side effects (flushing) can be minimized by raising the dose gradually and taking the niacin with meals. Should be taken only under medical supervision at doses >1 g/day because of rare but potentially serious side effects, including liver inflammation and hyperglycemia
To reduce risk of oxidation of blood cholesterol		
Vitamin C	1–2 g	Protects against fat oxidation; lowers tendency for platelet aggregation; lowers blood cholesterol.[14] May reduce frequency and severity of angina
Vitamin E and selenium	200–400 mg vitamin E, 200 µg selenium	Protects against LDL cholesterol oxidation; lowers tendency for platelet aggregation.[15–17] May reduce frequency and severity of angina
To reduce elevated cholesterol and blood pressure		
Calcium and magnesium	600 mg calcium; 300 mg magnesium. Can be taken as dolomite tablets	Calcium helps lower elevated cholesterol levels and may protect against atherosclerosis. Magnesium reduces cholesterol levels and raises HDLs; also reduces risk of dysrhythmias and reduces severity of angina.[18]
Omega-3 fatty acids	2–3 g EPA and DHA as fish oil capsules	Reduces risk of atherosclerosis by reducing blood cholesterol and triglycerides, lowering blood pressure, and reducing tendency for platelet aggregation.[3]
To improve myocardial energy metabolism		
Carnitine	1–2 g	Lowers total blood cholesterol while increasing HDLs. Reduces symptoms of angina by increasing efficiency of energy metabolism in the myocardium[19]
Coenzyme Q10	60–120 mg	Reduces symptoms of angina by increasing efficiency of energy metabolism in the myocardium. Supports heart function and cardic output in hearts weakened by atherosclerosis[20]

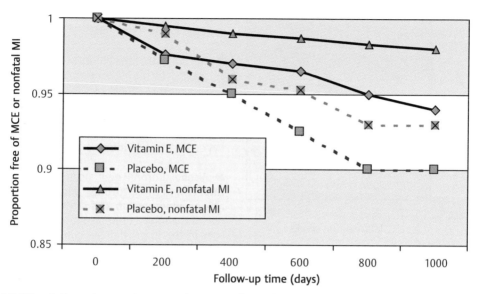

Fig. 5.**8**: **Vitamin E supplements in men with coronary heart disease (CHD).** 2002 men with CHD and a previous myocardial infarction were given 400–800 mg/day of vitamin E for 2–3 years. In the vitamin E group the risk of a major cardiovascular event (MCE) and nonfatal myocardial infarction (MI) was reduced 47 % and 68 %, respectively. (From Stephens NG, et al. Lancet. 1996;347:781)

Hypertension and Stroke

Hypertension (high blood pressure) is very common, affecting about one in four adults in industrialized countries. Hypertension over many years silently and progressively damages the heart, blood vessels, and kidneys. It is the major risk factor for stroke (cerebrovascular accident), the third leading cause of death in most industrialized countries.

Diet · Hypertension

The major dietary risk factors for hypertension and stroke are as follows:

● *Overweight.* Obesity is commonly associated with high blood pressure. Overweight hypertensive persons who lose weight often experience a significant reduction in blood pressure.[21]

● *Low intake of PUFAs.* Especially when combined with a high intake of saturated fat, low intake of essential PUFAs can increase risk of high blood pressure (see Fig. 5.9).

● *Salt.* Although for most people sodium in the diet plays only a minor role in determining blood pressure, some individuals are very sensitive to sodium in the diet. Individuals with a family history of hypertension or who are older than 55 years are most likely to be sodium sensitive.[22] In about one-third of cases of hypertension, blood pressure can be significantly lowered by limiting sodium intake, most of which comes from salt added to processed foods, such as bread, cheese, canned soups and salty snacks.

● *Potassium.* High sodium intake is a much stronger risk factor when combined with low potassium intake.[5] People with low intakes of potassium are nearly five times more likely to die from stroke than those with higher intakes. Achieving a balanced intake of sodium and potassium should be a goal for people with, or at risk for hypertension. High potassium/low sodium foods, such as potatoes,

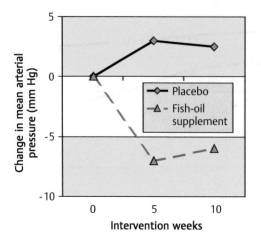

Fig. 5.9: Omega-3 fatty-acids in hypertension. 156 hypertensive adults were treated for 10 weeks with 5.1 g/day of omega-3 fatty acids (EPA and DHA). The mean systolic blood pressure decreased by 4.6 mm Hg and the diastolic pressure by 3.0 mm Hg in the group receiving the fish oil.
(From Bonaa KH, et al. N Engl J Med. 1990;322:795)

green vegetables, orange juice, apricots, and bananas can be beneficial.

● *Calcium.* Low dietary intake of calcium is associated with a higher risk of hypertension, and increasing intake of calcium (from supplements or calcium-rich foods such as low-fat milk products, sesame seeds, or dark green vegetables) can reduce blood pressure in hypertensive individuals.[23]

● *Alcohol.* Chronic high alcohol intake (more than two to three "drinks" per day) increases risk of hypertension and stroke.[11] Alcohol is one of the most common causes of hypertension in the industrialized countries. Individuals who drink regularly and have high blood pressure can often see a significant drop in blood pressure after a few days of abstention.

● *Antioxidants and other food components.* Rich intake of dietary antioxidants from high consumption of fruits and vegetables (particularly carrots and spinach) protects against high blood pressure and can reduce risk of stroke by 50% (see Fig. 5.**10**).[28]

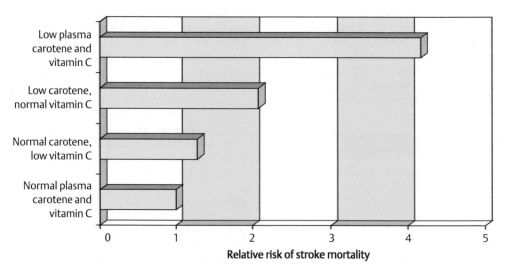

Fig. 5.10: Plasma antioxidants and risk of stroke. In a 12-year prospective study in nearly 3000 men, low plasma concentrations of vitamin C and carotenes were associated with a relative risk (RR) of death from stroke of 4.17 (95% CI 1.68–10.33, P = 0.002).
(Adapted from Gey KF, et al. Clin Invest. 1993;71:3)

Micronutrients · Hypertension

Nutrient	Suggested daily dose	Comments
To treat hypertension		
Calcium and magnesium	1.5 g calcium and 600 mg magnesium; can be taken as dolomit tablets	Dietary deficiencies of calcium and/or magnesium increase blood pressure; supplements can produce vasodilation and lower blood pressure[18,23]
Coenzyme Q10	60–120 mg	Lowers blood pressure in hypertension[24]
Omega-3 fatty acids	2–3 g EPA and DHA as fish-oil capsules	Lowers blood pressure in hypertension[25]
Taurine	3 g	Lowers blood pressure in hypertension[26]
In addition to the above, to prevent stroke		
Vitamin B complex	Should contain 0.8–1.0 mg folic acid, 25–50 mg vitamin B6 as part of a balanced formula	Reduces blood homocysteine levels and lowers risk of platelet aggregation,[2] thereby reducing risk of stroke
Vitamin E and selenium	200 mg vitamin E; 200 µg selenium	Reduces platelet aggregation[27] and helps protect against stroke

Peripheral Vascular Disease (Intermittent Claudication)

Poor blood circulation to the extremities can be a nagging problem, causing the hands and feet to be pale and cool and increasing sensitivity to cold. A common peripheral circulatory disorder is intermittent claudication. This occurs when atherosclerosis narrows the arteries in the legs, limiting blood supply to muscles in the calves and thighs. The first symptoms appear during walking or climbing stairs, as increased demand for oxygen and nutrients by the muscles cannot be met by the limited blood supply, producing pain, burning sensation, and cramping in the leg muscles.

Diet · PVD

The diet recommendations for atherosclerosis apply (see pp. 177). In general, saturated fat in the diet should be replaced with cold-pressed plant and seed oils that provide EFAs and can aid circulation. Eating fish two to three times per week provides omega-3 fatty acids that help maintain blood circulation. Refined carbohydrates should be replaced with complex carbohydrates from vegetables and whole grains to provide additional fiber.

Micronutrients · PVD

Nutrient	Suggested daily dose	Comments
Vitamin E	400 mg	Decreases tendency for platelet aggregation and improves circulation.[27] May reduce calf pain and cramping in peripheral vascular disease.
Niacin (in form of nicotinic acid)	100–200 mg	Lowers LDL cholesterol in the blood and raises HDL cholesterol, thereby reducing atherogenic risk.[13] Produces peripheral vasodilation that aids circulation.
Magnesium	400 mg	May help dilate blood vessels and improve circulation
Omega-3 fatty acids	2–3 g EPA and DHA (as fish-oil capsules)	Decreases platelet aggregation and improves circulation[3]

References

1. Clarke R, et al. Dietary lipids and blood cholesterol: quantitative meta-analysis of metabolic ward studies. BMJ. 1997;314:112.
2. Boushey CJ, at al. A quantitative assessment of plasma homocysteine as a risk factor for vascular disease. Probable benefits of increasing folic acid intakes. JAMA. 1995;274:1049.
3. Connor SL, Connor WE. Are fish oils beneficial in the prevention and treatment of coronary artery disease? Am J Clin Nutr. 1997;66:1020S.
4. Klatsky AL. Alcohol and hypertension. Clin Chim Acta. 1996;246:91.
5. Reusser ME, McCarron DA. Micronutrient effects on blood pressure regulation. 1994;52:367.
6. Steinberg D. Antioxidant vitamins and coronary heart disease. N Engl J Med. 1993;328:1487.
7. Ascherio A. Metabolic and atherogenic effects of trans fatty acids. J Intern Med. 1995;238:93.
8. Hunninghake DB, et al. Long term treatment of hypercholesterolemia with dietary fiber. Ann Intern Med. 1994;97:504.
9. Adler AJ, Holub BJ. Effect of garlic and fish-oil supplementation on serum lipid and lipoprotein concentrations in hypercholesterolemic men. Am J Clin Nutr. 1997;65:445.
10. Daviglus E, et al. Fish consumption and 30-year risk of myocardial infarction. N Engl J Med. 1997;336:1046.
11. Klatsky AL. Cardiovascular effects of alcohol. Sci Am Sci Med. 1995;2:28.
12. Peterson JC, Spence JD. Vitamins and progression of atherosclerosis in hyperhomocysteinemia. Lancet. 1998;351:263.
13. Luria MH. Effect of low-dose niacin on high density lipoprotein cholesterol and total cholesterol/high density lipoprotein cholesterol concentration. Arch Intern Med. 1988;148:2493.
14. Simon JA. Vitamin C and cardiovascular disease: A review. J Am Coll Nutr. 1992;11:107.
15. Rapola JM, et al. Effect of vitamin E and beta-carotene on the incidence of angina pectoris. JAMA. 1996;275:693.
16. Stephens NG, et al. Randomised controlled trial of vitamin E in patients with coronary disease. Lancet. 1996;347:781.
17. Kok FJ, et al. Decreased selenium levels in acute myocardial infarction. JAMA. 1989;261:1161.
18. Whelton PK, Klag MJ. Magnesium and blood pressure: Review of the epidemiologic and clinical trial experience. Am J Cardiol. 1989;63:26G.
19. Kamikawa T, et al. Effects of L-carnitine on exercise tolerance in patients with stable angina pectoris. Jpn Heart J. 1984;25:587.
20. Langsjoen PH, et al. Long-term efficacy and safety of coenzyme Q10 therapy for idiopathic dilated cardiomyopathy. Am J Cardiol. 1990;65:521.
21. Bronner LL, et al. Primary prevention of stroke. N Engl J Med. 1995;333:1392.
22. Morimoto A, et al. Sodium sensitivity and cardiovascular events in patients with essential hypertension. Lancet. 1997;350:1734.
23. Allender PS, et al. Dietary calcium and blood pressure: a meta-analysis of the randomized clinical trials. Ann Intern Med. 1996;124:825.
24. Digiesiv, et al. Effect of coenzyme Q10 on essential arterial hypertension. Curr Ther Res. 1990;47:841.
25. Bonaa KH, et al. Effect of EPA and DHA on blood pressure in hypertension. N Engl J Med. 1990;322:795.
26. Azuma J, et al. Therapeutic effect of taurine in congestive heart failure: A double-blind crossover trial. Clin Cardiol. 1985;8:276.
27. Jandak J, Steiner M, Richardson PD. Alpha tocopherol, an effective inhibitor of platelet adhesion. Blood. 1989;73:141.
28. Manson JE, Stampfer MJ, Willett WC, et al: Antioxidant vitamin consumption and incidence of stroke in women. Circulation. 1993;87:678.

Disorders of Blood Sugar Regulation

Diabetes

Diabetes is a chronic disease caused by inadequate secretion of, or peripheral resistance to, insulin. It is characterized by hyperglycemia and hyperlipidemia. Diabetes, when poorly controlled, causes widespread damage to blood vessels and nerves, which can result in blindness, kidney failure, or heart attack.

There are two main forms of diabetes. Type 1 diabetes appears suddenly in childhood and is caused by autoimmune destruction of the pancreatic beta cells and loss of insulin production. Type 2 diabetes appears gradually in older people and is characterized by loss of insulin sensitivity – that is, cells no longer respond to signals from insulin. More than 90% of diabetic patients have type 2 diabetes.

Diet · Diabetes

The best way to prevent type 2 diabetes is to avoid gaining weight. Overweight people are four times more likely to develop type 2 diabetes than those who maintain normal body weight. Overweight diabetic patients can often reduce their need for drugs and control their blood sugar by weight loss.

The glucose tolerance factor (GTF) is a naturally occuring compound that helps regulate blood sugar. It is found in rich amounts in brewer's yeast. Chromium is an essential component of GTF, and diets deficient in chromium produce glucose intolerance (see Fig. 5.**11**).[1–3] Diabetics who excrete glucose in their urine have increased urinary loss of minerals (such as magnesium, zinc, and chro-

mium). Deficiencies of these important minerals further impair the ability to control blood glucose. Therefore, diabetic diets should emphasize foods rich in these minerals.

The best diet for most diabetics is one low in refined sugars and high in complex carbohydrates and fiber (which slow absorption of dietary sugars, reducing peaks in blood glucose).[4] Foods such as vegetables, fruits, legumes, and whole grains should be emphasized, and adopting a mainly vegetarian diet can be beneficial. To reduce elevated blood lipids and lower risk of cardiovascular disease, saturated fat intake should be minimized and replaced by high-quality plant oils that supply essential PUFAs.

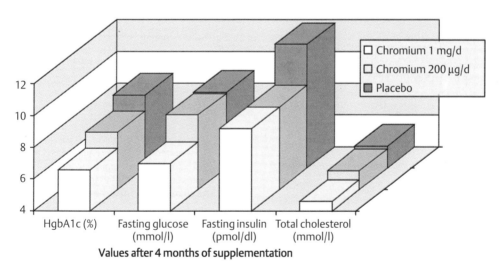

Fig. 5.**11**: **Chromium supplements in diabetes.** 180 subjects with type 2 diabetes were given either 1 mg chromium, 200 µg chromium, or placebo daily for 4 months. In the group receiving chromium there were significant decreases in HgbA1C, serum cholesterol, and fasting glucose and insulin values, compared with placebo. (Adapted from Anderson RA, et al. Diabetes. 1997; 46:1786)

Micronutrients · Diabetes

Nutrient	Suggested daily dose	Comments
To enhance the action of insulin and help control blood glucose		
Vitamin E	800 mg. Begin with 100 mg/day and gradually increase dose	Can enhance insulin sensitivity and reduce needs for oral hypoglycemics and/or insulin.[5-7] Reduces platelet aggregation and risk of thrombosis
Chromium	200–1000 µg chromium	As a component of GTF, helps control blood glucose and decrease need for insulin or hypoglycemic drugs.[1-3] Can be taken together with 5–10 g brewer's yeast
Vitamin C	1–2 g; can be taken as complex with bioflavonoids	Can help regulate blood glucose, strengthen small blood vessels, and reduce risk of early heart disease[8-10]
To prevent mineral deficiencies that impair glucose tolerance		
Magnesium	400–600 mg	Magnesium deficiency is common in diabetes. Supplements may help control blood glucose and protect against cardiovascular disease[11]
Multimineral supplement	Balanced formula containing at least 15 mg zinc	Helps replenish urinary losses
To treat diabetic neuropathy		
Omega-6 fatty acids	GLA as 1–4 g evening primrose oil	Beneficial in treating neuropathy[12]
Myo-inositol	1–2 g	Beneficial in treating neuropathy[13]
Vitamin B complex	High potency supplement containing at least 50 mg thiamin and vitamin B6	Neuropathic symptoms may respond to supplemental thiamin and vitamin B6[14]
To help control newly -diagnosed type 1 diabetes		
Niacinamide	1–3 g; begin with 500 mg/day and increase gradually	Supplements in newly diagnosed type 1 diabetes can reduce insulin requirements and extend the time before beginning insulin.[15] Avoid nicotinic acid, another form of niacin, which can be harmful in diabetics

Hypoglycemia

Oversecretion of insulin in response to meals produces a disorder termed "reactive hypoglycemia." In reactive hypoglycemia meals rich in simple sugars and refined carbohydrates stimulate a large insulin response; the insulin then pushes down blood glucose to below normal levels.[16] Symptoms most often occur mid-morning and mid-to-late-afternoon, usually 2–4 hours after eating a carbohydrate-rich meal. Because the brain depends on a steady supply of glucose, hypoglycemia impairs mentation, alertness, and concentration. Reactive hypoglycemia may cause fatigue and irritability.

Reactive hypoglycemia can produce the following symptoms:

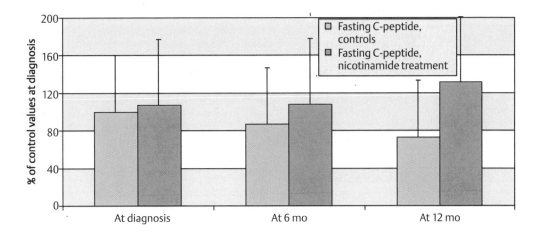

Fig. 5.**12**: **Nicotinamide in newly diagnosed type 1 diabetes.** Meta-analysis of 10 randomized trials involving more than 200 newly diagnosed, nicotinamide-treated type 1 diabetic patients. One year after diagnosis baseline C-peptide (a measure of beta-cell function) was significantly higher in nicotinamide-treated pateints, compared with controls.
(Adapted from Pozzilli P, et al. Diabetes Care. 1996;19:1357)

- Weakness, fatigue
- Faintness, dizziness
- Impaired concentration
- Headache
- Tachycardia
- Intense hunger
- Anxiety or panic attacks[17]
- Cold sweats, nausea
- Insomnia (if a meal is eaten late in the evening)
- Mood swings, personality changes

Diet · Hypoglycemia

A diet plan to reduce reactive hypoglycemia should include:

● Avoiding simple sugars and refined carbohydrates (such as white flour and white rice). These produce rapid rises in blood glucose that trigger oversecretion of insulin.

● Substituting foods high in complex carbohydrates and fiber (which slow absorption of dietary sugars, reducing glycemic peaks during meals) such as vegetables, legumes, oats, and whole grains.[16]

● Eating five to six small meals spaced throughout the day to provide a constant source of energy to maintain blood sugar. Each meal should include foods containing high-quality protein and moderate amounts of cold-pressed plant oils.

● Avoiding large amounts of alcohol and coffee, which can exacerbate reactive hypoglycemia.

The glycemic index measures a food's potential to rapidly elevate blood glucose. If vulnerable to reactive hypoglycemia, foods with a high glycemic index may stimulate insulin oversecretion and trigger low blood sugar. These foods should therefore be avoided in favor of foods with a low to moderate glycemic index.

Glycemic index of selected foods

Very high	High	Moderate	Low	Very low
Honey	Whole-wheat bread	Buckwheat	Sweet potatoes	Nuts
Potatoes	Brown rice	Oat flakes	Apples	Soybeans
Cornflakes	Raisins	Sweet corn	Milk	Kidney beans
White bread	Bananas	Green peas	Yoghurt	Lentils
White rice		Carrots	Tomatoes	
		Pasta	Fruit	

Micronutrients · Hypoglycemia

Nutrient	Suggested daily dose	Comments
Chromium	200–400 µg	May help regulate blood glucose levels.[18] Take with 5–10 g brewer's yeast (rich in GTF)
Multimineral supplement	Balanced supplement with 200 mg magnesium, 20 mg zinc, and 5 mg manganese	Deficiencies of zinc, magnesium,[19] and manganese increase risk of reactive hypoglycemia

References

1. Anderson R, et al. Chromium supplementation in type II diabetes. Diabetes. 1997;46:1786.
2. Jeejeebhoy KN, et al. Chromium deficiency, glucose intolerance and neuropathy reverses by chromium supplementation in a patient receiving long-term total parenteral nutrition. Am J Clin Nutr. 1977;3:531.
3. Lee NA, Reasner CA. Beneficial effects of chromium supplementation on serum triglyceride levels in NIDDM. Diabetes Care. 1994;17:1449.
4. Jenkins DJA, Jenkins AL. Nutrition principles and diabetes. Diabetes Care. 1995;18:1491.
5. Caballero B. Vitamin E improves the action of insulin. Nutr Rev. 1993;51:339.
6. Jain SK, et al. The effect of modest vitamin E supplementation on lipid peroxidation products and other cardiovascular risk factors in diabetic patients. Lipids. 1996;31:S87.
7. Salonen JT, et al. Increased risk of non-insulin dependent diabetes mellitus at low plasma vitamin E concentrations: A four year follow up study in men. BMJ. 1995;311:1124.
8. Will JC, Byers T. Does diabetes mellitus increase the requirement for vitamin C? Nutr Rev. 1996;54:193.
9. Ting HH, et al. Vitamin C improves endothelium-dependent vasodilation in patients with non-insulin-dependent diabetes mellitus. J Clin Invest. 1996;97:22.
10. Paolisso G, et al. Metabolic benefits deriving from chronic vitamin C supplementation in aged non-insulin dependent diabetics. J Am Coll Nutr. 1995;14:387.
11. Paolisso G, et al. Improved insulin response and action by chronic magnesium administration in aged NIDDM subjects. Diabetes Care. 1989;12:265.
12. The Gamma-linolenic Acid Multicenter Trial Group. Treatment of diabetic neuropathy with gamma-linolenic acid. Diabetes Care. 1993;16:8.
13. Salway JG, et al. Effect of myo-inositol on peripheral-nerve function in diabetics. Lancet. 1978;2:1281.
14. Rogers KS, Mohan C. Vitamin B6 metabolism and diabetes. Biochem Med Metab Biol. 1994;52:10.
15. Pozzilli P, et al. Meta-analysis of nicotinamide treatment in patients with recent-onset IDDM. Diabetes Care. 1996;19:1357.
16. Hofeldt FD. Reactive hypoglycemia. Endocrinol Metab Clin North Am. 1989;18:185.
17. Gorman JM, et al. Hypoglycemia and panic attacks. Am J Psychiatry. 1984;141:101.
18. Anderson RA, et al. Effects of supplemental chromium on patients with symptoms of reactive hypoglycemia. Metabolism. 1987;35:351.
19. Stebbing JB, et al. Reactive hypoglycaemia and magnesium. Magnesium Bull. 1982;4:131.

Anemia

Anemia is an abnormally low number of red blood cells (RBCs) circulating in the blood. Symptoms of anemia are fatigue, weakness, pallor, and shortness of breath on exertion. Anemic children have difficulty concentrating, have reduced memory, and learn poorly at school. Anemia can have many causes. Chronic blood loss (e.g., from heavy menstrual periods or a peptic ulcer) can produce anemia. A common cause is a micronutrient deficiency.

Diet · Anemia

RBCs are continually produced by the bone marrow, live about 90 days, and are then broken down. Growth of RBCs requires a steady supply of nutrients. The most common nutrient deficiencies that produce anemia are iron, folic acid, and vitamin B12.[1,2] Less commonly, inadequate dietary supply of vitamins A and C, several other B vitamins, and copper produces anemia.[2]

Anemia caused by iron and folic acid deficiency is very common among growing children and pregnant women, because their diets do not supply adequate iron and folate to meet their increased needs.[3,4] People with low iron stores should not drink coffee or tea with their meals, as these beverages sharply reduce absorption of iron from foods. Vitamin C strongly promotes absorption of iron, thus a glass of orange juice or other vitamin-C rich food included with meals can be beneficial.[5] In contrast, vitamin B12 deficiency is most often found in older people, many of whom absorb vitamin B12 poorly[6] because of reduced gastric function. Vitamin B12 deficiency can also occur in strict vegetarians whose diets contain little or no vitamin B12. See pages 66, 46, and 49 respectively for foods rich in iron, folate, and vitamin B12.

Micronutrients · Anemia

Nutrient	Suggested daily dose	Comments
To prevent anemia and promote healthy development of red blood cells		
Vitamin B Complex	Should contain at least 5 mg vitamin B6, 0.4 mg folate, and 5 µg B12	Lack of riboflavin, thiamin, folate, and vitamins B6 and B12 can all cause anemia. Particularly important during pregnancy and lactation, as well as in childhood and adolescence[2,4]
Multimineral supplement with iron	Containing balanced amounts of all essential minerals, including 5–10 mg iron	Particularly important during pregnancy and lactation, as well as in childhood and adoleseonce[1,3]
Vitamin A	800 µg	Deficiency can contribute to anemia. Helps to move iron from storage sites in the body to the bone marrow for use in erythrocyte production
Vitamin C	100 – 250 mg	Deficiency can cause anemia.[2,7] When taken with meals containing iron or with an iron supplement, vitamin C sharply increases absorption of iron
To treat anemia caused by a single nutrient deficiency		
Iron	100–150 mg iron (in a bioavailable form such as ferrous fumarate)	Iron supplements should be continued for 3–6 months after the hemoglobin level returns to normal, to refill iron stores.[3] High doses of iron can block absorption of other minerals, including zinc and copper. High doses of iron should always be taken with a multimineral supplement to maintain mineral balance

continued

| Folic acid | 1–5 mg[2] | Should be taken until hemoglobin returns to normal. Should be given along with a balanced vitamin B complex containing at least 5 µg vitamin B12 |
| Vitamin B12 | If caused by vitamin B12 malabsorption: 1 mg/day by intramuscular injection for 7 days, then 1 mg twice a week intramuscularly for 2 months.[2] If caused by dietary lack (vegetarianism): 1 mg oral vitamin B12/day for 3–6 months | After stores are replenished, vitamin B12 deficiency due to malabsorption usually requires lifelong monthly injections[8] or, in cases of mild malabsorption, 1 mg/day[2] oral vitamin B12 to maintain status For vegetarians a daily supplement of 2–5 µg vitamin B12 will usually maintain reserves |

References

1. Beard JL, et al. Iron metabolism: A comprehensive review. Nutr Rev. 1996;54:295.
2. Hoffbrand AV. Megaloblastic anemia and miscellaneous deficiency anemias. In: Weatherall DJ, Ledingham JGG, Warrell DA, eds. Oxford Textbook of Medicine. Oxford: Oxford Medical Publications; 1996:3484.
3. Oski FA. Iron deficiency in infancy and childhood. N Engl J Med. 1993;329:190.
4. Middleman AB, et al. Nutritional vitamin B12 deficiency and folate deficiency in an adolescent patient presenting with anemia, weight loss, and poor school performance. J Adolesc Health. 1996;19:76.
5. Hurrell RF. Bioavailabilty of iron. Eur J Clin Nutr. 1997;51:4S.
6. Lindenbaum J, et al. Prevalence of cobalamin deficiency in the Framingham elderly population. Am J Clin Nutr. 1994;60:2.
7. Ajayi OA, Nnaji UR. Effect of ascorbic acid supplementation on haematological response and ascorbic acid status of young female adults. Ann Nutr Metab. 1990;34:32.
8. Pruthi RK, Tefferi A. Pernicious anemia revisted. Mayo Clin Proc. 1994;69:144.

Musculoskeletal Disorders

Osteoarthritis

Osteoarthritis, also called degenerative joint disease, is characterized by gradual loss of the smooth articular cartilage that covers joint surfaces and by degenerative changes in the underlying bone. Osteoarthritis is common in people over 55 years (over two-thirds show evidence of this disorder). It is one of the most common causes of chronic disability in the industrialized countries. Symptoms are joint pain, deformity, and loss of mobility. The joints most often affected are the fingers, hips, knees, neck, and lower back. Although osteoarthritis mostly results from "wear and tear" of the joints, suboptimum nutrition can also be a contributing factor.

Diet · OA

Aspirin and other NSAIDs taken for arthritis disrupt the integrity of the gastrointestinal mucosa and may increase the ability of food allergens to cross into the bloodstream. This may increase the risk of food sensitivities that can exacerbate joint symptoms. The most commonly implicated foods belong to the nightshade family – potato, tomato, eggplant, and peppers. Overweight places a greater load on joints and can contribute to osteoarthritis in the hips, back, and knees. Fruits and vegetables are good sources of vitamins C and E; high intake of these antioxidant nutrients is associated with lower risk of osteoarthritis (see Fig. 5.**13**).[1]

Rheumatoid Arthritis

Rheumatoid arthritis (RA), a chronic, often progressive inflammatory disorder of the joints, is caused by autoimmune damage to synovial tissues. Release of cytokines and oxidants by white blood cells in the joint produces swelling, inflammation, and destruction. The autoimmune reaction can also damage other tissues including the digestive tract. Nutrition can play a central role in prevention and treatment of RA.

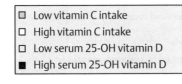

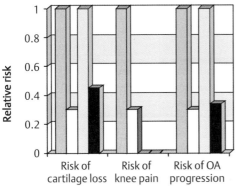

Fig. 5.**13**: **Vitamin C intake, serum 25-OH vitamin D, and progression of osteoarthritis (OA).** In a study in 640 adults for 7–10 years, the upper tertiles of vitamin C intake and serum 25-OH vitamin D were associated with a two to three fold reduced risk of cartilage loss, pain, and disease progression in osteoarthritis of the knee, compared with the lower tertiles. Average upper and lower tertiles for vitamin C intake were 430 mg/day and 81 mg/day.
(Adapted from McAlindon TE, et al. Arthritis Rheum. 1996;39:648, and McAlindon TE, et al. Ann Intern Med. 1996;125:353)

Diet · RA

Food sensitivities are a common cause of rheumatoid arthritis.[6] An elimination diet should be used to determine the presence of food sensitivities (see pp. 205). Identification and avoidance of offending foods can produce dramatic improvements in symptoms and function. Aspirin and other NSAIDs damage the gastrointestinal mucosa and increase the ability of allergens to cross into the bloodstream, thereby aggravating food sensitivities that often contribute to RA. Diets high in essential polyunsaturated fat and low in saturated fat can increase tissue production of anti-inflammatory prostaglandins and leukotrienes that reduce pain and swelling. Cold-water fish should be eaten two to three times per week to provide omega-3 fatty acids to reduce inflammation (see Fig. 5.**14**).[7]

Micronutrients · OA

Nutrient	Suggested daily dose	Comments
Vitamin E	400–800 mg	Can help reduce pain and stiffness and improve joint mobility.[2] May slow progression of osteoarthritis
Vitamin D	5–10 µg	May slow progression of osteoarthritis[3]
Multimineral supplement	Balanced formula containing generous amounts of calcium, magnesium, and 100–200 µg selenium[4]	Supports repair of articular cartilage and underlying bone
Vitamin B Complex	Complete formula containing at least 0.8 mg folic acid and 25 µg vitamin B12	May help provide relief of symptoms[5]
Niacinamide	500 mg – 1 g	May help reduce inflammation and pain

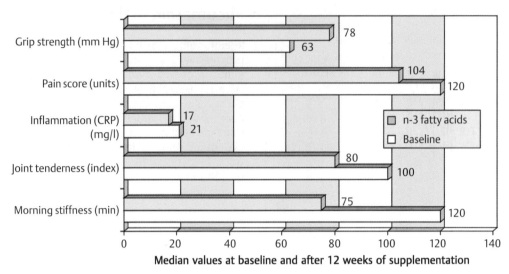

Fig. 5.**14**: **Omega-3 fatty acids and rheumatoid arthritis.** 51 subjects with rheumatoid arthritis were given 3.2 g/day EPA and DHA for 12 weeks. Compared with placebo, there was significant improvement in morning stiffness and joint tenderness as well as a significant reduction in C-reactive protein (CRP) (a marker of inflammation).
(Adapted from Nielsen GL, et al. Eur J Clin Invest. 1992;22:687)

For some patients, a semi-vegetarian diet (including fish, but no meat, milk, or eggs) can significantly reduce inflammation and halt progression of RA.[8] In advanced cases of RA, because nutrient absorption is impaired (due to the autoimmune reaction in the intestine), nutrient deficiencies – particularly of the B vitamins and trace minerals – are common.[9]

Micronutrients · RA

Nutrient	Suggested daily dose	Comments
Omega-3 fatty acids	2–3 g EPA (as fish-oil capsules)	Reduces inflammation and may lessen stiffness and pain.[7,10] Supports healing of damaged synovium
Vitamin E	400–800 mg	Protects against oxidative damage, reduces inflammation, and may provide effective pain relief[11]
Omega-6 fatty acids	1–2 g GLA as evening primrose oil	May reduce inflammation, pain, and swelling[12]
L-histidine	0.5–1.5 g	May help reduce joint pain and stiffness[13]
Multimineral formula	High-dose formula with 2–6 mg copper, 15–30 mg zinc, 100–200 μg selenium	Copper stimulates the enzyme superoxide dismutase (SOD) that can reduce oxidative damage, stiffness, and pain.[14] Zinc[15,16] and selenium may reduce inflammation and help relieve symptoms[17]

In severe RA treated with methotrexate, supplemental folic acid may be beneficial (methotrexate interferes with folate metabolism).[18]

Osteoporosis

Aging bones tend to lose minerals and density, gradually becoming thinner and more fragile. In osteoporosis, loss of bone mineral has progressed to the point where fractures can occur with minimal or no trauma. Although both men and women can develop osteoporosis, it is much more common in older women. This is because loss of endogenous estrogens during menopause sharply accelerates bone loss. In severe cases, up to 20% of the mineral content of the skeleton can be lost in the 3–5 years of the menopause. Osteoporosis progresses silently, and often the first indication of its presence is a fracture of the hip or spine. Optimum nutrition can substantially reduce risk of osteoporosis.[19]

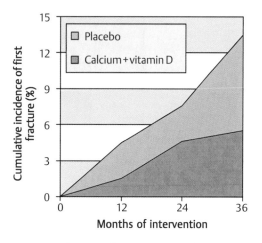

Fig. 5.**15**: **Calcium and vitamin D supplementation and bone fractures in older adults.** 389 men and women 65 years of age or older were given 500 mg calcium plus 700 IU vitamin D3 daily for 3 years. In the supplemented group there were significant increases in bone mineral density and a 60% reduction in nonvertebral fractures.
(Adapted from Dawson-Hughes B, et al. N Engl J Med. 1997;337:670)

Diet · Osteoporosis

Although osteoporotic fractures occur in the elderly, prevention begins early in life. Achieving peak bone mass during childhood, teenage, and early adult years ensures that reserves of bone mineral will be available to draw on in later years (see pp. 147).[20] Foods rich in the nutrients needed to build bone – particularly calcium, magnesium, manganese, and vitamins A and D – should be consumed regularly during childhood and adolescence. During adulthood, low-fat milk products enriched with vitamin D should be consumed daily to provide calcium and minerals (see Fig. 5.**15**). Even in women taking postmenopausal estrogen, additional calcium will help maintain bone density (see Fig. 5.**16**).[21] Foods rich in boron, a trace element that can conserve calcium stores in bone,[22] should also be emphasized.

Boron-rich foods

- Cabbage
- Dates
- Peas
- Almonds
- Beans
- Hazelnuts
- Apples
- Raisins

Diets in the industrialized countries contain large amounts of food components that increase calcium loss and risk of osteoporosis. Phosphorus (in meats, processed foods, soft drinks) can interfere with bone remodeling and increase calcium loss. Similarly, high intakes of protein, sodium, caffeine, and alcohol increase loss of body calcium.[19] Together with widespread dietary deficiencies of vitamin D,[23,24] calcium, and minerals, these dietary patterns contribute to the epidemic of osteoporosis among older individuals in the industrialized countries.

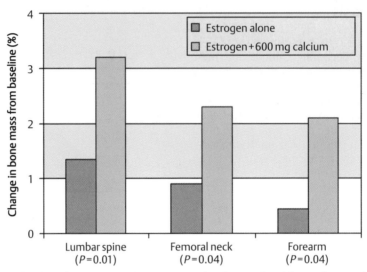

Fig. 5.**16**: **Enhanced effect of estrogens on bone mass with calcium.** The addition of 600 mg/day calcium to the diets of women on estrogen replacement therapy (ERT) (with baseline calcium intakes of 500–600 mg/day) resulted in a significant two to three fold increase in bone mass, when compared with ERT alone. (Adapted from Nieves JW, et al. Am J Clin Nutr. 1998; 67:18)

Micronutrients · Osteoporosis

Nutrient	Suggested daily dose	Comments
Calcium	1 g; for postmenopausal women 1.5 g	Supplemental calcium should be taken in divided doses during the day, with about half the total dose taken at bedtime[25,26]
Vitamin D	10–20 µg	Increases absorption of calcium and maintains bone density.[27,28] Regular exposure to sunshine helps maintain vitamin D levels. Supplements are especially valuable in dark, winter months or for housebound people
Vitamin C	100–250 mg	Needed for synthesis of the proteins in bone; even marginal deficiency can contribute to bone loss
Magnesium	300–500 mg	Activates enzymes essential in bone formation. Deficiency is common in osteoporosis[29]
Multimineral preparation	Should contain ample amounts of manganese, zinc, and copper	The trace minerals manganese, copper, and zinc are important in bone maintenance[30]

Muscle Cramps

Muscle cramps are painful, sudden, involuntary contractions of muscles. They may be triggered by overuse or strain of the muscle. Muscle cramps that occur during strenuous exercise, working in hot weather, or fever may also be a sign of dehydration. Poor circulation with inadequate blood and nutrient supply to an exercising muscle will produce muscle cramping. Nighttime cramps, in the calves and feet are common, particularly in growing children, pregnant women, and older people.[31]

Diet · Cramps

Diets in the industrialized countries are often low in magnesium, calcium, and potassium, and many commonly used drugs, including diuretics and laxatives, increase loss of these important minerals. Low levels of potassium, magnesium, and/or calcium in muscles can trigger spasm and cramps.[31] Daily consumption of fruits, vegetables, low-fat milk products, and whole grains will provide generous amounts of these minerals. Adequate intake of fluid during hot weather and exercise will eliminate cramping caused by dehydration.

Micronutrients · Cramps

Nutrient	Suggested daily dose	Comments
Vitamin E	200–400 mg	Reduces night-time leg cramps.[32] Also helps reduce muscle cramps during pregnancy. During strenuous exercise, oxidative stress contributes to muscle fatigue and cramps; vitamin E helps protect against oxidative stress
Calcium and magnesium	1000 mg and 400 mg	Low levels of calcium increase irritability of nerves and muscles and can produce muscle cramps. Particularly effective for pregnancy-associated leg cramps[31]
Vitamin B complex	Balanced supplement containing 25–50 mg thiamin, niacin, and pantothenic acid	Supports optimum energy metabolism in muscles and helps clear byproducts of exercise (such as lactate) that cause muscles to cramp

References

1. McAlindon TE, et al. Do antioxidant nutrients protect against development and progression of knee osteoarthritis? Arthritis Rheum. 1996;39:648.
2. Machtey I, Ouaknine L. Tocopherol in osteoarthritis: a controlled pilot study. J Am Geriat Soc. 1978;26:328
3. McAlindon TE, et al. Relation of dietary intake and serum levels of vitamin D to progression of osteoarthritis of the knee among participants of the Framingham study. Ann Intern Med. 1996;125:353.
4. Jameson S, et al. Pain relief and selenium balance in patients with connective tissue disease and osteoarthrosis: A double-blind selenium tocopherol supplementation study. Nutr Res Suppl. 1985;1:391.
5. Flynn MA The effect of folate and cobalamin on osteoarthritic hands. J Am Coll Nutr. 1994;13:351.
6. Darlington LG, Ramsey NW. Review of dietary therapy for rheumatoid arthritis. Compr Ther. 1994;20:490.
7. Sperling RI. Eicosanoids in rheumatoid arthritis. Rheum Dis Clin North Am. 1995;21:741.
8. Kjeldsen Kragh J, et al. Vegetarian diet for patients with rheumatoid arthritis–status: two years after introduction of the diet. Clin Rheumatol. 1994;13:475.
9. Kremer JM, Bigaouette J. Nutrient intake of patients with rheumatoid arthritis is deficient in pyridoxine, zinc, copper, and magnesium. J Rheumatol. 1996;23:990.
10. Belch JJF, et al. Effects of altering dietary essential fatty acids on requirements for non-steroidal antiinflammatory drugs in patients with rheumatoid arthritis: A double-blind placebo controlled study. Ann Rheum Dis. 1988;47:96.
11. Kolarz GO, et al. High dose vitamin E in chronic polyarthritis. Aktuelle Rheumatol. 1990;15:233.
12. Zurier RB, et al. Gamma-linolenic acid treatment of rheumatoid arthritis. A randomized, placebo-controlled trial. Arthritis Rhem. 1996;39:1808–17.
13. Pinals RS, et al. Treatment of rheumatoid arthritis with L-histidine: A randomized, placebo-controlled, double-blind trial. J Rheumatol. 1977;4:414.
14. Honkanen VEA, et al. Plasma zinc and copper concentrations in rheumatoid arthritis: Influence of dietary factors and disease activity. Am J Clin Nutr. 1991;54:1082.
15. Peretz A, et al. Effects of zinc supplementation on the phagocytic functions of polymorphonuclears in patients with inflammatory rheumatic diseases. J Trace Elem Electrolytes Health Dis. 1994;8:189.
16. Simkin PA. Treatment of rheumatoid arthritis with oral zinc sulphate. Agents Action Suppl. 1981;8:587.
17. Tarp U. Selenium in rheumatoid arthritis. A review. Analyst. 1995;120:877.
18. Morgan SL. Supplementation with folic acid during methotrexate therapy for rheumatoid arthritis. A double blind, placebo-controlled trial Ann Intern Med. 1994;121:833.

19. Heaney RP. Bone mass, nutrition and other lifestyle factors. Nutr Rev. 1996;54:S3.
20. Teegarden D, Weaver CM. Calcium supplementation increases bone density in adolescent girls. Nutr Rev. 1994;52:171.
21. Nieves JW, et al. Calcium potentiates the effect of estrogen and calcitonin on bone mass: Review and analysis. Am J Clin Nutr. 1997;67:18.
22. Nielsen FH, et al. Boron enhances and mimics some effects of estrogen therapy in postmenopausal women. J Trace Elem Exp Med. 1992;58:237.
23. Villareal DT, et al. Subclinical vitamin D deficiency in postmenopausal women with low vertebral bone mass. J Clin Endocrinol Metab. 1991;72:628.
24. Thomas MK, et al. Hypovitaminosis D in medical inpatients. N Engl J Med. 1998;338:777.
25. Reid IR. Therapy of osteoporosis: Calcium, vitamin D, and exercise. Am J Med Sci. 1996;312:278.
26. Dawson-Hughes B. Calcium supplementation and bone loss: A review of the controlled clinical trials. Am J Clin Nutr. 1991;54:274S.
27. Chapuy MC, et al. Vitamin D_3 and calcium to prevent hip fractures in elderly women. N Engl J Med. 1992;327:1637.
28. Dawson-Hughes B, et al. Effect of vitamin D supplementation on wintertime and overall bone loss in healthy postmenopausal women. Ann Int. Med. 1991;115:505.
29. Münzenberg KJ, Koch W. Mineralogic aspects in the treatment of osteoporosis with magnesium. J Am Coll Nutr. 1989;8:461.
30. King J. Does poor zinc nutriture retard skeletal growth and mineralization in adolescents? Am J Clin Nutr. 1996;64:375.
31. Hammar M, et al. Calcium treatment of leg cramps in pregnancy. Effect on clinical symptoms and total serum and ionized serum calcium concentrations. Acta Obstet Gynecol Scand. 1981;60:345.
32. Cathcart RF. Leg cramps and vitamin E. JAMA. 1972;219:216.

Infectious Diseases

The Immune System

The physical barriers of the skin and epithelia lining the respiratory, digestive, and urinary tracts are the first lines of immune defense. The epithelium of the digestive tract forms a remarkably effective barrier against bacteria: it normally prevents the more than 500 species of bacteria that colonize the colon from invading the body.[1] Similarly, intact skin forms a nearly impenetrable barrier to potential pathogens. Epithelial tissues are very active: cells are continuously shed and replaced with newly developing cells. The entire lining of the small intestine turns over every 4 to 5 days.[1] This rapid growth and turnover of epithelial tissues requires a rich and steady supply of nutrients. Therefore, the skin and the mucosae of the respiratory, digestive, and urinary tracts are highly vulnerable to nutritional deficiencies. After several weeks of a diet lacking in folic acid, the mucosa of the digestive tract will begin to weaken and atrophy. One of the first signs of vitamin A deficiency is abnormal development and function of the cells in the skin, the conjunctiva, and the mucosa of the respiratory tree.

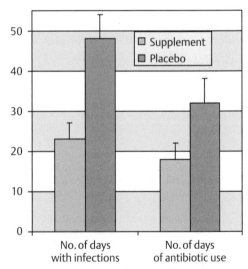

Fig. 5.**17: Decreased risk of infection in older adults with micronutrient supplementation.** 96 healthy elderly people were given a multivitamin/mineral supplement or placebo for 1 year. After 1 year the immune function of the supplement group had significantly improved, and the group had fewer days of infection-related illness and antibiotic use.
(Adapted from Chandra RK. Lancet. 1992;340:1124)

This causes the epithelium to become dry and brittle, and produces microscopic breaks that allow invasion of pathogenic bacteria and viruses. Optimum micronutrition plays a central role in maintaining the health of the epithelial tissue barrier.

Inside the body, both the humoral and cellular components of the immune system are dependent on nutrition. About one out of every 100 cells in the body is a white blood cell. This enormous "defensive army" of white cells is very sensitive to nutrient supply. It can be weakened by even marginal deficiencies of vitamins A, E, C, B6, B12, and folate, as well as lack of the minerals iron, zinc, manganese, copper, and selenium.[2-5] Deficiencies can impair production of new white cells and their and activity against foreign substances and cells. Certain micronutrients (such as vitamins E,[6,7] C,[7] and B6,[8] and selenium and zinc[9]) can boost the immune system, enhance white cell activity, and increase resistance to infection (see Fig. 5.17).

Diet · Immunity

Diets high in refined carbohydrate and saturated fat weaken the immune system. Regular heavy alcohol intake also impairs function of the immune system and increases risk of infection. To maintain immune strength, the diet should supply ample protein, EFAs, and micronutrients. It should emphasize lean meats and low-fat milk products, whole grains, and fresh fruits and vegetables. In addition, certain dietary components – such as garlic and onions – may increase resistance to infection.

Micronutrients · Immunity

Nutrient	Suggested daily dose	Comments
Vitamin A	3000–6000 µg to prevent infection. Up to 30 000 µg to treat active infection. Can be taken as beta-carotene[11]	Enhances immune system function.[10] Deficiency sharply increases risk of infection. Maintains health of skin and mucosal barriers to pathogens. High doses of vitamin A should only be taken under medical supervision
Vitamin C	100–500 mg to prevent infection. Up to 5 g to treat active infection	Enhances immune cell function.[12] May be effective in reducing severity of infections, particularly those caused by viruses[13]
Vitamin E	100–200 mg to prevent infection	Enhances immune cell function[6,7] and may increase reastance to infection, particularly among the elderly
Vitamin B6	25–50 mg to prevent infection. 250–500 mg to treat active infection	Deficiency increases risk of infection. Enhances immune cell function and may increase resistance to infection[8,14]
Zinc	10–20 mg to prevent infection. Up to 100 mg to treat active infection	Deficiency increases risk of infection.[4] Enhances immune cell function and may increase reastance to infection[9]
Selenium	100 µg to prevent infection. 200–400 µg to treat active infection	Deficiency increases risk and severity of infections, particularly those caused by viruses[15,16]

Colds and Influenza

A cold is caused by a viral infection (usually a rhinovirus or coronavirus) of the the nose and throat. The virus produces a self-limited syndrome with symptoms of nasal congestion, discharge, sore throat, sneezing, and cough. On average, children have approximately six to eight colds per year and adults two to three per year. Although colds and influenza are common, especially during wintertime, nutritional support of the immune system may reduce the chances of catching a cold and shorten the duration and severity of symptoms if a cold develops.

Diet · Colds

See the recommendations on pages 196. Drinking plenty of hot fluids usually helps relieve congestion and clear secretions from the nose and throat.

Micronutrients · Colds

Nutrient	Suggested daily dose	Comments
Zinc	15–30 mg to prevent colds. At the first sign of a cold developing, 60–90 mg as 15 mg doses four to six times a day. Particularly effective in the form of tablets or lozenges that dissolve slowly in the mouth before swallowing	Can effectively shorten the duration of a cold and reduce severity of symptoms[17]
Vitamin C	250–500 mg to protect against colds. 1 g to treat a cold	Can help reduce severity and shorten the duration of a cold[12,13]

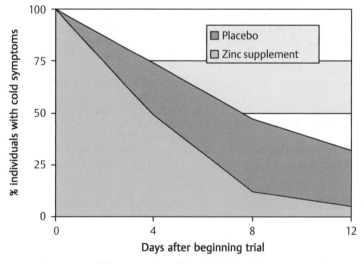

Fig. 5.**18**: **Zinc supplements and the common cold.** 100 adults with acute onset of cold symptoms were given lozenges containing 13.3 mg zinc and told to dissolve a lozenge in their mouth every 2 hours while awake. Treatment with zinc significantly accelerated healing and resolution of symptoms. Median time to resolution of all symptoms was 4.4 days in the zinc group compared with 7.6 days with placebo.
(Adapted from Mossad S, et al. Ann Intern Med. 1996; 125:81)

Viruses that cause colds and influenza can survive for several hours on the skin and other surfaces (such as clothes, towels, and dishes). The virus is usually picked up on the hands and then transferred to the nose, mouth, or eyes where it causes the infection. To help prevent colds, wash the hands thoroughly after shaking hands with a person with a cold or touching objects that have recently been handled by a person with a cold.

Herpes Simplex Infection

There are two main types of herpes simplex viruses (HSV). HSV type 1 infects the tissues around the lips and mouth (and rarely the eye), while HSV type 2 causes genital infections. Herpes produces recurrent clusters of small, painful blisters containing the virus. HSV infections are common: it is estimated that 20–40% of the US population have recurrent infections of one or both forms. HSV type 1, in otherwise healthy adults, is not dangerous, but genital herpes occuring during pregnancy and delivery can produce a life-threatening infection in the newborn. Although most people are exposed to herpes viruses (contact with HSV type 1 is nearly universal), not everyone develops a recurrent infection. Optimum nutrition and stress reduction may help reduce the frequency and severity of infections.

Diet · HSV

See the recommendations on pages 196 for maintaining the strength of the immune system. The dietary ratio of two amino acids may influence herpes infections. High intakes of arginine promote growth of the virus (the herpes virus requires arginine for growth), while higher intakes of lysine may inhibit growth,[18] mainly by reducing the amount of arginine available to the virus. Therefore, a lysine-rich, arginine-poor diet can help reduce recurrence and severity of herpes infections. Foods that have a particularly high ratio of arginine/lysine should be avoided by individuals with recurrent herpes. These include:

● Nuts (particularly almonds, hazelnuts, cashews, and peanuts)

● Chocolate

● Seeds and certain grains (wheat, oats)

● Raisins, gelatin

Micronutrients · HSV

Nutrient	Suggested daily dose	Comments
Lysine	500 mg to help prevent recurrences, 2–4 g during active infection	Along with supplemental lysine, reduce intake of arginine-rich foods. May reduce severity and frequency of outbreaks[18]
Vitamin C	250–500 mg to help prevent recurrences. 1 g to help treat active infections	Has anti-viral action and may help reduce the severity and shorten the duration of recurrent infections[19]
Vitamin E	Apply topically to blisters several times a day)	May help reduce pain and enhance healing
Zinc	15–30 mg to help prevent recurrences, 60–100 mg during active infection. Can also be applied topically in zinc-containing creams or lotions	Has anti-viral action and may help reduce the severity and shorten the duration of recurrent infections[20]

HIV Infection and Acquired Immunodeficiency Syndrome (AIDS)

AIDS is caused by the human immunodeficiency virus (HIV). It can be transmitted during unprotected sex, from contaminated needles shared by intravenous drug users, and from a pregnant mother to her baby. HIV invades white blood cells (T cells), multiplies, and then destroys the cells. As T cell counts fall, the cellular immune response weakens, increasing vulnerability to infection and cancer. Many people infected with HIV carry the virus for years without developing AIDS: only about one in four HIV-infected people develop AIDS in the first 5 years after initial infection. Many remain healthy carriers of HIV, while others progress quickly to AIDS. In HIV disease, a critical determinant of progression is nutritional status. A combination of carefully selected diet, prudent micronutrient supplementation, moderate exercise, and a supportive social environment can maintain optimum immune function and, along with effective drug therapy, can slow progression of the disease.[21–23]

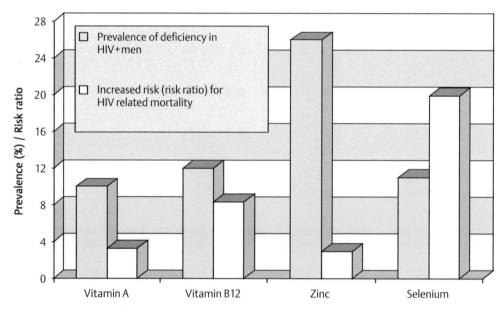

Fig. 5.**19**: **Micronutrient deficiencies and HIV-related mortality.** A high prevalence of micronutrient deficiencies is found in HIV-positive adults: 89% are deficient in at least one micronutrient and 41% have multiple abnormalities. An increased risk of HIV-related mortality was associated with micronutrient deficiencies in 125 HIV-positive men and women followed for 3.5 years. Particularly dramatic was the nearly 20-fold increase in risk of mortality in selenium-deficient individuals.
(Adapted from Baum MK, et al. Nutr Rev. 1998; 56:S135)

Diet · HIV

See recommendations on pages 196 for a healthy immune system. The diet should emphasize whole grains and fresh fruits and vegetables. Intake of refined carbohydrates, sugar, saturated fat, and alcohol should be reduced. Foods rich in vitamins A, C, E, B6, and the minerals zinc and selenium should be eaten regularly.[22,23]

Micronutrients · HIV

Nutrient	Suggested daily dose	Comments
Vitamin A	3000–8000 µg as retinol or beta-carotene	Maintains health of the skin and digestive-tract epithelium. Can help reduce risk of respiratory infection[24]
Vitamin C	0.5 g-1.0 g	May help inhibit viral growth and maintain immune strength[6,25]
Vitamin B6	100–250 mg	Can enhance immune function[8] and resistance to infection
Vitamin E	200–400 mg	May reduce oxidant damage from infection and help maintain immune response to the virus[7,25]
Zinc	30–60 mg	Can enhance immune function and resistance to infection[26]
Selenium	200–300 µg	Deficiency sharply increases risk of progression and disease severity[16,27]
Arginine plus glutamine	2–3 g arginine, 3–5 g glutamine	Arginine stimulates production of white blood cells,[28] glutamine supports the immune system and increases white blood cell function[29]

References

1. Mainous MR, Deitch EA. The gut barrier. In: Zaloga GP, ed. Nutrition in Critical Care. St. Louis: Mosby; 1994:557.
2. Grimble RF. Effect of antioxidative vitamins on immune function with clinical applications. Internat J Vit Nutr Res. 1997;67:312.
3. Lesourd BM, et al. The role of nutrition in immunity in the aged. Nutr Rev. 1998;56:S113.
4. Solomons NW. Mild zinc deficiency produces an imbalance between cell-mediated and humoral immunity. Nutr Rev. 1998;56:27.
5. Dallman PR. Iron deficiency and the immune response. Am J Clin Nutr. 1987;46:329.
6. Jeng KCG, et al. Supplementation with vitamins C and E enhances cytokine production by peripheral blood mononuclear cells in healthy adults. Am J Clin Nutr. 1996;64:960.
7. Meydani SN, Beharka AA. Recent developments in vitamin E and immune response. Nutr Rev. 1998;56:S49.
8. Rall LC, Meydani SN. Vitamin B6 and immune competence. Nutr Rev. 1993;51:217.
9. Bogden JD, et al. Effects of one year of supplementation with zinc and other micronutrients on cellular immunity in the elderly. J Nutr. 1990;3:214.
10. Semba RD. The role of vitamin A and related retinoids in immune function. Nutr Rev. 1998;56:S38.
11. Bendich A. Carotenoids and the immune response. J Nutr. 1989;119:112.
12. Anderson R. The immunostimulatory, anti-inflammatory and anti-allergic properties of ascorbate. Adv Nutr Res. 1984;6:19.
13. Hemilia H. Vitamin C intake and susceptibility to the common cold. Br J Nutr. 1997;77:59.
14. Talbott MC, et al. Pyridoxine supplementation: Effect on lymphocyte responses in elderly persons. Am J Clin Nutr. 1987;46:659.
15. Kiremidjian-Schumacher L, Stotzky G. Selenium and immune responses. Environ Res. 1987;42:277.
16. Baum MK, et al. High risk of HIV-related mortality is associated with selenium deficiency. J Acquir Immune Def Syndr Hum Retrovirol. 1997;15:370.
17. Mossad SB, et al. Zinc gluconate lozenges for treating the common cold. Ann Intern Med. 1996;125:81.
18. Griffith RS, et al. Success of L-lysine therapy in frequently recurrent herpes simplex infection. Dermatologica. 1987;175:183.
19. Terezhalmy GT, et al. The use of water-soluble bioflavonoid-ascorbic acid complex in the treatment of recurrent herpes labialis. Oral Surg. 1978;45:56.
20. Eby G. Use of topical zinc to prevent recurrent herpes simplex infection: Review of literature and suggested protocols. Med Hypotheses. 1985;17:157.
21. Tang AM, et al. Effects of micronutrient intake on survival in HIV-1 infection. Am J Epidemiol. 1996;143:1244.

22. Gorbach SL, et al. Interactions between nutrition and infection with HIV. Nutr Rev. 1993;51:226.
23. Baum MK, Shor-Posner G. Micronutrient status in relationship to mortality in HIV-1 disease. Nutr Rev. 1998;56:S135.
24. Ross AC, Stephenson CB. Vitamin A and retinoids in antiviral responses. FASEB J. 1996;10:979.
25. Allard JP, et al. Oxidative stress and plasma antioxidant micronutrients in humans with HIV infection. Am J Clin Nutr. 1998;67:143.
26. Faluz J, Tsoukas C, Gold P. Zinc as a cofactor in human immunodeficiency virus-induced immunosuppression. JAMA. 1988;259:2850.
27. Kalebic T, et al. Suppression of human immunodeficiency virus expression in chronically infected monocytic cells by glutathione, glutathione ester, and N-acetylcysteine. Proc Natl Acad Sci USA. 1991;88:986.
28. Barbul A. Arginine and immune function. Nutr. 1990;6:53.
29. Calder PC. Glutamine and the immune system. Clin Nutr. 1994;13:2.

Cancer

Cell division is normally carefully controlled, but in cancer a cell breaks free from normal regulation and begins dividing out of control. Many cancers begin when the DNA of the cell is damaged by a carcinogen. About one in three people will develop cancer during their lifetime. A major factor contributing to the high rates of cancer in the industrialized countries is the combination of increased exposure to carcinogens – enviromental chemicals, air pollution, food additives, cigarette smoke, radiation – together with a highly processed diet high in fat and low in protective micronutrients. Dietary factors, as initiators or promoters of cancer, are estimated to play a role in about 50% of all cases.[1] With healthy dietary choices and prudent micronutrient supplementation, risk of cancer can be reduced significantly (see Fig. 5.**20**).[2]

Diet · Cancer

Different dietary factors have been identified as either promoters (encouraging cancer growth) or inhibitors (discouraging cancer growth).

Dietary substances that promote cancer and should be avoided[1,3]

- High intake of fat, especially saturated fat from meat products
- Burned or darkly browned foods, such as heavily roasted or barbecued meats
- Nitrites and nitrates (food preservatives used to give processed meats a pink color)
- Pesticides and other agrochemicals
- Regular heavy alcohol intake
- Processed meats (such as sausages, luncheon meats, smoked, pickled, or salt-cured meats)
- Rancid (oxidized) fats, such as fat used repeatedly for deep-fat frying
- Old, mouldy foods; particularly potatoes, peanuts, mushrooms, sprouts
- Artificial food dyes
- Heavily chlorinated drinking water

Dietary substances that reduce risk of cancer and should be eaten regularly[1,2,4]

- Fiber-rich foods (whole grains, bran, fruits, vegetables, legumes, seeds)
- Dark-green and yellow-orange vegetables
- "Cruciferous" vegetables: broccoli, Brussels sprouts, cabbage, cauliflower
- Fresh beet, carrot, asparagus, and cabbage juices
- Onions and garlic
- Calcium-rich foods (see Fig. 5.**21**)
- Fresh fruit and fruit juices

Maintaining a reasonable body weight is important: obesity increases risk of cancer of the breast, colon, prostate, and uterus.

Micronutrients · Cancer

Nutrient	Suggested daily dose	Comments
Selenium	200 µg	Supplementation reduces risk of cancer.[5,6] An essential component of antioxidant enzyme systems that can protect cells and DNA from oxidant damage. Deficiency increases risk of cancer
Vitamin A	1000 µg	Regulates development of the epithelium of the oropharynx, the digestive and respiratory tracts, and the skin.[7-9] Supplementation may reduce risk of cancer
Vitamin C	250–500 mg	An antioxidant that protects cells and DNA from oxidant damage.[10] Particularly effective in reducing risk of lung cancer[11] and stomach cancer from processed meats containing nitrites[12]
Vitamin E	200 mg	An antioxidant that protects cell membranes and DNA from oxidant damage. May reduce risk of cancer[6,13-15]
Folic acid plus vitamin B12	0.4 mg folic acid; 10–20 µg vitamin B12	Maintains healthy development of digestive and respiratory epithelium. May reduce risk of cancer of the bronchi and lung, particularly in smokers[16]
Calcium plus vitamin D	1 g calcium; 10 µg vitamin D	May reduce risk of colon cancer[17-19]

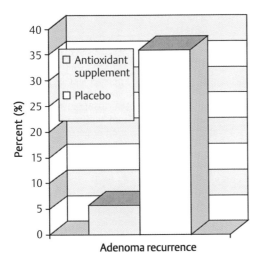

Fig. 5.**20**: **Antioxidant vitamins and colonic polyps.** In 209 patients with a history of a precancerous adenoma, a daily supplement containing vitamin E (70 mg), vitamin C (1 g), and vitamin A (30 000 IU) given for 18 months sharply reduced the recurrence rate (5.7% compared with 35.9% in the placebo group).
(Adapted from Roncucci L, et al. Dis Colon Rectum. 1993;36:227)

Very high doses of vitamins A, C, E, and selenium are potentially beneficial as adjuvants in cancer treatment.[20] In addition, high-dose supplements of niacin, vitamin E, and coenzyme Q10 can be beneficial in reducing toxicity of chemotherapy and radiation therapy. These treaments require expertise and should be considered only with an oncologist.

References

1. Trichopoulos D, et al. What causes cancer? The top two causes–tobacco and diet–account for almost two-thirds of all cancer deaths and are among the most correctable. Sci American. 1996;9:50.
2. Dwyer JT. Diet and nutritional strategies for cancer risk reduction. Focus on the 21st century. Cancer. 1993;72:1024.
3. Fontham ETH. Prevention of upper gastrointestinal tract cancers. In: Bendich A, Deckelbaum RJ, eds. Preventive Nutrition. Torowa, New Jersey: Humana; 1997:33.
4. Steinmetz KA, Potter JD. Vegetables, fruit and cancer prevention: A review. J Am Diet Assoc. 1996;96:1027.
5. Clark LC, et al. Effects of selenium supplementation for cancer prevention in patients with carcinoma of the skin. JAMA. 1996;276:1957.
6. Blot WJ, et al. Nutrition intervention trials in Linxian, China. Supplementation with specific vitamin/mineral combinations, cancer incidence and disease spe-

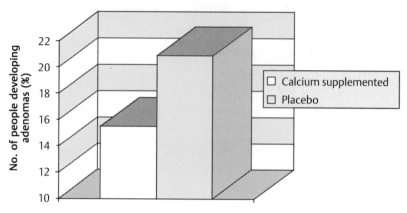

Fig. 5.**21**: **Calcium supplementation and colon adenomas.** In a study of 552 adults, treatment with calcium (2 g/day) reduced risk of developing precancerous adenomas by 34% compared to placebo. Source: Bonithon-Kopp C, et al. Lancet 2000; 356:1300

cific mortality in the general population. J Natl Cancer Inst. 1993;85:1483.

7. De Luca LM, et al. Vitamin A in epithelial differentiation and skin carcinogenesis. Nutr Rev. 1994;52:45.

8. Stich HF, et al. Remission of precancerous lesions in the oral cavity of tobacco chewers and maintenance of the protective effect of beta-carotene or vitamin A. Am J Clin Nutr. 1991;53:S298.

9. Willet WC, Hunter DJ. Vitamin A and cancers of the breast, large bowel and prostate: Epidemiologic evidence. Nutr Rev. 1994;52:53.

10. Block G. Epidemiologic evidence regarding vitamin C and cancer. Am J Clin Nutr. 1991;54:S1310.

11. Comstock GW, Helzlouser KJ. Prevention of upper gastrointestinal tract cancers. In: Bendich A, Deckelbaum RJ, eds. Preventive Nutrition. Torowa, New Jersey: Humana; 1997:109.

12. Kim Y, Mason JB. Nutritional chemoprevention of gastrointestinal cancers. Nutr Rev. 1996;54:259.

13. DeCosse JJ, et al. Effect of wheat fiber and vitamins C and E on rectal polyps in patients with familial adenomatous polyposis. J Natl Can Inst. 1989;81:1290.

14. Garewal HS, Schantz S. Emerging role of beta-carotene and antioxidant nutrients in prevention of oral cancer. Arch Otolaryngol Head Neck Surg. 1995;121:141.

15. Trickler D, Shikler G. Prevention by vitamin E of experimental oral carcinogenesis. J Natl Can Inst. 1987;78:165.

16. Heimburger DC, et al. Improvement in bronchial squamous metaplasia in smokers treated with folate and vitamin B12. JAMA. 1988;259:1525.

17. Rozen P, et al. Oral calcium suppresses increased rectal epithelial proliferation of persons at risk of colorectal cancer. Gut. 1989;30:650.

18. Garland CF, et al. Can colon cancer incidence and death rates be reduced with calcium and vitamin D? Am J Clin Nutr. 1991;54:S193.

19. Bostick RM. Diet and Nutrition in the etiology and primary prevention of colon cancer. In: Bendich A, Deckelbaum RJ, eds. Preventive Nutrition. Torowa, New Jersey: Humana; 1997:57.

20. Cameron E, Pauling L. Supplemental ascorbate in the supportive treatment of cancer: Prolongation of survival times in terminal human cancer. Proc Natl Acad Sci USA. 1976;73:3685.

Allergic Disorders

Allergic Rhinitis

Allergic rhinitis is an allergic reaction in the lining tissues of the nose and eyes, usually triggered by airborne environmental allergens. Symptoms include nasal congestion, red and itchy conjunctiva, sneezing, and a watery discharge. Pollens (trees, grass, flowering plants), dust, animal hairs, and feathers are common triggers. Less commonly, allergic rhinitis can be a manifestation of food sensitivity.[1]

Micronutrients · Rhinitis

Nutrient	Suggested daily dose	Comments
Vitamin C	250–750 mg	Increases breakdown of histamine produced by the allergic response[2] and thereby reduces symptoms
GLA	As 1–2 g evening primrose oil	Reduces inflammation and congestion,[3] rebalances the immune response

Asthma

Asthma is a common atopic disorder characterized by airway inflammation, hyperresponsiveness, and reversible airway obstruction. Asthma causes episodes of wheezing, coughing, and shortness of breath. It can be triggered by inhaled allergens, stress, exercise, cold air, or can be a symptom of food sensitivity.[1]

Diet · Asthma

Asthma may improve if food sensitivities are diagnosed and offending foods eliminated.[1,4] Diets high in sodium may increase reactivity of the bronchi to histamine, thus asthmatics should minimize salt intake. Asthmatics should also avoid foods containing sulfite additives. Sulfites are added as preservatives to certain fresh vegetables, salads, potatoes, and wine and can trigger asthma.[5]

Micronutrients · Asthma

Nutrient	Suggested daily dose	Comments
Vitamin C	1–2 g	Increases breakdown of histamine produced in the asthmatic response and reduces frequency and severity of asthma.[2,6] Particularly effective against asthma triggered by exercise
Omega-3 fatty acids	2–4 g as fish-oil capsules	Reduces inflammation and may decrease symptoms[12,13]
Magnesium	400 mg	Can reduce severity of attacks and improve lung function.[7,8] Magnesium deficiency is common among asthmatics
Vitamin B6	50–100 mg	May reduce frequency and severity of asthmatic attacks[9–11]
Vitamin B12	50–100 µg	May reduce frequency and severity of asthmatic attacks, particularly those triggered by sulfites in foods[5]

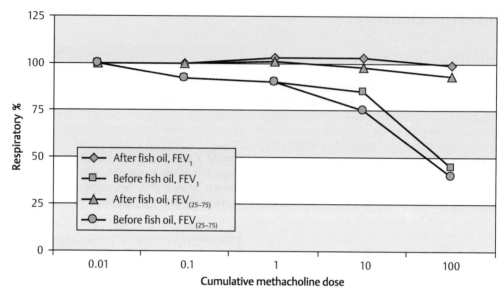

Fig. 5.**22**: **Fish-oil supplements in asthma.** A trial in 26 atopic asthmatics compared respiratory function in response to a methacholine challenge before and after 4 weeks of supplemental fish oil (3.3 g EPA and DHA). In 40% of the subjects, treatment with fish oil significantly reduced bronchoconstriction (as measured by improved forced expiratory volume for 1 sec (FEV_1) and forced expiratory flow 25–75% (FEF_{25-75}). (From Broughton KS, et al. Am J Clin Nutr. 1997; 65:1011)

Food Allergies and Sensitivities

Food sensitivities occur when a component of the diet triggers an allergic reaction or an abnormal, "overzealous" immune response.[14,15] Food sensitivities can cause histamine-mediated allergic reactions resulting in itching, swelling, and hives. They can also trigger autoimmune reactions, where immune cells activated by exposure to the food component cross-react with and harm the body's own tissues. Sensitivity can develop to foods or food additives and can produce a wide variety of symptoms. Symptoms can be confined to the digestive tract, such as bloating, cramping, diarrhea, or irritable bowel syndrome.[1,15] They can also occur in parts of the body far away from the digestive tract, such as the joints (arthritis), skin (swelling and hives) and brain (headache).[1,4,15] Symptoms can occur immediately after eating the food, or may be delayed for hours.

Diet · Allergies

Food sensitivity can develop at any age but is particularly common in infants and young children. About 7–10% of children exhibit food allergies during their growing years.[1] Colic in babies may be caused by sensitivity to a food – a common allergen is the protein in cow's milk. Adults can also develop sensitivity reactions, particularly when the immune system is knocked "off-balance" by stress, illness, food additives, and poor nutrition.

Food allergies are often difficult to identify. Although many diagnostic tests have been tried, none is entirely satisfactory. Elimination of suspected foods from the diet is the most direct and reliable method; if one of the eliminated foods was causing the reaction, improvement will occur.[1,4,14] Foods must be eliminated for at least 5 days (and often for 2–4 weeks) to allow time for their adverse effects to completely disappear. If improvement occurs, the eliminated foods should be reintroduced one at a time to pinpoint the specific problem food. To discriminate between the effects of different foods, one food should be reintroduced about every 3 days. Keeping a food diary – recording the days and times foods are reintroduced and recording changes in symptoms is helpful to keep things straight.

Foods that continue to be eaten during an elimination diet should be those least suspected of triggering symptoms. If there is uncertainty over which foods to eliminate and which to continue eating, the most practical approach is the common food elimination diet. In this diet, only foods that are normally eaten more than twice a week are eliminated. More difficult is a two-food diet, such as the lamb-and-pear diet, where only two less commonly eaten foods – one supplying protein and fat, the other carbohydrate – are eaten. The remaining foods are then gradually reintroduced, one by one. Clearly, elimination diets can be difficult, and food reintroduction may take several months. However, they remain the "gold standard" test of food sensitivity.[1,4,14]

Because a food once caused a sensitivity reaction doesn't mean it will continue to do so. More than three-quarters of children with food allergies grow out of them. Reducing stress can reduce susceptibility to allergies. Nutritional deficiencies may increase vulnerability to food sensitivity reactions, which can gradually clear with proper diet and prudent nutritional supplementation.

Potential Symptoms[1,15]

- Acne

- Arthritis

- Asthma

- Abdominal pain and bloating

- Diarrhea

- Fatigue

- Swelling and fluid retention

- Headaches

- Nasal congestion

- Poor memory and concentration

- Repeated colds, sinus and inner ear problems

- Itchy, watery eyes

Most Common Dietary Triggers of Food Sensitivity Reactions[1,4,14,15]

- Wheat, oats, corn

- Eggs

- Milk products

- Beef and pork

- Fish and shellfish

- Citrus fruits

- Peanuts

- Tomatoes

- Chocolate, tea, coffee

- Alcohol

- Food colorings, additives, and preservatives
    - Monosodium glutamate (MSG)
    - Sulfites
    - Colorings, tartrazine (yellow dye)
    - Benzoates
    - Vanillin

Micronutrients · Allergies

Nutrient	Suggested daily dose	Comments
Vitamin C	1–2 g	Increases breakdown of histamine produced by the allergic response[2], thereby reducing symptoms
Vitamin B6	50–100 mg	May reduce food sensitivities, particularly to additives such as monosodium glutamate
Omega-3 fatty acids	2–4 g as fish-oil capsules	Reduces inflammation and may decrease symptoms[12,13]
Vitamin B12	50–100 µg	May reduce food sensitivity, particularly to sulfites[5]

References

1. Bruijnzeel-Koomen C, et al. Adverse reactions to foods: European Academy of Allergology and Clinical Immunology Position Paper. Allergy. 1995;50:623.
2. Bucca C, et al. Effect of vitamin C on histamine bronchial responsiveness of patients with allergic rhinitis. Ann Allergy. 1990;65:311.
3. Melnik BC, Plewig G. Is the origin of atopy linked to deficient conversion of omega-6-fatty acids to prostaglandin E1? J Am Acad Dermtol. 1989;21:557.
4. Terho EO, Savolainen J. Review: Diagnosis of food hypersensitivity. Eur J Clin Nutr. 1996;50:1.
5. Anonymous. Vitamin B12 confirmed as effective sulfite allergy blocker. Allergy Observ. 1987;4:1.
6. Bielory L, Gandhi R. Asthma and vitamin C. Ann Allergy. 1994;73:89.
7. Monem GF, et al Use of magnesium sulfate in asthma in childhood. Pediatr Ann. 1996;25:139.
8. Rolla G, et al. Reduction of histamine-induced bronchoconstriction by magnesium in asthmatic subjects. Allergy. 1987;42:286.
9. Anonymous. Can B6 add to asthma therapy? Med World News. 1986;8:63.
10. Reynolds RD, Natta CL. Depressed plasma pyridoxal phosphate concentrations in adult asthmatics. Am J Clin Nutr. 1985;41:684.
11. Shimizu T, et al. Theophylline attenuates circulating vitamin B6 levels in children with asthma. Pharmacology. 1994;49:392.
12. Arm J, et al. The effects of dietary supplementation with fish oil on asthmatic responses to antigen. J Clin Allergy. 1988;81:183.
13. Blok WL. Modulation of inflammation and cytokine production by dietary (n-3) fatty acids. J Nutr. 1996;126:1515.
14. Bock SA, Atkins FM. Patterns of food hypersensitivity during sixteen years of double-blind, placebo-controlled foood challenges. J Pediatrics. 1990;117:561.
15. Wüthrich B, et al.: Food allergy. Internist. 1995;36:1052.

Insomnia

Individual needs for sleep vary. A good night's sleep is whatever allows a person to feel rested, refreshed, and alert during the day. Some people need 9 to 10 hours, while others only 6 hours. Insomnia is a persistent difficulty in obtaining adequate sleep. Symptoms can include difficulty in falling asleep, frequent awakenings with difficulty falling back asleep, or poor quality, light sleep. Between 25% and 30% of adults suffer from insomnia. Insomnia can have many causes, including stress, depression, anxiety, or poor nutrition.

Diet · Insomnia

For the evening meal, foods that contain a high tryptophan to total protein ratio should be eaten. Tryptophan is the precursor for brain synthesis of serotonin, a sleep-inducing neurotransmitter (see pp. 109).[1] Eating a tryptophan-rich supper (or late-evening snack) together with ample carbohydrate can improve sleep quality. Carbohydrates stimulate production of insulin, and insulin enhances uptake of tryptophan into the brain.

Although alcohol has a sedative effect that can hasten sleep onset, heavy alcohol intake often produces light, unsettled sleep and increases nighttime awakening. Because alcohol can interfere with deep sleep, alcoholic "nightcaps" should generally be avoided A better bedtime drink is a glass of warm milk. Milk is rich in tryptophan and calcium, both of which have a calming effect and may improve sleep quality.

The more caffeine consumed during the day, the higher the risk of insomnia. Consumption of coffee, tea, or cola drinks should be avoided within 6 hours of bedtime and minimized during the day. Some individuals are sensitive to small amounts of natural stimulants found in aged cheeses, bacon, ham, sausages, sauerkraut, eggplant, spinach, and tomatoes, and these foods may contribute to insomnia if eaten in the evening. Low nighttime blood-sugar levels can cause frequent or early awakening and may be a sign of reactive hypoglycemia (see pp. 185.)[2]

Foods with a high tryptophan: protein ratio

- Walnuts
- Milk and milk products
- Soybeans and soy products
- Eggs
- Bananas
- Fish

Micronutrients · Insomnia

Nutrient	Suggested daily dose	Comments
Tryptophan	1–3 g 30 min before bedtime	Helps improve sleep patterns[1,3,4]
Melatonin	1–5 mg 30–60 min before bedtime	Particularly effective in individuals over 50 years with chronic insomnia[5]
Calcium	600 mg 30 min before bedtime	Has calming effects and may improve sleep quality

References

1. Young SN. Behavioral effects of dietary neurotransmitter precursors: basic and clinical aspects. Neurosci Biobehav Rev. 1996;20:313.
2. Hofeldt FD. Reactive hypoglycemia. Endocrinol Metab Clin North Am. 1989;18:185.
3. Wyatt RJ, et al. Effects of L-tryptophan (a natural sedative) on human sleep. Lancet. 1970;1:842.
4. Hartman E, Spinweber CL. Sleep induced by L-tryptophan: Effect of dosages within the normal dietary intake. J Nerv Ment Dis. 1979;167:497.
5. Garfinkel D, et al. Improvement of sleep quality in elderly people by controlled release melatonin. Lancet. 1995;346:541.

Nervous System Disorders I

Migraine

Migraine headaches appear to be caused by abnormal constriction and dilation of blood vessels supplying the brain. First, blood vessels narrow, producing the "aura" of migraine, typically accompanied by visual disturbances or the appearance of sparkling lights in the visual field. Then, the vessels dilate, producing headache, nausea, and sensitivity to bright lights and noise. Migraines can also occur without a discernable aura. The pain is usually throbbing and located on one side of the head. Many different factors can trigger migraine, including stress, illness, weather changes, nutrient imbalances, and food sensitivities.[1]

Diet · Migraine

Foods are often triggers for migraine. Potential food sensitivities should try to be identified; elimination diets can pinpoint the offending foods (see pp. 205).[1] Reactive hypoglycemia may also trigger migraines (see pp. 185).[2]

Substances that may trigger migraine	Food sources
Vasoactive amines are substances that cause blood vessel dilation (tyramine and phenylethylamine are the most common forms)	Red wine, aged cheese, chicken liver, pickled herring, sausage and processed meat, sour cream, chocolate, bananas, pork, onions
Lactose (milk sugar) in people who are lactose intolerant	Dairy products
Ethanol	Alcoholic beverages
Aspartame	Artificially swetened products
Nitrites (meat preservatives and colorings)	Sausage, salami, processed meats
Caffeine	Coffee, soft drinks, chocolate, tea
Copper (foods with high copper content can dilate blood vessels and stimulate migraine)	Chocolate, nuts, shellfish, wheat germ
Monosodium glutamate (flavor enhancer)	Processed foods

Micronutrients · Migraine

Nutrient	Suggested daily dose	Comments
Magnesium plus vitamin B6	400–600 mg magnesium; 50 mg vitamin B6	Low levels of magnesium in the body may increase risk of blood vessel constriction and spasm.[3,4] Particularly effective in women who have migraines associated with the menstrual period or during pregnancy
Omega-3 fatty acids	2–4 g EPA (as fish-oil capsules	May reduce frequency and intensity of migraines[5]
Vitamin D plus calcium	10 µg vitamin D; 600 mg calcium	May reduce frequency and intensity of migraines[6]
Riboflavin	200–400 mg	May reduce frequency and intensity of migraines[6]

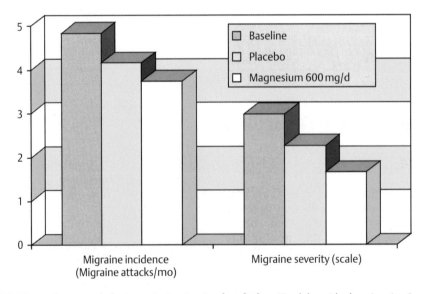

Fig. 5.23: **Magnesium prophylaxis against migraine headache.** 43 adults with chronic migraines received either 600 mg/day magnesium or placebo for 2 months. The severity and incidence of migraines was significantly reduced in the magnesium group vs. placebo.
(Adapted from Taubert K. Forschrit Ther. 1994; 112:328)

Carpal Tunnel Syndrome

Carpal tunnel syndrome (CTS) is a painful disorder of the wrist and hand caused by compression of the median nerve as it enters the hand through the narrow "tunnel" formed by the wrist bones. Repeated movements of the hand and wrist – such as typing, working on an assembly line, or piano playing – can cause inflammation of the tissues surrounding the nerve and compression of the nerve. This causes pain and stiffness in the hand and wrist, along with weakness, numbness, and tingling in the fingers. Fluid retention during menstrual periods or pregnancy can also compress the nerve and cause CTS.

Diet · CTS

Food sensitivities are an occasional cause of swelling in the wrists and can trigger CTS. An elimination diet (see pp. 205) can identify food sensitivities; avoiding the offending foods may provide significant relief.

Micronutrients · CTS

Nutrient	Suggested daily dose	Comments
Vitamin B6 plus magnesium	100–200 mg vitamin B6, 400–600 mg magnesium	May reduce inflammation, swelling, and symptoms[7]
Thiamine	50–100 mg	May reduce inflammation and pain[8,9]
Vitamin E	400–800 mg	May reduce inflammation and symptoms[10]

Learning Disabilities (see also hyperactivity)

Children are termed "learning disabled" when their academic level is 2 years or more behind normal for their age. Dyslexia is a learning disorder in which mastering words and symbols is difficult. Learning requires intelligence, motivation, and the ability to concentrate, all of which can be influenced by nutrition during childhood.

Diet · Learning Disabilities

Suboptimum micronutrient intake during childhood can be a cause of learning disability.[11] Deficiencies of iron, magnesium, iodine, and zinc can reduce learning ability, and even marginal deficiencies can have subtle adverse effects. For example, moderate iron deficiency during early childhood and adolescence can decrease IQ and mental development.[12,13] Along with minerals and vitamins, a rich supply of essential PUFAs is important. The omega-3 fatty acids (found in fish and shellfish) are critical to the formation of neurons and their supporting tissues in the brain during early childhood.[14] Food sensitivities can play a role in learning disabilities in children, particularly sensitivities to food ad-

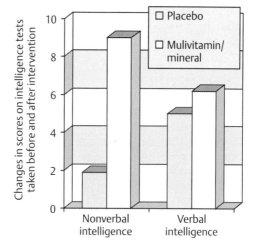

Fig. 5.**24**: **Multivitamin/mineral supplementation and intelligence in schoolchildren.** 60 12-year-old British schoolchildren were given a multivitamin/mineral supplement or placebo for 8 months. In the group receiving treatment, scores on a test of nonverbal intelligence (Calvert test) increased significantly, compared with placebo.
(Adapted from Benton D, et al. Lancet. 1988;1:140)

ditives (see pp. 205). [15] Children have only limited body stores of glucose (the sugar used by the brain for energy) and are thus sensitive to missed meals. Skipping breakfast can im-

pair concentration and learning ability at school.[16] A nutritious breakfast restores energy stores used up overnight and maintains energy levels and ability to concentrate.

Micronutrients · Learning Disabilities

Nutrient	Suggested daily dose	Comments
Multimineral supplement	Balanced supply of all the essential minerals and trace elements, including 5–10 mg iron	Iron deficiency is common among children and adolescents, and deficiencies of iron and other minerals can reduce learning ability [11–13]
Omega-3 fatty acids	1–2 g EPA (as fish-oil capsules)	Critical for optimum brain development and mental function[14]
Vitamin B Complex	Complete formula containing 10 mg thiamin and vitamin B6, 25 µg vitamin B12, and 0.4 mg folic acid	Deficiencies of the B vitamins, particularly thiamin (B1), folic acid, vitamin B6 and B12, can interfere with the ability to concentrate and learn[11,17,18]

Chronic environmental exposure to trace amounts of lead during childhood can impair intelligence and learning ability.[19] Lead is a common contaminant of water and food. Another source is older housepaints (which produce small paint chips and dust that can be ingested by small children), containing very high amounts of lead (see pp. 146).

Hyperactivity

Hyperactivity (attention-deficit hyperactivity disorder or ADHD) is a behavioral disturbance characterized by short attention span, restlessness, and distractability. It usually develops before age 6–7 years, and although the majority of children grow out this disorder, in rare cases it can continue into adulthood. Hyperactivity can seriously impair function and learning at home and at school.

Diet · Hyperactivity

Breakfast is the crucial meal for children with ADHD. Skipping breakfast can cause drops in blood sugar that can trigger restlessness and irritability.[16] Breakfasts high in protein and calcium have a calming influence in many

children and improve learning capability in ADHD. Children may be sensitive to high amounts of phosphates present in certain foods, including sausages, processed foods, milk products, and soft drinks. Food sensitivites can produce or aggravate ADHD.[15, 20,21] Artificial food colors and flavors, as well as foods containing natural salicylates may trigger ADHD, and the Feingold Diet may be helpful in some children with hyperactivity.[22]

Foods to be avoided in children with ADHD (the Feingold Diet)[22]:

● Foods containing natural salicylates

almonds	apple cider and vinegar
apricots	blackberries
cherries	cloves
cucumbers	pickles
grapes	raisins
mint flavors	nectarines
oranges	peaches
plums	strawberries
tomatoes	wine vinegar
raspberries	

● All foods containing artificial colors, sweeteners, and flavors

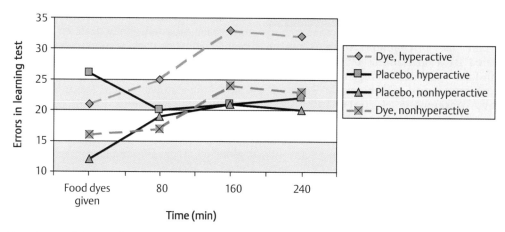

Fig. 5.**25**: **Food dyes and hyperactivity.** 40 children (20 hyperactive and 20 nonhyperactive) were challenged with 100–150 mg of a blend of artificial food dyes or placebo. On learning tests administered over the next 4 hours, the behavior of the hyperactive children significantly deteriorated when challenged with the dyes, compared with the nonhyperactive children and placebo.
(Adapted from Swanson JM, et al. Science. 1980; 207:1485)

Micronutrients · Hyperactivity

Nutrient	Suggested daily dose	Comments
Vitamin B Complex	Complete formula emphasizing thiamin (B1) and vitamin B6	May produce improvement in behavior and attention[1]
Essential PUFAs	Omega-3 fatty acids (1–2 g EPA as fish-oil capsules) plus GLA as 1–2 g evening primrose oil	PUFA metabolism may be abnormal in children with ADHD,[23] and deficiencies of omega-3 and omega-6 fatty acids are found in many children with ADHD[23]
Multimineral supplement	Balanced supplement containing ample amounts of zinc and magnesium	Deficiencies of magnesium and zinc may aggravate ADHD

Epilepsy

Epilepsy is a disease characterized by recurrent seizures. Seizures occur when large numbers of brain neurons fire simultaneously and uncontrollably. Although risk for epilepsy may be inherited, susceptibilty to seizures can be increased by high fever, brain injury, or certain metabolic defects, some of which are responsive to nutritional therapy.[24] In addition to traditional anticonvulsants, micronutrients can play important adjuvant roles in seizure control.

Diet · Epilepsy

Certain types of childhood seizures can be treated by a specialized low-carbohydrate, high-fat diet (termed a ketogenic diet) that requires careful medical supervision.[25] Chronic heavy consumption of alcohol can trigger seizures, as can abruptly stopping alcohol in- take after prolonged heavy use. The artificial sweetener aspartame may produce seizures in children when consumed in high doses. In rare cases, food sensitivities can produce seizures in epileptic children with a history of atopy.[26] An elimination diet (see pp. 205) may identify food sensitivities that can contribute to epilepsy.

Micronutrients · Epilepsy

Nutrient	Suggested daily dose	Comments
Taurine	0.5–2.0 g	May reduce severity and frequency of seizures[27,28]
Vitamin E plus selenium	200–400 mg vitamin E; 100 µg selenium	Can reduce frequency of seizures when added to regular anticonvulsant therapy in children with epilepsy[29,30]
Vitamin B6	50–250 mg	In some cases, seizures can be caused by inadequate production of the inhibitory neurotransmitter gamma-aminobutyric acid (GABA). Vitamin B6 may stimulate production of GABA in the brain and reduce severity of seizures [31–33]
Multimineral supplement	Complete formula containing 300–400 mg magnesium and 10–20 mg manganese	Deficiency can cause seizures; epileptics often have low levels of body magnesium and manganese[34]

References

1. Vaughan TR. The role of food in the pathogenesis of migraine headache. Clin Rev Allergy. 1994;12:167.
2. Dexter JD, et al. The five hour glucose tolerance test and effect of low sucrose diet in migraine. Headache. 1978;18:91.
3. Peikert A, et al. Prophylaxis of migraine with oral magnesium: results from a prospective, multicenter, placebo-controlled and double-blind randomized study. Cephalalgia. 1996;16:257.
4. Taubert K. Magnesium in migraine. Results of a multicenter pilot study. Fortschr Med. 1994;112:328.
5. Glueck CJ, et al. Amelioration of severe migraine with omega-3 fatty acids: A double-blind, placebo-controlled clinical trial. Am J Clin Nutr. 1986;43:710.
6. Thys-Jacobs S. Alleviation of migraines with therapeutic vitamin D and calcium. Headache. 1994;34:590.
7. Jacobson MD. Vitamin B6 therapy for carpal tunnel syndrome. Hand Clin. 1996;12:253.
8. Skelton WP, Skelton NK. Thiamine deficiency neuropathy: It's still common today. Postgrad Med. 1989;85:301.
9. Hanck A, Weiser H. Analgesic and anti-inflammatory properties of vitamins. Int J Vitam Nutr Res. 1985;27:S189.
10. Traber MG, et al. Lack of tocopherol in peripheral nerves of vitamin E-deficient patients with peripheral neuropathy. N Engl J Med. 1987;317:262.
11. Benton D. Vitamin-mineral supplements and the intelligence of children: A review. J Orthomol Med. 1992;7:31.
12. Bruner AB, et al. Randomised study of cognitive effects of iron supplementation in non-anemic iron-deficient adolescent girls. Lancet. 1996;348:992.
13. Idjradinata P, Pollitt E. Reversal of developmental delays in iron-deficient infants treated with iron. Lancet. 1993;341:1.
14. Wainwright PE. Do essential fatty acids play a role in brain development? Neurosci Biobehav Rev. 1992;16:193.
15. Boris M, Mandel FS. Foods and additives are common causes of the attention deficit hyperactive disorder in children. Ann Allergy. 1994;72:462.
16. Simeon DT, Grantham-McGregor S. Effects of missing breakfast on the cognitive functions of school children of differing nutritional status. Am J Clin Nutr. 1989;49:646.
17. Pfeiffer SI, et al. Efficacy of vitamin B6 and magnesium in the treatment of autism: A methodology review and summary of outcomes. J Autism Dev Disord. 1995;25:481.

18. Middleman AB, et al. Nutritional vitamin B12 deficiency and folate deficiency in an adolescent patient presenting with anemia, weight loss, and poor school performance. J Adolesc Health. 1996;19:76.

19. Baghurst PA, et al. Environmental exposure to lead and children's intelligence at age of seven years. N Engl J Med. 1992;327:1279.

20. Egger J, et al. Controlled trial of oligoantigenic treatment in the hyperkinetic syndrome. Lancet. 1985;1:540.

21. Schulte-Korne G, et al. Effect of an oligo-antigen diet on the behavior of hyperkinetic children. Kinder Jugenpsychiatr. 1996;24:176.

22. Feingold BF. Why Your Child is Hyperactive. New York: Random House; 1974.

23. Stevens LJ, et al. Essential fatty acid metabolism in boys with attention-deficit hyperactivity disorder. Am J Clin Nutr. 1995;62:761.

24. Allan RB. Nutritional aspects of epilepsy–a review of the potential of nutritional intervention in epilepsy. Int Clin Nutr Rev. 1983;3:3.

25. Carroll J, Koenigsberger D. The ketogenic diet: A practical guide for caregivers. J Am Diet Assoc. 1998;98:316.

26. Egger J, et al. Oligoantigenic diet treatment of children with epilepsy and migraine. J Pediatr. 1989;114:51.

27. Durelli L, Tutani R. The current status of taurine in epilepsy. Clin Neuropharmacol. 1983;6:37.

28. Takahashi R, Nakane Y. Clinical trial of taurine in epilepsy. In: Barbeau A, Huxtable RJ, eds. Taurine and Neurological Disorders. New York: Raven Press; 1978.

29. Raju GB, et al. Randomized, double-blind, placebo-controlled, clinical trial of vitamin E as add-on therapy in uncontrolled epilepsy. Epilepsia. 1994;35:368.

30. Ramaekers VT, et al. Selenium deficiency triggering intractable seizures. Neuropediatrics. 1994;25:217.

31. Bernstein AL. Vitamin B6 in neurology. Ann N Y Acad Sci. 1990;585:250.

32. Crowell GF, Roach ES. Pyridoxine-dependent seizures. Am Fam Physician. 1983;27:183.

33. Goutieres F, Aicardi J. Atypical presentations of pyridoxine dependant seizures: A treatable cause of intractable epilepsy in infants. Ann Neurol. 1985;17:117.

34. Carl GF, et al. Association of low blood manganese concentration with epilepsy. Neurology. 1986;36:1584.

Nervous System Disorders II

Parkinson's Disease

Parkinson's disease is a chronic and progressive brain disorder that affects 1–2% of people older than 60 years. It results from the degeneration of nerve cells in the center of the brain that normally produce dopamine, an important neurotransmitter. Inadequate dopamine "signalling" in the brain results from loss of these cells. The disease typically begins as trembling in the arms and hands, but as it progresses muscle rigidity develops, trembling worsens, and simple movements become difficult. L-dopa, an amino acid that can be converted into dopamine in the brain, is often used in the medical treatment of Parkinson disease.

Diet · Parkinson's

A low-protein diet can be beneficial in Parkinson's disease.[1] L-dopa is one of several amino acids that compete for uptake into the brain from the bloodstream. During L-dopa therapy, restricting dietary protein reduces competition from other amino acids and allows more L-dopa to enter the brain. One limitation of L-dopa therapy is that its beneficial effects unpredictably wax and wane through the day. Protein restriction can reduce these daily fluctuations and make L-dopa therapy more effective, particularly if most of the daily protein is eaten with the evening meal.[1] Free-radical damage (see pp. 115) appears to play a role in Parkinson's disease. Diets high in natural antioxidants (such as vitamins E and C and carotenoids) may reduce risk of Parkinson's disease or slow down its progression.[2,3]

Micronutrients · Parkinson's

In Parkinson's disease high doses of vitamin B6, iron, and manganese should be avoided. High doses of vitamin B6 may decrease the effectiveness of of L-dopa therapy, and high doses of iron and manganese can aggravate the disease.

Nutrient	Suggested daily dose	Comments
Vitamin E and selenium	800–2400 mg vitamin E; 200–400 µg selenium	Antioxidants may protect against nerve-cell degeneration. Begin with 400 IU and gradually increase over several weeks.[2,3]
Vitamin C	1–4 g	May improve symptoms, especially alongside treatment with L-dopa
Vitamin B complex	Balanced formula containing 0.4 mg folic acid, 50 mg niacin	Deficiencies of niacin and folic acid often develop in Parkinson disease, and low body stores of these B vitamins can worsen symptoms
GLA	As evening primrose oil, 2–4 g/day	May be effective in reducing trembling
L-methionine	1–5 g	Start with 1 g/day and increase dose over several weeks. Can increase ease of movement and strength and improve mood and sleep[4]

Multiple Sclerosis

Multiple sclerosis (MS) is a chronic and progressive disorder in which the the myelin sheath that surrounds and protects many neurons degenerates, and the nerves are damaged. Depending on which nerves are affected, symptoms can include walking difficulties, vision problems, dizziness, numbness, weakness, slurred speech, or paralysis. The disease usually develops in people aged 25–40, and tends to wax and wane over many years. The cause is not clear; however, increased stress or poor nutrition may increase risk of MS.

Diet · MS

Especially when instituted at the onset of the disease, a diet low in fat (< 15 g fat/day) may slow down progression and reduce severity of MS. In addition to reducing total fat intake, polyunsaturated fats (cold-pressed nut and seed oils) should be substituted for saturated fats.[5] Because oxidative damage from free radicals (see pp. 115) may play a role in MS, diets should be high in natural antioxidants (e.g., vitamin E, vitamin C, beta carotene and other carotenoids, and selenium). [6] Food sensitivities may aggravate MS (common offending foods are milk and chocolate), and an elimination diet (see pp. 205) with identification and avoidance of offending foods may be beneficial.

Micronutrients · MS

Nutrient	Suggested daily dose	Comments
Vitamin E plus selenium	400–1200 mg vitamin E; 200 µg selenium	Antioxidants may protect against myelin degeneration[6]
Omega-3 fatty acids	1–2 g EPA (as fish-oil capsules)	May slow down progression and reduce severity[7]
Vitamin B complex	Balanced formula containing 50 mg B6, 50 mg thiamin, and 0.4 mg folic acid	Deficiencies of vitamin B6, niacin, and folic acid can aggravate symptoms
Vitamin B12	1 mg/week by intramuscular injection	Vitamin B12 is essential for production of fatty acids that make up myelin. Deficiency can aggravate MS[8]
GLA	As 1–4 g evening primrose oil	Supplementation may be beneficial, particularly as part of a diet low in saturated fat

Memory and Concentration Loss

During the aging process the number of functioning brain cells gradually decreases and smaller amounts of neurotransmitters are produced. These changes may impair memory and concentration. However, like most age-associated changes in function, there is great variability in the rate and degree of decline among people. The brain is very sensitive to proper nutrition, and needs a high blood flow and oxygen supply. Poor intake of micronutrients can interfere with mentation and memory and may accelerate functional losses associated with aging.[9]

Diet · Memory

Diets high in saturated fat, salt, alcohol, and cholesterol and low in polyunsaturated fats and fiber can produce hypertension and atherosclerosis of the cerebral arteries that gradually reduce flow of nutrients and oxygen.[9] Foods high in antioxidant nutrients (see pp. 115) may reduce free-radical damage to brain cells and reduce risk of atherosclerosis.[10] In older people decreased digestive function leads to poor absorption of certain nutrients from the diet. Even marginal deficiencies of several of the B vitamins – particularly thiamin, niacin, folate, and vitamin B12 – can impair mental function.[9,11] Reactive hypoglycemia (see pp. 185), triggered by high intakes of refined carbohydrate and sugar, can also interfere with brain function. Brain levels of acetylcholine, a neurotransmitter that is vital to memory, can be maintained by regular consumption of choline-rich foods, such as eggs, nuts, and cauliflower. Over time, regular consumption of a nutritious, well-balanced diet – low in saturated fat, alcohol, and salt, and rich in choline, antioxidant nutrients, minerals, and B vitamins – can help maintain optimum mental function.

Micronutrients · Memory

Nutrient	Suggested daily dose	Comments
Vitamin B complex	Balanced formula containing 50 mg thiamin, niacin, and vitamin B6, 50 µg vitamin B12, and 0.4 mg folic acid	Mild deficiencies of vitamin B12,[11] thiamin, and folic acid are common in older adults and can impair memory. Niacin may help maintain blood circulation through small blood vessels in the brain. In older people who absorb vitamin B12 poorly, vitamin B12 may need to be given by intramuscular injection
Choline plus pantothenic acid	5 g (as high-quality lecithin) with 50 mg pantothenic acid	A building block for brain synthesis of acetylcholine.[12] Pantothenic acid is essential for synthesis of acetylcholine
Multimineral supplement	Containing ample amounts of iron and zinc	Deficiencies of iron,[13] zinc, and other minerals can impair brain function
Vitamin E plus selenium	400 mg vitamin E; 200 µg selenium	Antioxidants may protect against the age-associated decline in brain cells

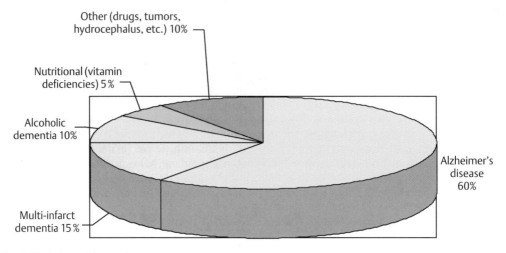

Other (drugs, tumors, hydrocephalus, etc.) 10%

Nutritional (vitamin deficiencies) 5%

Alcoholic dementia 10%

Multi-infarct dementia 15%

Alzheimer's disease 60%

Fig. 5.**26**: Causes of dementia.

Dementia and Alzheimer's Disease

Dementia is a disorder in which loss of brain cells severely impairs mentation and produces slowness of thought, memory loss, confusion, and disorientation. Advanced dementia can also cause personality changes. Dementia is common among older people – 10% of people over the age of 65 have dementia and over 30% of those over 85 are affected. Alzheimer's disease is the most common cause of dementia. It is marked by loss of brain cells that produce acetylcholine, an important neurotransmitter. Another common cause of dementia is decreased blood supply to the brain, termed "multi-infarct dementia." This type of dementia is the result of multiple, small strokes, each one damaging a small section of the brain. The strokes occur in an unpredictable, random pattern over months or years and, as more and more brain cells are damaged and lost, dementia develops.

Diet · Dementia

It is estimated that about one-quarter of all dementias are caused by nutritional factors that are, at least partially, reversible.[9] Deficiencies of several B vitamins – niacin, vitamin B12, thiamin, and folate – can cause dementia.[9,14,15] Chronic heavy alcohol consumption can also produce dementia – large amounts of alcohol have a direct toxic effect on brain cells. Because multi-infarct dementia is caused by small strokes, the same dietary changes that were recommended for prevention of high blood pressure and stroke (see pp. 180) can decrease risk of this disorder and also slow down progression of the disease in affected individuals by preventing more strokes.[16,17] Often, because of their disability and poor dietary habits, demented patients develop nutritional deficiencies that can sharply accelerate their disease.[9]

Micronutrients · Dementia

Nutrient	Suggested daily dose	Comments
Vitamin E plus selenium	800–1200 mg vitamin E; 200 μg selenium	Antioxidants can protect against brain cell loss and may slow down progression of the diease[18]
L-Carnitine	1.5–2.0 g	May slow down progression of the disease. Induces release of acetylcholine in the brain[19]
Choline plus pantothenic acid	10–15 g (as high-quality lecithin); 100 mg pantothenic acid	May enhance synthesis and release of acetylcholine[12]
Vitamin B12	1 mg/day for 1 week, then 1 mg/week, by intramuscular injection	Deficiency in the brain may produce dementia despite normal blood levels.[11] Absorption of dietary vitamin B12 is poor in many older people and in younger people with digestive disorders
Vitamin B complex	Containing ample amounts of thiamine, niacin, and folic acid	Vitamin B deficiencies can produce dementia, particularly in older people, those with chronic illnesses, and heavy consumers of alcohol[9]

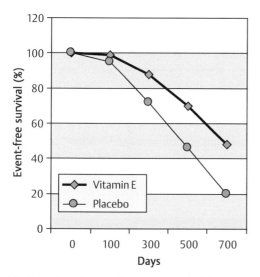

Fig. 5.**27**: **Supplemental vitamin E and Alzheimer's disease.** 341 subjects with Alzheimer's disease of moderate severity were given either 2000 mg/day vitamin E or placebo for 2 years. In the treated group there were significant delays in time to death, institutionalization, loss of ability to perform daily functions, or severe dementia: a median of 670 days for the vitamin E group, compared with 440 days for the placebo group. Treatment with vitamin E slows progression of moderate-severity Alzheimer's disease. (Adapted from Sano M, et al. N Engl J Med. 1997; 336:1216)

References

1. Kempster PA, Wahlqvist ML. Dietary factors in the management of Parkinson's disease. Nutr Rev. 1994;52:51.
2. Fahn S. An open trial of high-dosage antioxidants in early Parkinson's disease. Am J Clin Nutr. 1991;53:S380.
3. Grimes JD, et al. Prevention of progression of Parkinson's disease with antioxidative therapy. Prog Neuropsychopharmacol Biol Psychiatry. 1988;12:165.
4. Smythies JR, Halsey JH. Treatment of Parkinson's disease with L-methionine. South Med J. 1984;77:1577.
5. Swank RL, Dugan BB. Effect of low saturated fat diet in early and late cases of multiple sclerosis. Lancet. 1990;336:37.
6. Mai J, et al. High dose antioxidant supplementation to multiple sclerosis patients. Biol Trace Element Res. 1990;24:109.
7. Cendrowski W. Multiple sclerosis and MaxEPA. Br J Clin Prac. 1986;40:365.
8. Ransohoff RM, et al. Vitamin B12 deficiency and multiple sclerosis. Lancet. 1990;335:1285.
9. Gray GE. Nutrition and dementia. J Am Diet Assoc. 1989;89:1795.
10. Steinberg D. Antioxidant vitamins and coronary heart disease. N Engl J Med. 1993;328:1487.
11. Lindenbaum J, et al. Neuropsychiatric disorders caused by cobalamin deficiency in the absence of anemia or macrocytosis. N Engl J Med. 1988;318:1720.
12. Canty DJ, Zeisel SH. Lecithin and choline in human health and disease. Nutr Rev. 1994;52:327.
13. Bruner AB, et al. Randomised study of cognitive effects of iron supplementation in non-anemic iron-deficient adolescent girls. Lancet. 1996;348:992.

14. Geldmacher DS, Whitehouse PJ. Evaluation of dementia. N Engl J Med. 1996;335:330.
15. Blass JP, et al. Thiamine and Alzheimer's disease: A pilot study. Arch Neurol. 1988;45:833.
16. Perry IJ, et al. Prospective study of serum total homocysteine concentration and risk of stroke in middle-aged British men. Lancet. 1995;346:1395.
17. Bronner LL, et al. Primary prevention of stroke. N Engl J Med. 1995;333:1392.
18. Sano M, et al. A controlled trial of selegiline, alpha-tocopherol, or both as treatment for Alzheimer's disease. N Engl J Med. 1997;336:1216.
19. Bowman B. Acetyl-carnitine and Alzheimer's disease. Nutr Rev. 1992;50:142.

Psychiatric Disorders

Anxiety and Nervous Tension

Anxiety is a feeling of disquiet, nervousness, or fear without a clear or realistic cause. It can manifest as apprehensiveness, trembling, sweating, and difficulty sleeping. Although some anxiety is a normal human emotion, when it becomes chronic or severe it is not only uncomfortable but can interfere with a person's life and ability to function. Sudden episodes of extreme anxiety are called panic attacks.

Diet · Anxiety

In people susceptible to reactive hypoglycemia (see pp. 185), consumption of refined carbohydrates or sugar may trigger increased anxiety and, in rare cases, panic attacks.[1] In individuals prone to nervousness and anxiety, consumption of caffeine can worsen their symptoms.[2]

Depression

Depression can range from normal sadness triggered by loss or mourning to a severe feeling of overwhelming hopelessness. Depression is often accompanied by loss of appetite, fatigue, sleeping problems, poor concentration, inability to enjoy normally pleasurable activities, and low self-esteem. Many cases of severe depression appear to be caused by imbalanced chemistry in the brain. Low levels of certain neurotransmitters, including serotonin and norepinephrine, can produce depression. Synthesis of these neurotransmitters is dependent on both amino acid precursors and enzyme systems that contain essential micronutrients.[3,5] Therefore, optimum diet and nutrition can enhance neurotransmitter levels in the brain and influence mood.

Diet · Depression

Poor eating habits can contribute to depression by failing to provide the nutrients necessary for synthesis of important neuro-

Micronutrients · Anxiety

Nutrient	Suggested daily dose	Comments
Tryptophan	1–3 g	Tryptophan can increase levels of serotonin, a brain neurotransmitter that has a calming effect.[3] Should be taken together with 50 mg vitamin B6
Magnesium	400–600 mg	May decrease anxiety and nervous tension.[4] Medications, illness, and stress can deplete magnesium stores and produce agitation and irritability

transmitters.[3,5] In turn, depression can then aggravate nutrient deficiencies by causing lack of appetite. Food sensitivities can interfere with brain chemistry and alter mood. People with mood swings, which fluctuate according to food habits, should investigate possible sensitivities and eliminate the offending foods (see pp. 205). Although small amounts of caffeine can have mood-elevating properties, chronic high intake of coffee and black teas may aggravate anxiety and depression.[2]

Micronutrients · Depression

Nutrient	Suggested daily dose	Comments
L-phenylalanine	0.5 g-3.0 g. Begin with 0.5 g/day and increase gradually to a dose that produces improvement	The amino acid precursor to norepinephrine, a mood-elevating neurotransmitter.[6,7] Should be taken with 50 mg vitamin B6
Tryptophan	1–3 g	Can increase levels of brain serotonin, a mood-elevating neurotransmitter.[3,5,8] Should be taken with 50 mg vitamin B6
Folic acid	0.8 mg-5.0 g	Can increase methylation reactions in the brain that may elevate mood.[9,10] May increase response to serotonin-uptake inhibitors[10]
Vitamin B complex	Containing at least 25 mg of thiamin, riboflavin, niacin, and pyridoxine	Marginal deficiencies of thiamin, riboflavin, niacin, and pyridoxine can produce depression[11,12]
Vitamin B12	1 mg/week by intramuscular injection	Particularly effective in older people with fatigue and depression[13,14]

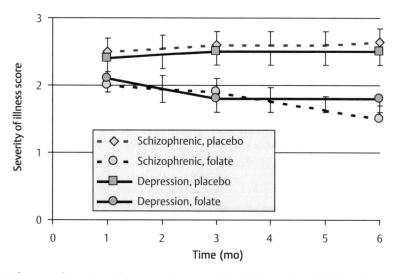

Fig. 5.**28**: **Folate supplements and recovery from psychiatric illness.** 41 psychiatric patients with folate deficiency were given 15 mg/day of methylfolate in addition to standard psychotropic treatment. In both schizophrenic and depressed subjects, folate significantly improved clinical and social recovery.
(Adapted from Godfrey PSA, et al. Lancet. 1990; 336:392)

References

1. Gorman JM, et al. Hypoglycemia and panic attacks. Am J Psychiatry. 1984;141:101.
2. Garattini S. Caffeine, Coffee, and Health. New York: Raven Press; 1993.
3. Young SN. Behavioral effects of dietary neurotransmitter precursors: Basic and clinical aspects. Neurosci Biobehav Rev. 1996;20:313.
4. Seelig MS. Consequences of magnesium deficiency on the enhancement of stress reactions; Preventive and therapeutic implications (a review). J Am Coll Nutr. 1994;13:429.
5. Crowdon, JM. Neuro-transmitter precursors in the diet: Their use in the treatment of brain diseases. In. Wurtman RJ, Wurtman JJ, eds. Nutrition and the Brain. Vol 3. New York: Raven Press; 1979.
6. Beckman V, Ludoph E. DL-phenylalanine as antidepressant. Arzneimit Forschung. 1978;28:1283.
7. Kravitz HM, et al. Dietary supplements of phenylalanine and other amino acid precursors of brain neuroamines in the treatment of depressive disorders. J Am Osteopath Assoc. 1984;84:119.

8. Thomson J, Rankin H, Ashcroft GW, et al. The treatment of depression in general practice; a comparison of L-tryptophan, amitriptyline, and a combination of L-tryptophan and amitriptyline with placebo. Psychol Med. 1982;12:741.
9. Reynolds EH, et al. Methylation and mood. Lancet. 1984;2:196.
10. Alpert JE, Fava M. Nutrition and depression: the role of folate. Nutr Rev. 1997;55:145.
11. Adams PW, et al. Effect of pyridoxine hydrochloride (vitamin B6) upon depression associated with oral contraception. Lancet. 1973;1:897.
12. Brozek J. Psychological effects of thiamin restriction and deprivation in normal young men. Am J Clin Nutr. 1951;5:104.
13. Oren DA, et al. A controlled trial of cyanocobalamin (vitamin B12) in the treatment of winter seasonal affective disorder. J Affect Disord. 1994;32:197.
14. Bottiglieri T. Folate, vitamin B12 and neuropsychiatric disorders. Nutr Rev. 1996;54:382.

Women's Health

Premenstrual Syndrome (PMS)

Premenstrual syndrome (PMS) is a group of symptoms that generally appear 4 to 10 days before menstruation and end, often abruptly, as menstruation begins. The most common symptoms are irritability, nervous tension, depression, mood swings, craving for sugary foods, breast tenderness, water retention, and weight gain.[1] The symptoms of PMS can be mild or severe: about one in five women have severe symptoms that interfere with daily activities. In many women, an imbalance of too much estrogen and too little progesterone triggers the symptoms of PMS.

Diet · PMS

Many women with PMS experience cravings for refined carbohydrates and sugar. Carbohydrates may improve mood by enhancing production of the neurotransmitter serotonin in the brain.[2] However, eating large amounts of sugar and refined carbohydrate can increase water retention and weight gain. Increasing intake of tryptophan-rich foods (the amino acid tryptophan is converted to serotonin in the brain, see pp. 109), can reduce cravings for carbohydrate. Heavy alcohol and caffeine intake during the 2 weeks leading up to menstruation can aggravate headache and irritability associated with PMS. A diet low in salt may reduce fluid retention. High intakes of magnesium may help reduce the symptoms of PMS.[3] Rich sources are seeds, nuts, whole grains, and vegetables. Iron deficiency is especially likely in women who have heavy bleeding during their periods. Women with heavy periods should consume rich dietary sources of iron (lean meats, liver, raisins, clams, dark green leafy vegetables) to replace losses of iron in bleeding.

Micronutrients · PMS

Nutrient	Suggested daily dose	Comments
GLA	As 2–4 g evening primrose oil	May reduce severity of symptoms[4]
Vitamin B6 plus magnesium	50–100 mg vitamin B6, 400 mg magnesium	Marginal deficiency can aggravate symptoms. Supplements can reduce nervous tension, menstrual cramps, breast pain, and weight gain.[5,6,7]
Omega-3 fatty acids	EPA as 1–3 g fish oil	May help reduce painful menstrual cramping[8,9]
Vitamin C with bioflavonoids	100–250 mg vitamin C with a bioflavonoid complex	May help reduce heavy bleeding during menstrual periods[10]
Vitamin E	400 mg	May help reduce severity of breast tenderness and menstrual cramps[11]

Fibrocystic Breast Disease

Fibrocystic breast disease (FBD) is characterized by breast swelling, lumpiness, and tenderness and is often worse during the menstrual period. In FBD, small fluid-filled cysts surrounded by fibrous tissue form in the breast tissue. When the cysts expand under the influence of hormonal changes of the menstrual cycle, they stretch the surrounding tissues, causing pain and tenderness. Between 20% and 40% of women aged 25–50 are affected to some degree.

the diet (so that only 15–20% of calories come from fat) can reduce breast swelling and tenderness in FBD.[12] Together with a low-fat diet, reducing or eliminating caffeine and theobromine (a substance similar to caffeine found in black tea) can significantly improve symptoms.[13]

Sources of caffeine and theobromine

- Coffee
- Black teas
- Colas and other soft drinks
- "Energy" or "alertness" drinks
- Diuretics
- Over-the-counter analgesic, allergy, and cold/flu preparations

Diet · FBD

The more fat in the diet, the greater the risk of developing FBD. Reducing the fat content of

Micronutrients · FBD

Nutrient	Suggested daily dose	Comments
Vitamin E	200–400 mg	Supplementation can reduce or eliminate symptoms in many women[14,15]
GLA	As 1–3 g evening primrose oil	May reduce lumpiness and tenderness, especially when symptoms are perimenstrual[16]
Vitamin A	5000–8000 µg	Supplementation can reduce swelling and tenderness.[17] Large doses of vitamin A should be taken under medical supervision only
Iodine	150–250 µg	Can relieve pain and swelling and reduce lumpiness. Kelp supplements are a rich source of iodine

Oral Contraceptives

Oral contraceptive pills contain mixtures of the female hormones estrogen and progesterone and prevent pregnancy by preventing ovulation. Although effective as birth control, they can have adverse side effects, including headache, weight gain, and fluid retention. Oral contraceptive pills can also adversely affect nutritional status.[18]

The nutritional impact of oral contraceptive pills (OCPs)

Increase requirements for:	
Thiamin, riboflavin, and vitamin B12	Interfere with metabolism and increase requirements for these B vitamins[18,19]
Vitamin B6	Interfere with metabolism.[20] Vitamin B6 requirements are 2 to 10 times higher when taking OCPs
Folic acid	Interfere with metabolism and increase requirements. Women taking OCPs are often deficient in folate.[19] Folate deficiency is particularly dangerous for the fetus during early pregnancy and can cause birth defects (see pp. 122). Women should wait 3–6 months after stopping OCPs before attempting pregnancy, and during these months a vitamin B complex with 0.8 mg folic acid should be taken to replenish body stores
Vitamin C	May lower tissue and blood levels[18]
Zinc and magnesium	May interfere with metabolism and increase requirements for these minerals.[18] Many women taking OCPs are deficient in zinc and magnesium.
May lower requirements for:	
Vitamin A	Increase levels of the vitamin A transport protein and vitamin A in the blood. High doses of vitamin A should be avoided because OCPs can potentially increase the chances of vitamin A toxicity
Vitamin K	Increase levels of the vitamin K-dependent clotting proteins in the blood, increasing risk of blood clots
Copper	Increase circulating copper levels in the blood

Diet · OCPs

Oral contraceptive pills may impair a woman's ability to control levels of blood lipids and glucose, and hyperlipidemia and impaired glucose tolerance may develop. These women need to be particularly careful to minimize consumption of saturated and hydrogenated fats, as well as refined carbohydrates and sugar, to help keep blood lipid and glucose levels in a healthy range.

Micronutrients · OCPs

Vitamin B complex	Complete formula containing at least 5 mg thiamin and riboflavin, 25 mg vitamin B6, 0.4 mg folate, and 10 µg vitamin B12
Vitamin C	100–250 mg
Multimineral supplement	Should contain at least 250 mg magnesium and 15 mg zinc

Menopause

Menopause is the permanent cessation of the menstrual periods that occurs around age 50 in most women. As a woman moves into her late 40s, her body's estrogen production slows down, and she gradually stops ovulating. Symptoms of the menopause include hot flashes, headaches, fatigue, vaginal irritation, mood swings, and depression. These symptoms can range from mild to severe: about one in five women seek medical attention for symptoms of the menopause. A major concern at the menopause is the loss of bone mineral (mainly calcium) from the skeleton due to the loss of estrogens.[21] Up to 20% of the bone mineral density can be lost at menopause, which can sharply increase risk of osteoporosis and bone fractures. The loss of estrogen at menopause also causes LDL cholesterol levels in the blood to rise and levels of HDL cholesterol to fall, increasing risk of heart attack and stroke.[22]

Diet · Menopause

Women going through menopause should increase intake of rich food sources of calcium, magnesium, and vitamins D and K to maintain integrity of the skeleton.[23,24] In addition, high amounts of phosphorus (found in red meat, processed foods, and cola drinks) should also be avoided; too much phosphorus in the diet accelerates loss of minerals from bones. Reducing sodium, caffeine, and protein intake can also help maintain body stores of calcium. To keep levels of blood fats in the healthy range, the saturated fat content of the diet should be reduced (by eating less meat, eggs, and whole-fat milk products).

Micronutrients · Menopause

Nutrient	Suggested daily dose	Comments
Vitamin E	400 mg. Vitamin E in creams can be used topically in the vagina to reduce itching and irritation	Can significantly improve hot flashes, fatigue, depression, and vaginal irritation[25]
GLA	As 2–4 g evening primrose oil	Can be effective in reducing hot flashes, vaginal irritation, and mood swings[26]
Calcium plus vitamin D	800–1000 mg calcium; 10 µg vitamin D	Reduces loss of mineral content of bones and helps maintain bone integrity[23,24]

Cervical Dysplasia (Abnormal Pap Smear)

If a Pap smear shows cervical dysplasia (precancerous cells), effective intervention is needed to prevent development of cancer. Untreated cervical dysplasia (depending on its severity) will typically develop into cervical cancer over the next 2–8 years. Unlike many other cancers that appear at older ages, cervical cancer most often occurs in younger women (ages 30–45). A healthy diet can reduce risk of cervical dysplasia, and supplementation with micronutrients after an abnormal Pap smear may help the dysplastic cells revert to normal.[27]

Diet · Cervical Dysplasia

A diet high in fat (particularly saturated fat from meat and whole-milk products) increases risk of cervical dysplasia, whereas a diet rich in fresh fruits and vegetables offers significant protection, probably due to its high content of vitamin C, carotenes, and fiber. Female smokers are three to ten times more likely to develop cervical dysplasia than female nonsmokers.

Micronutrients · Cervical Dysplasia

Nutrient	Suggested daily dose	Comments
Vitamin A	3000 µg for women who have an abnormal Pap smear showing cervical dysplasia; 800 µg for prevention	May help reverse dysplasia.[27,28] High doses of vitamin A should only be taken with the advice of a physician
Folic acid	5 mg for women who have an abnormal Pap smear; 0.4 mg for prevention	May reverse dysplasia.[29–31] Should be taken as part of a vitamin B complex
Antioxidant formula	Should contain ample beta-carotene, vitamin E, and vitamin C, as well as selenium (see pp. 118 for recommended levels of antioxidants)	May help reverse cervical dysplasia. Low intake of antioxidants increases risk[28,32,33]

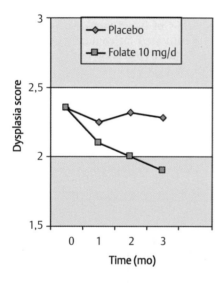

Fig. 5.**29: Folic acid supplementation and cervical dysplasia.** 47 women taking oral contraceptives with dysplasia of the uterine cervix were given folic acid (10 g/day) or placebo for 3 months. At the end of treatment cytology scores from the folate group were significantly better than for the placebo group. Cervical dysplasia asociated with oral contraceptive use may, in some cases, be arrested or reversed by folate supplementation.

(Adapted from Butterworth CE, et al. Am J Clin Nutr. 1982;35:73)

Breast Cancer

Breast cancer is the most common cancer in women. About one in ten women will develop the disease, many at a young age (about one-third of cases occur in women below 50 years). High levels of estrogens in the body are thought to be a contributing factor in many cases of breast cancer. There is a strong hereditary component: a woman whose mother or sister develops breast cancer has about twice the normal risk. Dietary changes and nutritional supplementation in women at increased risk may significantly reduce the chance of developing breast cancer.

Diet · Breast Cancer

High intakes of saturated fat may increase risk of breast cancer, whereas intake of monounsaturated fats (such as in olive oil and avocados) reduces the risk.[34,35] Higher intakes of dietary fiber (> 25–30 g/day) may also help protect against breast cancer.[36,37] Regular consumption of vegetables, particularly cabbages, brocolli, and cauliflower, reduces estrogen activity in the body and risk of breast cancer.[35] Foods rich in isoflavonoids, such as soy products like tofu and soy milk, are also protective. It is important for women to maintain a normal weight; women who are overweight are much more likely to develop breast cancer. Alcohol should be consumed only in moderation. Women who drink more than 2–3 "drinks" per day increase their chances of developing breast cancer by about 50%.[38,39] Heavy, chronic alcohol intake nearly triples the risk.

Guidelines for reducing overall cancer risk are discussed on pages 201.

Micronutrients · Breast Cancer

To reduce the chances of developing breast cancer:

Nutrient	Suggested daily dose	Comments
Antioxidant formula	Should contain ample beta-carotene, vitamin E, and selenium (see pp. 115 for recommended levels of antioxidants)	Low intake of antioxidants increases risk of developing breast cancer[36,40]
Vitamin C	0.5 g–1.0 g	Higher intakes can sharply reduce risk of breast cancer[41]

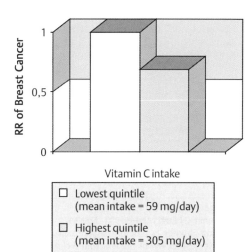

Vitamin C intake

☐ Lowest quintile (mean intake = 59 mg/day)

☐ Highest quintile (mean intake = 305 mg/day)

Fig. 5.**30**: **Vitamin C intake and risk of breast cancer.** In 12 studies of diet and breast cancer, vitamin C intake had the most consistent and significant inverse association with breast cancer risk. The risk was nearly one-third lower with the highest intakes of vitamin C, compared with lower intakes. The mean intake of the lowest quintile was the current recommended dietary allowance for vitamin C.
(Adapted from Howe GR, et al. J Natl Cancer Inst. 1990;82:561)

References

1. Abraham GE. Management of the premenstrual tension syndromes: Rationale for a nutritional approach. In: Bland J, ed. 1986 A Year in Nutritional Medicine. New Canaan: Keats Publishing; 1986.
2. Young SN. Behavioral effects of dietary neurotransmitter precursors: Basic and clinical aspects. Neurosci Biobehav Rev. 1996;20:313.
3. Fontana-Klaiber H, Hogg B. Therapeutic effects of magnesium in dysmenorrhea. Schweiz Rundsch Med Prax. 1990;79:491.
4. Budeiri D, et al. Is evening primrose oil of value in the treatment of premenstrual syndrome? Control Clin Trials. 1996;17:60.
5. Kendall KE, Schnurr PP. The effects of vitamin B6 supplementation of premenstrual symptoms. Obstet Gynecol. 1987;70:145.
6. Doll H. Vitamin B6 and the premenstrual syndrome: A randomized cross-over trial. J R Coll Gen Pract. 1989;39:364.
7. Facchinetti F, et al. Oral magnesium successfully relieves premenstrual mood changes. Obstet Gynecol. 1992;78:177.
8. Deutch B. Menstrual pain in Danish women correlated with low n-3 polyunsaturated fatty acid intake. Eur J Clin Nutr. 1995;49:508.
9. Harel Z, et al. Supplementation with omega-3 polyunsaturated fatty acids in the management of dysmenorrhea in adolescents. Am J Obstet Gynecol. 1996;174:1335.
10. Cohen JD, Ruben HW. Functional menorrhagia: Treatment with bioflavonoids and vitamin C. Curr Ther Res. 1960;2:539.
11. London RS. Efficacy of alpha-tocopherol in the treatment of the premenstrual syndrome. J Reprod Med. 1987;32:400.
12. Boyd NF, et al. Effect of a low-fat high-carbohydrate diet on symptoms of cyclical mastopathy. Lancet. 1988;2:128.
13. Boyle CA, et al. Caffeine consumption and fibrocystic breast disease: A case-control epidemiologic study. J Natl Canc Inst. 1984;72:1015.
14. Ernster VL, et al. Vitamin E and benign breast "disease": a double-blind, randomized clinical trial. Surgery. 1985;97:490.
15. London RF, et al. The effect of vitamin E on mammary dysplasia: A double-blind study. Obstet Gynecol. 1985;65:104.

16. Preece P, et al. Evening primrose oil for mastalgia. In: Horrobin DF, ed. Clinical Uses of Essential Fatty Acids. London: Eden Press; 1982.

17. Band PR, et al. Treatment of benign breast disease with vitamin A. Prev Med. 1984;13:549.

18. Thorp VJ. Effect of oral contraceptive agents on vitamin and mineral requirements. J Am Diet Assoc. 1980;76:581.

19. Prasad AS, et al. Effect of oral contraceptives on nutrients: vitamin B6, B12 and folic acid. Am J Obstet Gynaecol. 1976;125:1063.

20. Leklem JE. Vitamin B6 requirement and oral contraceptive use-a concern? J Nutr. 1986;116:475.

21. Reid IR. Therapy of osteoporosis: calcium, vitamin D, and exercise. Am J Med Sci. 1996;312:278.

22. Wenger NK, et al. Cardiovascular health and disease in women. N Engl Med J. 1993;329:247.

23. Dawson-Hughes B. Calcium supplementation and bone loss: a review of the controlled clinical trials. Am J Clin Nutr. 1991;54:274S.

24. Chapuy MC, et al. Vitamin D₃ and calcium to prevent hip fractures in elderly women. N Engl J Med. 1992;327:1637.

25. Finkler RS. The effect of vitamin E in the menopause. J Clin Endocrinol Metab. 1949;9:89.

26. Chenoy R. Effect of evening primrose oil on menopausal flushing. BMJ. 1994;308:501.

27. Shimizu H, et al. Decreased serum retinol levels in women with cervical dysplasia. Br J Cancer. 1996;73:1600.

28. Giuliano AR, Gapstur S. Can cervical dysplasia and cancer be prevented with nutrients? Nutr Rev. 1998;56:9.

29. Butterworth CE, et al. Improvement in cervical dysplasia associated with folic acid therapy in users of oral contraceptives. Am J Clin Nutr. 1982;35:73.

30. Whitehead N, et al. Megaloblastic changes in the cervical epithelium associated with oral contraceptive therapy and reversal with folic acid. JAMA. 1973;226:1421.

31. Childers JM, et al. Chemoprevention of cervical cancer with folic acid. Cancer Epidemiol Biomarkers Prev. 1995;4:155.

32. Palan PR, et al. Plasma levels of antioxidant beta-carotene and alpha-tocopherol in uterine cervix dysplasias and cancer. Nutr Cancer. 1991;15:13.

33. Romney SL, et al. Plasma vitamin C and uterine cervical dysplasia. Am J Obstet Gynecol. 1985;151:976.

34. Willett WC. Specific fatty acids and risks of breast and prostate cancer: Dietary intake. Am J Clin Nutr. 1997;66:1557S.

35. Franceschi S, et al. Intake of macronutreints and risk of breast cancer. Lancet. 1996;347:1351.

36. Howe GR. Nutrition and breast cancer. In: Bendich A, Deckelbaum RJ, eds. Preventive Nutrition. Torawa, New Jersey: Humana press; 1997:97–106.

37. Rohan T, et al. Dietary fiber, vitamins A, C, and E, and risk of breast cancer: A cohort study. Cancer Causes Control. 1993;4:29.

38. Longnecker MP, et al. A meta-analysis of alcohol consumption in relation to rate of breast cancer. JAMA. 1988;652:260.

39. Holmberg L, et al. Alcohol intake and risk of breast cancer. JAMA. 1998;279:535.

40. Vant-Veer P, et al.Tissue antioxidants and postmenopausal breast cancer: The European Community Multicentre Study on Antioxidants. Cancer Epidemiol Biomark Prev. 1996;5:441.

41. Howe GR, et al. Dietary factors and risk of breast cancer: combined analysis of 12 case-control studies. J Natl Cancer Inst. 1990;82:561.

Urinary Tract Disorders

Prostate Enlargement (Benign Prostatic Hyperplasia)

The prostate gland produces the fluid that surrounds and nourishes the sperm in semen. A common condition of older men is enlargement of the prostate gland (benign prostatic hyperplasia): three-quarters of men undergo some enlargement by their seventh decade. The prostate gland surrounds the urethra just below the bladder, and enlargement of the gland constricts flow of urine out of the bladder. This results in a frequent need to urinate, a slow, diminished stream of urine, and inability to fully empty the bladder. Although prostate enlargement can rarely be due to a cancer in the gland, in most cases, the process is benign and the cause unknown.

Diet · Prostate

High-fat diets, particularly saturated fat from animal sources (meat, eggs, dairy products), promotes enlargement of the prostate and may also increase risk of prostate cancer.[1,2] Diets high in fruits and vegetables, particularly those rich in lycopene (a carotenoid found in large amounts in tomatoes), reduce risk of prostate enlargement and cancer.[1] Overactivity of certain prostaglandins within the prostate gland may contribute to enlargement. Substituting high-quality, cold-pressed plant oils for saturated fat in the diet, along with eating fresh fish two to three times per week, will provide important essential PUFAs. The EFAs and their metabolites – GLA, EPA, and DHA – can decrease activity of these prostaglandins (see pp. 89) and may reduce enlargement and improve symptoms.

Micronutrients · Prostate

Nutrient	Suggested daily dose	Comments
Zinc	30–60 mg	Impaired zinc metabolism within the prostate gland may contribute to enlargement. Supplementation may reduce gland size and improve symptoms[3]
Vitamin E	200–400 mg	Supplementation may reduce risk of enlargement and prostate cancer[1]
EFAs	GLA as 1–2 g evening primrose oil; 1–3 g EPA and DHA as fish-oil capsules	Overactivity of certain prostaglandins within the prostate gland may contribute to enlargement. Supplementation can reduce activity of these substances and may reduce gland size and improve symptoms
Amino acids	Combination of three amino acids, L-glycine, L-alanine and L-glutamic acid, each taken at a dose of 500 mg/day	May reduce size of the gland and improve symptoms[4]

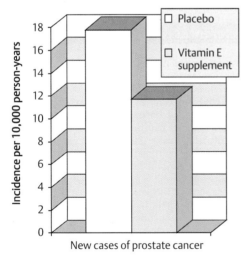

Fig. 5.**31**: **Vitamin E supplementation and risk of prostate cancer.** 30,000 50–69-year-old Finnish men were given 50 mg/day alpha-tocopherol or placebo for 5–8 years. There were 151 new cases of prostate cancer in the placebo group, compared with only 99 new cases in the treatment group.
(Source: The ATBC Cancer Prevention Group. N Engl J Med. 1994;330:1029)

Nephrolithiasis (Kidney Stones)

Nephrolithiasis is a disorder in which small stones – usually formed from calcium and oxalate – precipitate in the kidney. If they pass into the ureter they cause irritation, spasm, and may block the flow of urine. The pain of a kidney stone is intense: it typically starts suddenly in the lower back and radiates down and around toward the groin. In general, the more calcium and oxalate in the urine, the greater the chances of developing kidney stones. Uric acid in the urine can be the "seed" around which calcium oxalate stones develop. The risk of kidney stones can be strongly influenced by dietary factors.[5]

Diet · Nephrolithiasis

Individuals with a tendency to form kidney stones can reduce the risk by:

● Eating less animal protein. Animal protein increases the amount of calcium, oxalate, and uric acid in the urine.

● Increasing the fiber content of the diet, which can reduce urinary calcium excretion. Diets high in fat and salt and low in fiber increase risk of developing stones.

● Reducing caffeine intake, as high intakes increase calcium excretion into the urine and may promote stone formation. Heavy alcohol consumption also increases the chance of developing kidney stones.

● Drinking plenty of water and other fluids, which increases urinary volume and decreases the concentration of stone-forming substances. Drinking at least 2 l of fluid throughout the day.

● Minimizing intake of foods high in oxalate, as these increase risk of stone formation.[5]

Foods high in oxalates:

● Beans

● Carrots

● Chocolate

● Celery

● Instant coffee

● Cucumbers

● Parsley

● Grapefruit

● Rhubarb

● Peanuts

● Spinach

● Sweet potatoes

● Tea

● Pepper

Because vitamin C can be metabolized to oxalate, it has been suggested that high intakes of vitamin C might increase risk of kidney stones. However, oxalate in the urine generally does not increase unless the daily dose of vitamin C is greater than 6 g, and even then only rarely. In individuals susceptible to stone formation who are taking high doses of vitamin C, supplemental vitamin B6 and magnesium can reduce risk of increased oxalate in the urine.

Micronutrients · Nephrolithiasis

Nutrient	Suggested daily dose	Comments
Vitamin B6	50–100 mg	Required for breakdown of oxalate. Reduces chance of stone formation in people with high amounts of urinary oxalate, [6,7]
Magnesium	400 mg	Binds with oxalate and decreases risk of stone formation[7,8]

References

1. Giles G, Ireland P. Diet, nutrition and prostate cancer. Int J Cancer. 1997;10:13S.
2. Giovanucci E, Rimm EB, Colditz GA, et al. A prospective study of dietary fat and risk of prostate cancer. J Natl Cancer Inst. 1993;85:1571.
3. Fahim MS, et al. Zinc treatment for the reduction of hyperplasia of the prostate. Fed Proc. 1976;35:361.
4. Dumrau F. Benign prostatic hyperplasia: Amino acid therapy for symptomatic relief. Am J Geriatr. 1962;10:426.
5. Robertson WG. Diet and calcium stones. Miner Electrolyte Metab. 1987;13:228.
6. Mitwalli A, et al. Control of hyperoxaluria with large doses of pyridoxine in patients with kidney stones. Int Urol Nephrol. 1988;20:353.
7. Prien EL, Gershoff SF. Magnesium oxide-pyridoxine therapy for recurrent calcium oxalic calculi. J Urol. 1974;112:509.
8. Labeeuw M, et al. Magnesium in the physiopathology and treatment of renal calcium stones. Presse Med. 1987;16:25.

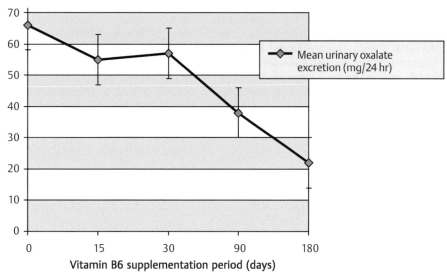

Fig. 5.**32**: **Supplemental vitamin B6 and oxalate excretion in urine.** Supplementation of vitamin B6 (10 mg/day) significantly decreased oxalate excretion in the urine after 90 days. (Adapted from Murthy MSR, et al. Int J Clin Pharmacol Ther. 1982;20:434)

Stress and Fatigue

Often the daily stress of modern lifestyles – a job, financial pressures, deadlines, and family responsibilities – build up to a point where it is difficult to manage. A common complaint of many adults, fatigue is excessive tiredness, inability to concentrate, and lack of energy. Fatigue can be caused by chronic stress, lack of exercise, and poor sleep patterns, often combined with an inadequate and erratic eating pattern. Prolonged fatigue and stress can have serious adverse health effects. Along with adequate rest and regular exercise, a balanced and nutritious diet can help manage stress and prevent fatigue.

Disorders linked to psychological stress

- Angina and heart attack
- Asthma
- Immune weakness (increased colds, influenza, other infections)
- Migraine and tension headaches
- Anxiety and depression
- High blood pressure
- Premenstrual syndrome
- Ulcerative colitis
- Arthritis
- Ulcers
- Eczema

Diet · Stress

Modern, affluent diets are typically high in energy, refined carbohydrate, salt, and saturated fat, but low in complex carbohydrates and fresh fruits and vegetables. This dietary pattern produces chronic, marginal deficiencies of several micronutrients – the B vitamins, magnesium, iron, and zinc – important for maintaining energy and fighting fatigue. Moreover, during periods of increased workload and stress, requirements for these micronutrients are higher. Increasing intake of whole grains and lean sources of protein, together with fresh fruits and vegetables will provide ample amounts of the B vitamins and minerals needed to combat fatigue.

Many people make the mistake of relying on large amounts of sugar and coffee during times of stress. Although they may supply short bursts of energy, too much caffeine and refined carbohydrate ultimately worsens chronic fatigue and produces headaches, irritability, and concentration difficulties. Because control of blood glucose is more difficult during times of stress, it is important to minimize intake of refined carbohydrates, which may trigger periods of reactive hypoglycemia (see pp. 185).

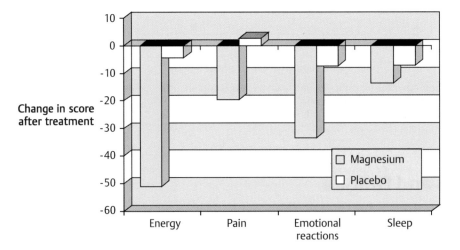

Fig. 5.**33**: **Magnesium supplementation and chronic fatigue.** 32 adults with chronic fatigue received either placebo or 50% magnesium sulfate (1 g in 2 ml) intramuscularly every week for 6 weeks. In the treatment group there was significant improvement in energy level, pain perception, and emotional state, compared with placebo. (Adapted from Cox IM, et al. Lancet. 1990;337:757)

Micronutrients · Stress

Nutrient	Suggested daily dose	Comments
Multimineral supplement	Balanced formula with 5–10 mg iron and 10–20 mg zinc	Especially prevalent in women and vegetarians, iron and zinc deficiencies can cause chronic fatigue[1,2]
Vitamin B complex	Complete formula providing 10–25 mg of thiamin, riboflavin, niacin, and pantothenic acid, and 0.8 mg folic acid	Deficiencies of the B vitamins, because of their central role in energy production, produce fatigue. Requirements are higher during times of increased activity and energy expenditure[3]
Magnesium	400–600 mg	Can reduce fatigue and increase alertness
Vitamin B12	25–50 µg (In people with intestinal malabsorption, 1 mg by intramuscular injection)	Vitamin B12 deficiency produces anemia, fatigue, and depression[4] and is particularly common among the elderly[5]

References

1. Beard JL, et al. Iron metabolism: A comprehensive review. Nutr Rev. 1996;54:295.
2. Cousins RJ. Zinc. In: Ziegler E, Filer L, eds. Present Knowledge in Nutrition. Washington DC: ILSI Press; 1997:293–306.
3. Recommended Dietary Allowances. Subcommittee on the 10th edition of the RDAs. Food and Nutrition Board; National Research Council. 10th ed. Washington DC: National Academy Press; 1989:125.
4. Middleman AB, et al. Nutritional vitamin B12 deficiency and folate deficiency in an adolescent patient presenting with anemia, weight loss, and poor school performance. J Adolesc Health. 1996;19:76.
5. Lindenbaum J, et al. Prevalence of cobalamin deficiency in the Framingham elderly population. Am J Clin Nutr. 1994;60:2.

Infertility

Fertility is the biologic ability to conceive and have children. Couples are generally considered infertile when pregnancy does not occur after a year of regular intercourse. About 10–15% of couples in the USA and Europe are infertile. Nutritional and dietary factors can influence both male and female fertility.[1,2]

Females

Diet · Infertility

In women, being overweight or underweight can impair fertility.[3] Excessive thinness from vigorous dieting or strenuous exercise is a common cause of infertility in women in the industrialized countries. In underweight women with body fat content lower than 16–18% of their body weight (women normally have about 25% body fat), ovarian production of estrogen is reduced. This can impair ovulation, interrupt the menstrual cycle, and produce infertility. On the other hand, too much body fat can also interfere with ovulation and cause infertility. About one in ten overweight women have irregular menstrual cycles. Weight loss in overweight, infertile women can cause a return of ovulation and fertility. Women who are trying to become pregnant to maintain or attain a normal body weight.[2,3]

High intakes of alcohol and caffeine may reduce fertility in women. Women trying to conceive should limit their alcohol intake to less than two glasses of wine or beer per day and minimize their coffee intake. Deficiencies of vitamin E, vitamin B12, and folate, as well as iron and zinc, can reduce fertility.[4,5] A high body burden of toxic metals (such as lead, mercury, and cadmium) may also impair fertility.

Micronutrients · Infertility

Nutrient	Suggested daily dose	Comments
Multimineral supplement	Balanced formula containing 10–20 mg zinc and 10 mg iron	Deficiencies of iron or zinc may impair fertility[4,5]
Vitamin B Complex	Balanced supplement containing 0.4–0.8 mg folic acid and 2.5 µg vitamin B12	Deficiencies of folate and vitamin B12 may impair fertility

Males

Diet · Infertility

In men, poor nutrition – a diet high in refined carbohydrates, saturated fat, and processed foods and low in important micronutrients – may reduce sperm number and motility. To help increase sperm quality, the diet should emphasize high-quality protein, whole grains, and fresh fruits and vegetables. Heavy alcohol consumption (more than 3 "drinks" per day) can impair fertility.[6] Overweight men are more likely to have low testosterone levels and lower numbers of sperm.

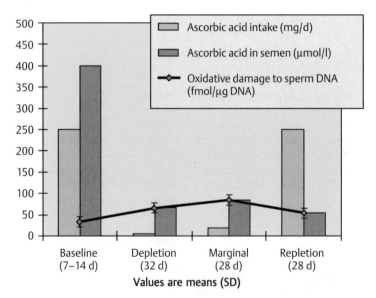

Fig. 5.**34: Dietary ascorbic acid intake and oxidative damage to DNA in semen.** Ascorbic acid is present in high concentrations in seminal fluid and may play a role in protecting sperm from oxidative damage. Depletion of seminal ascorbic acid in male volunteers on a control diet significantly increased sperm cell 8-OH-deoxyguanosine levels, a marker of oxidative damage to DNA.
(Adapted from Fraga CG, et al. Proc Natl Acad Sci USA. 1991;88:11003)

Micronutrients · Infertility

Nutrient	Suggested daily dose	Comments
Vitamin C	0.5 g-1.0 g	Reduces abnormal clumping of sperm that can cause infertility; may improve sperm motility[7]
Arginine	2–4 g	Can improve sperm number and quality[8]
Zinc	60 mg	Essential for sperm production and synthesis of testosterone. Supplementation may improve sperm count[9,10]
Multimineral supplement	Balanced supplement with 50–100 µg selenium and 100–200 µg chromium	Deficiencies of selenium and chromium can reduce sperm count

References

1. Calloway DH. Nutrition and reproductive function of man. Nutr Abstr Rev Rev Clin Nutr. 1983;53:361.
2. Wynn A, Wynn M. The need for nutritional assessment in the treatment of the infertile patient. J Nutr Med. 1990;1:315.
3. Shoupe D. Effect of body weight on reproductive function. In: Mishell DR, Darajan V, Lobo R, eds. Infertility, Contraception and Reproductive Endocrinology. Boston: Blackwell; 1991.
4. Keen CL, Bendich A, Wilhite CC, eds. Maternal Nutrition and Pregnancy Outcome. Ann NY Acad Sci. 1993;678:1–372.
5. Rushton DH. Ferritin and fertility. Lancet. 1991;337:1554.
6. Anderson RA, Jr, et al. Male reproductive tract sensitivity to ethanol: A critical overview. Pharmacol Biochem Behav. 1983;18:S305.
7. Dawson EB, et al. Effect of ascorbic acid on male fertility. Ann N Y Acad Sci. 1987;498:312.
8. Schachter A, et al. Treatment of oligospermia with the amino acid arginine. J Urol. 1973;110:311.
9. Piesse J. Zinc and human male infertility. Internat Clin Nutr Rev. 1983;3:4.
10. Takihara H, et al. Zinc sulfate therapy for infertile males with or without varicocelectomy. Urology. 1987;29:638.

Cigarette Smoking

Cigarette smoke contains multiple toxins, carbon monoxide, and cancer-causing substances. It is estimated that smoking contributes to about one-third of all cancers, fatal heart attacks, and strokes worldwide. On average, regular cigarette smoking reduces life span by about 10–15 years. Although it is the single most important preventable cause of death in many countries, 20–25% of adults in the USA and Europe continue to smoke. Moreover, many nonsmokers, at work or at home, are exposed to smoke from nearby smokers. "Passive" smoke can cause asthma, headaches, and many other health problems, and people chronically exposed to passive smoke (such as living with a smoker) increase their risk of cancer by 50–60%. Children are particularly vulnerable to harm from passive smoking. If unable to stop smoking or regularly exposed to passive smoke, the following nutritional guidelines may help reduce the dangers.

Diet · Smoking

Smoking can increase blood LDL cholesterol levels as well as increase oxidant damage to cholesterol and increase risk of heart attack and stroke. Smokers need to minimize intake of saturated fat and hydrogenated fat to help control their blood cholesterol level. Metabolism and breakdown of vitamin C in smokers is sharply increased[1] (a pack of cigarettes uses up about 300 mg of the body's stores). Smokers need more than double the amount of vitamin C that nonsmokers need to maintain body levels of the vitamin.[2] Chronic vitamin C deficiency in smokers can promote unhealthy, bleeding gums and premature wrinkling of skin, and increase the susceptibilty of LDL cholesterol to oxidation. Smoking also impairs metabolism of vitamin A, folate, and vitamin B12.[3,4] Poor folate and vitamin B12 status in smokers increases their already high risk of lung cancer (see Fig. 5.**36**).[3] Smoking interferes with conversion of vitamin B6 to its active form.[5] Smoking also increases loss of calcium from the skeleton and may increase risk of osteoporosis.

When people stop smoking, their basal metabolic rate falls, they often eat more, and many gain weight. Fear of weight gain, particularly in women, may make some reluctant to stop smoking. However, an average person will gain only between 2–3 kg, with half of those who stop gaining only 1 kg or less. This is a small price to pay for the enormous health benefits of stopping smoking, including halving the risk of a heart attack. Smokers trying to stop need to carefully watch their diets to keep their weight steady and avoid weight gain.

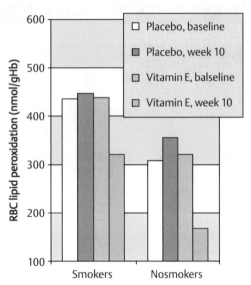

Fig. 5.**35**: **Reduced lipid peroxidation through vitamin E supplementation in smokers.** 30 male smokers and 30 male nonsmokers were given either 280 mg/day vitamin E or placebo for 10 weeks. Treatment significantly reduced peroxidation in both smokers and nonsmokers compared with placebo. RBC lipid peroxidation in smokers after treatment was similar to pretreatment levels in the nonsmokers, suggesting that vitamin E requirements are substantially higher in smokers than nonsmokers.
(Adapted from Brown KM, et al. Eur J Clin Nutr. 1998; 52:145)

Micronutrients · Smoking

To reduce damage from cigarette smoke

Nutrient	Suggested daily dose	Comments
Antioxidant supplement (containing ample amounts of vitamins A, C, E and zinc and selenium)	(See pp. 115 for antioxidant nutrients and suggested doses.) Should contain at least 100 mg vitamin E	Cigarette smoke is a powerful oxidant causing widespread cell damage and may accelerate atherosclerosis and other degenerative changes in the skin, lungs, and other organs.[6–8] Vitamin E requirements are higher in smokers; supplementation may help reduce oxidative damage[9,10]
Vitamin B Complex	Complete formula containing 0.4–0.8 mg of folic acid and 25–50 μg vitamin B12	Supplements of folate and vitamin B12 can reduce severity of the precancerous changes in the lungs of regular smokers[3]
Vitamin C	500 mg	Smokers break down body stores of vitamin C rapidly.[2] May help reduce oxidative damage and loss of respiratory function[11]

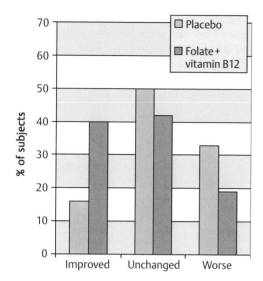

Fig. 5.**36: Reduced bronchial metaplasia in smokers supplemented with vitamin B12 and folate.** 73 chronic smokers with metaplasia (precancerous cells) in their bronchi were given either 10 mg folate plus 0.5 mg vitamin B12 or placebo for 4 months. Direct cytological comparison at 4 months showed significantly greater reduction of metaplasia in the treated group.
(Adapted from Heimburger DC, et al. JAMA. 1988; 259:1525)

References

1. Preston AM. Cigarette smoking; nutritional implications. Prog Food Nutr Sci. 1991;15:183.
2. Schectman G. Estimating ascorbic acid requirements for cigarette smokers. Ann NY Acad Sci. 1993;686:335.
3. Heimburger DC, et al Improvement in bronchial squamous metaplasia in smokers treated with folate and B12. JAMA. 1988;259:1525.
4. Paiva SAR, et al. Assessment of vitamin A status in chronic obstructive pulmonary disease patients and healthy smokers. Am J Clin Nutr. 1996;64:928.
5. Vermaak WJH, et al. Vitamin B6 status and cigarette smoking. Am J Clin Nutr. 1990;51:1058.
6. Marangon K, et al. Diet, antioxidant status and smoking habits in French men. Am J Clin Nutr. 1998;67:231.
7. Stryker WS. The relation of diet, cigarette smoking and alcohol consumption to plasma beta-carotene and alpha-tocopherol levels. Am J Epidemiol. 1988;127:283.
8. Anderson R, et al. Regulation by the antioxidants ascorbate, cysteine and dapsone of the increased extracellular and intracellular generation of reactive oxidants by activated phagocytes from cigarette smokers. Am Rev Respir Dis. 1987;135:1027.
9. Van Antwerpen VL, et al. Vitamin E, pulmonary functions and phagocyte-mediated oxidative stress in smokers and nonsmokers. Free Rad Biol Med. 1995;18:935.
10. Brown KM, et al. Erythrocyte membrane fatty acid composition of smokers and non-smokers: Effects of vitamin E supplementation. Eur J Clin Nutr. 1998;52:145.
11. Ness AR, et al. Vitamin C status and respiratory function. Eur J Clin Nutr. 1996;50:573.

Heavy Alcohol Consumption

For most adults, occasional moderate alcohol drinking (one to two "drinks" per day) is not harmful, and may have health benefits. Moderate alcohol drinking can increase the HDL-cholesterol level in the blood, decrease risk of blood clots, and reduce risk of heart attack.[1] However, regular heavy drinking (more than three to four "drinks" per day) is a health hazard. (A "drink" is considered a 180-ml glass of wine, 360-ml glass of beer, or 30–45 ml of spirits.) Heavy drinking increases risk of high blood pressure, stroke, liver disease, immune weakness, and cancer.[2,3] Moreover, about one in ten people who drink alcohol become physically addicted.

Diet · Alcohol

Heavy alcohol intake causes inflammation of the lining of the stomach and intestines, reducing absorption of vitamins and minerals.[4-6] It also damages the pancreas, which impairs production of digestive enzymes and further lowers nutrient absorption from foods. The liver is particularly vulnerable to alcohol – more than three "drinks" a day causes inflammation and accumulation of fat in the liver. This impairs liver function, reducing the ability to detoxify chemicals and drugs. Because the liver is important for blood sugar control, alcohol-induced liver damage can produce hypoglycemia, leading to fatigue, irritability, and concentration difficulties. Alcohol increases urinary losses of many minerals, including zinc, calcium, and magnesium.[5] Because of these effects, a diet rich in fresh fruits and vegetables, whole grains, lean meats, and low-fat milk products should be carefully chosen.

Alcoholic beverages are high in calories (a glass of beer or wine contains 120–150 cal), and alcoholic drinks have little nutritional value otherwise. If a person drinks three to four glasses of wine or beer each day, alcohol will provide 15–20% of the energy in the diet. When trying to maintain a steady weight or lose weight, limiting alcohol intake is one of the best ways to cut calories.

Heavy alcohol intake during pregnancy, especially during the first 3 months, can cause birth defects and mental retardation in the infant.[7] No one knows how much alcohol is safe during pregnancy, and many experts feel even one "drink" per day is harmful. The safest course for a pregnant women is probably complete abstention during early pregnancy and only very rare intake in later pregnancy.

Micronutrients · Alcohol

Nutrient	Suggested daily dose	Comment
Antioxidant supplement (containing vitamins A, C, E, and zinc and selenium)	(See pp. 115 for antioxidant nutrients and suggested doses)	Alcohol can cause widespread cell damage and fat peroxidation in the liver.[8] Supplements may help protect against oxidative damage. Vitamin C may help detoxify alcohol[9]
GLA	As 1–2 g evening primrose oil	May help reduce damage to the liver and lessen symptoms related to alcohol withdrawal in heavy drinkers[12]
Carnitine	0.5–1.5 g	May help reduce hepatic damage and development of fatty liver[13]
Niacinamide	1–1.5 g	May help reduce damage to hepatic protein metabolism[14]
Vitamin B complex	Complete formula containing at least 25 mg vitamins B1, B2, B3, and B6, 0.4–0.8 mg folic acid, and 25 µg vitamin B12	B vitamins are poorly absorbed and their activation is impaired by alcohol. Most heavy drinkers are deficient in many B vitamins
Magnesium	400 mg	Deficiency is very common in heavy drinkers and can produce heart and neuromuscular problems
Zinc	30–45 mg	The main enzymes that detoxify alcohol are dependent on zinc, thus zinc deficiency impairs ability to breakdown alcohol, increasing potential harm[4]

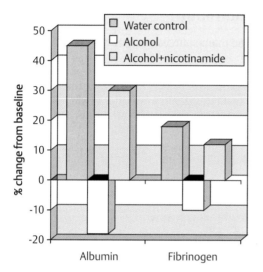

Fig. 5.**37**: **Counteracting the toxic effects of ethanol with nicotinamide.** In a controlled trial 15 healthy males were fed a test meal accompanied by either water, 750 ml wine (12% ethanol), or 750 ml wine plus 1.25 g nicotinamide. Over the 8-hour postprandial period, alcohol-induced impairment of hepatic protein synthesis was measured by determination of plasma albumin and fibrinogen. Nicotinamide treatment prevented the alcohol-induced fall in hepatic albumin and fibrinogen synthesis, suggesting that nicotinamide may help counteract the acute hepatotoxic effects of ethanol.
(From Volpi E, et al. J Nutr. 1997;127:2199)

References

1. Doll R, et al. Mortality in relation to consumption of alcohol: 13 years observations on male British doctors. BMJ. 1994;309:911.
2. Shaw S, Lieber CS. Nutrition and diet in alcoholism. In: Shils ME, Young VR, eds. Modern Nutrition in Health and Disease. Philadelphia: Lea & Febiger; 1994.
3. Seitz H, Pöschl G. Review: Alcohol and gastrointestinal cancer; pathogenic mechanisms. Add Biol. 1997;2:19.
4. McClain CJ, Su L. Zinc deficiency in the alcoholic: A review. Alcohol Clin Exp Res. 1983;7:5.
5. Odeleye OE, Watson RR. Alcohol-related nutritional derangements. In: Watson RR, Watzl B, eds. Nutrition and Alcohol. Boca Raton: CRC Press; 1992.
6. Salaspuro M. Nutrient intake and nutritional status in alcoholics. Alcohol Alcoholism. 1993;28:85.
7. Beattie JO. Alcohol exposure and the fetus. Eur J Clin Nutr. 1992;46:S7.
8. Tanner AR, et al. Depressed selenium and vitamin E levels in an alcoholic population: Possible relationship to hepatic injury through increased lipid peroxidation. Dig Dis Sci. 1986;31:1307.
9. Chen MF, et al. Effect of ascorbic acid on plasma alcohol clearance. J Am Coll Nutr. 1990;9:185.
10. Ravel JM, et al. Reversal of alcohol toxicity by glutamine. J Biol Chem. 1955;214:497.
11. Fincle LP. Experiments in treating alcoholics with glutamic acid and glutamine. Biochemical and Nutritional Aspects of Alcoholism. The University of Texas, Austin, 1964.
12. Segarnick DJ, et al. Gamma-linolenic acid inhibits the development of the ethanol-induced fatty liver. Prostaglandins Leukot Med. 1985;17:277.
13. Sachan DS, et al. Ameliorating effects of carnitine and its precursors on alcohol-induced fatty liver. Am J Clin Nutr. 1984;39:738.
14. Volpi E, et al. Nicotinamide counteracts alcohol-induced impairment of hepatic protein mezabolism in humans. J Nutr. 1997;127:2199.

Exposure to Heavy Metals

Toxic metals (lead, cadmium, mercury, aluminum) are naturally present in only trace quantities in the earth's crust. Modern industry has extracted these metals from the earth, concentrated them in various forms, and then dispersed them throughout the environment. Over the past century, soil, water, and air have become tainted with these metals. Once ingested, they tend to accumulate in the body – depositing in the skeleton, liver, and kidneys. Today, the average city-dweller has a body toxic metal burden 500–1000 times greater than that of people living in the preindustrial age. Even at low levels of exposure, toxic metals are potent poisons. They are thought to contribute to many modern ailments, including cancer, high blood pressure, and learning impairments in children.[1,2]

Lead

The main sources of lead pollution are[1,3,4]:

● Auto exhaust (foods grown near cities, industry, or busy roads)

● Industrial smoke from coal burning

● Pottery and glassware with lead-containing glaze or paint

● House paint (many older paints are very high in lead), house dust

● Canned foods (some canning processes use lead sealants)

● Car batteries, lead-shot, certain hair dyes, inks

● Lead plumbing (lead leaches into drinking water)

● Milk from animals grazing on grass containing traces of lead

● Cigarette smoke

The potential effects of low-level lead exposure include[2,5,6]:

● Learning problems, reduced intelligence, and hyperactivity in children, (exposure to lead during pregnancy can lead to permanent mental impairment of the infant)

● Anorexia and diarrhea

● Increased risk of cancer

● Headache, fatigue, irritability

● Depression, insomnia

● Increased risk of high blood pressure and heart disease (see Fig. 5.**38**)

Aluminum

The main sources of aluminum are[7,8]:

● Cookware. Use of aluminum pots and pans should be avoided, particularly when cooking vegetables, fruit, and other acidic foods that leach large amounts of aluminum from cookware

● Household and industrial utensils

● Aluminum-containing antacids

● Aluminum cans

● Deodorants, antiperspirants, cosmetics, toothpastes

● Refined white flour (aluminum-containing compounds are often used to bleach the flour)

● Anti-clumping additives in salt and spices, baking powder

The potential effects of low-level aluminum exposure include[7-9]:

● Disorders of the central nervous system: impaired memory, increased risk of Alzheimer's disease

● Impaired bone metabolism and increased risk of osteoporosis

● Liver and kidney toxicity

● Arthritis triggered by accumulation of aluminium in joints

Mercury

The main sources of mercury are:

● Amalgam dental fillings[10,11]

● Pesticides, fungicides, industrial waste

● Fish and shellfish from contaminated waters (they tend to concentrate mercury)

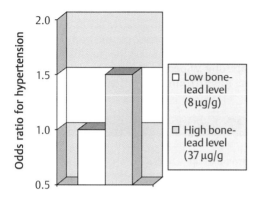

Fig. 5.**38**: **Lead exposure and risk of hypertension.** In 590 men, long-term exposure to lead was associated with increased risk of hypertension. An increase in bone lead from 8 µg/g of bone mineral to 37 µg/g increased risk of high blood pressure by 50%. (Adapted from Hu, H, et al. JAMA. 1996;275:1171)

The potential effects of low-level mercury exposure include[12]:

● Mental impairment, difficulty concentrating, headache

● Nerve damage that mimics multiple sclerosis

● Cerebral palsy, mental retardation, and birth defects if babies are exposed in utero

● Skin rash

● Increased risk of cancer

Cadmium

The main sources of cadmium are[13]:

● Metal coatings (cadmium is an anticorrosive) on metal pails, cans, refrigerator ice trays, water tanks

● Cigarette smoke (a concentrated source, containing about 20 g per cigarette). Smokers generally have body levels five times those of nonsmokers

● Insecticides

● Certain foods: instant coffee, canned foods, gelatin, some cola drinks, kidneys from animals given cadmium-containing worm-killing drugs

● Fish and shellfish from contaminated waters

● Pigments (especially red and yellow colors)

The potential effects of low-level cadmium exposure include[13]:

● Increased risk of high blood pressure[14]

● Increased risk of cancer

● Impaired immune function

Minimizing Exposure to Toxic Metals

Environmental sources. Exposure at home and work should be avoided. Cigarette smoke especially should be avoided (including "passive smoke" in cafes, restaurants, and at work), as well as exhaust fumes and areas where air pollution is high. Alternative dental filling materials should be substituted for amalgam fillings.

Water. Contamination from plumbing can be minimized by installing new plumbing if the old pipes are corroded or contain lead or galvanized coatings rich in cadmium. "Soft" water leaches more heavy metals from pipes than "hard" water. Another benefit of hard water is that it is richer in calcium and magnesium. High-quality water filters can minimize intake from drinking water. Water for cooking and drinking should not be taken from the hot-water tap if the plumbing is old (hot water leaches more metals from pipes). Water pipes should be flushed out before drawing water for drinking, especially in the morning or after periods of non-use when water has stood in them.

Food. Food and wine grown in gardens or vineyards located near heavily-trafficked roads should be avoided, as well as produce displayed outdoors near heavily-trafficked roads. Use of aluminum pots and pans for cooking should be avoided; they should be substituted by stainless-steel or enamel pots. Canned foods, particularly acidic foods such as fruits and tomatoes, should be avoided. The lip of newly-opened wine bottles should be carefully wiped to remove lead traces from the foil surrounding the cork.

Micronutrients · Heavy Metals

To speed elimination of toxic metals from the body and prevent accumulation

Nutrient	Suggested daily dose	Comments
Vitamin E plus selenium	200–400 mg vitamin E; 200 μg selenium	Helps reduce the adverse effects of lead and mercury[15,16]
Vitamin C	250 mg	May enhance excretion of toxic metals, protects against oxidative damage
Calcium plus magnesium	400 mg calcium; 200 mg magnesium	Reduces lead and cadmium absorption
Zinc	15–30 mg	May reduce absorption of cadmium; may enhance excretion of lead[17]

References

1. Folinsbee LJ. Human health effects of air pollution. Environ Health Perspect. 1993;100:45.
2. Baghurst PA, et al. Environmental lead exposure and children's intelligence at the age of seven years. N Engl J Med. 1992;327:1279.
3. Needleman HL. Preventing childhood lead poisoning. Prev Med. 1994;23:634.
4. Weiss ST, et al. The relationship of blood lead to blood pressure in a longitudinal study of working men. Am J Epidemiol. 1986;123:800.
5. Singh B, et al. Impact of lead pollution on the status of the other trace elements in blood and alterations in hepatic functions. Biol Trace Elem Res. 1994;40:21.
6. Ehle AL, Mckee DC. Neuropsychological effect of lead in occupationally exposed workers: A critical review. Crit Rev Toxicol. 1990;20:237.
7. Cooke K, Gould M. The health effects of aluminum: A review. J R Soc Health. 1991;111:163.
8. Doll R. Review: Alzheimer's disease and environmental aluminum. Age Ageing. 1993;22:138.
9. Exley C, et al. Aluminum toxicokinetics. J Toxicol Environ Health. 1996;48:569.
10. Stoz F, et al. Is a generalized amalgam ban justified? Studies of mothers and their newborn infants. Z Geburtshilfe Perinatol. 1995;199:35.
11. Pleva J. Dental mercury: A public health hazard. Rev Environ Health. 1994;10:1.
12. Ratcliffe HE, et al. Human exposure to mercury: A critical assessment of the evidence of adverse health effects. J Toxicol Environ Health. 1996;49:221.
13. Robards K, Worsfold P. Cadmium: Toxicology and analysis: A review. Analyst. 1991;116:549.
14. Nakagawa H, Nishijo M. Environmental cadmium exposure, hypertension, and cardiovascular risk. J Cardiovasc Risk. 1996;3:11.
15. Dhawan M, et al. Preventive and therapeutic role of vitamin E in chronic plumbism. Biomed Environ Sci. 1989;2:335.
16. Cuvin-Aralar ML, Furness RW. Mercury and selenium interaction: A review. Ecotoxicol Environ Safety. 1991;21:348.
17. Flora SJS, Tandon SK. Adjuvants for therapeutic chelating drugs in lead intoxication. Trace Elem Electrol. 1995;12:131.

Exercise and Sport

Regular training sharply increases an athlete's need for energy, protein, and many micronutrients, and dietary choices can have a profound impact on performance and endurance. Along with proper training, optimum nutrition will allow those who exercise to attain their "personal best."

Energy Sources: Carbohydrate and Fat

Energy needs for exercise vary considerably depending on the intensity and duration of the activity and on the size of the individual.[1] The more strenuous the exercise and the higher the body weight, the more energy is required. For example, the average 60-kg man running at a moderate pace (14.5 km/hr) will expend about 750 kcal/hr, whereas a 90-kg man, running for the same time period, would burn over 1200 kcal.

Both fat and carbohydrate are oxidized to provide energy during exercise. Whether the body uses predominantly fat or carbohydrate depends on the intensity of the activity.[1] Fat is particularly important as a source of energy during long, endurance events that last for several hours, such as cycling or distance running. Marathon runners derive over 75% of their energy needs from metabolism of fat. However, as exercise intensity increases, glucose stored in muscle and liver cells as glycogen becomes more important than fat as a fuel source. Sprinters burn mostly glucose in muscle during short, high-intensity exercise.

Body stores of glycogen are limited and contain only about 1200 kcal. Used alone, glycogen can provide energy for only short periods (about 60 mins). Therefore, most exercise – such as tennis, soccer, and cycling – is fueled by mixtures of fat and carbohydrate.[1] Because glucose stores are relatively small (compared with fat stores), during endurance events, glucose stores are depleted long before fat stores. When glucose stores are used

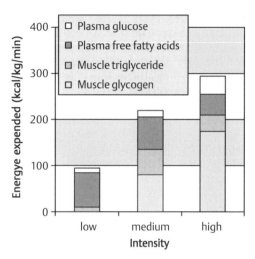

Fig. 5.**39**: **Energy fuels during exercise of different intensity.** Contribution of the major substrates for energy after 30 min exercise at 25%, 65%, and 85% of maximal oxygen uptake.
(Adapted from Romijn JA, et al. Am J Physiol. 1993; 265:E380)

up, muscles become fatigued and the athlete begins to feel exhausted. Highly trained athletes can store more glycogen in their muscles and are able to preserve these stores by using more energy from fat during exercise.[1]

Along with proper training, dietary choices have a strong influence on the amount of glucose stored in muscle. Diets high in carbohydrate stimulate muscles to store more glucose and can increase endurance.[2,3] Athletes consuming 60–70% of calories as carbohydrates are better able to build large reserves of muscle glycogen than those consuming 40% of calories as carbohydrate (the normal amount of carbohydrate in the typical diet is about 45%).[2]

For endurance athletes, at least two-thirds of total calories should come from carbohydrate. This means eating 500–600 g of carbohydrate each day. Emphasis should be on eating complex carbohydrates because, compared with simple carbohydrates, they contain more of the nutrients needed by athletes (they are richer in B vitamins, minerals, and fiber). Fat intake should be only 20–30% of total calories. Body fat stores, even in very lean athletes, contain much more fat than is needed during training or competition. For example, because each half kilo of fat contains approximately 3500 kcal, a 70-kg athlete with only 15% body fat has over 80000 kcal stored as fat.

For several hours after a strenuous workout, muscle cells are "hungry" for glucose, and depleted glycogen stores can be quickly and efficiently replenished.[4] Therefore, athletes should try to drink three to four cups of fruit juice or eat the equivalent of about five slices of bread within 2 hours after exercise. This carbohydrate will be used to replenish glycogen stores, and recovery from the exercise will be enhanced.[4]

Carbohydrate "Loading"

A good way to maximize glycogen stores in preparation for competition is to "load" carbohydrate.[3] One week before the event the athlete should train long and hard over the course of a day in an attempt to completely drain muscle glucose stores. This is followed by 3 days of only light to moderate training and a diet that minimizes replacing the depleted muscle glycogen – one very low in carbohydrate and higher in fat and protein. Finally, in the 3 days prior to the event, the athlete stops training and consumes a diet very high in carbohydrate (70% of calories). This cycle – intense depletion, limited glucose supply, then sudden abundance – triggers glucose stores in muscle to rebound to three to four times the normal level.[3,4] This can significantly increase endurance, particularly in events lasting longer than 90 minutes.

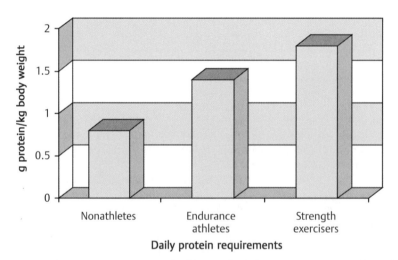

Fig. 5.**40**: **Increased protein requirements of athletes.** The daily protein requirement for endurance athletes is 1.2–1.4 g protein/kg body weight and for strength exercisers 1.7–1.8 g/kg body weight. This represents an increase of 150–175% and 212–225%, respectively, over the current recommended dietary allowance for nonathletes. (From Lemon PR. Nutr Rev. 1996;54:S169)

The Pre-Event Meal

Allowing for personal preferences, the pre-event meal should consist mainly of easily digestible carbohydrates and very low levels of fat and protein. Fat and protein-rich foods slow down stomach emptying and should be avoided just before competition; exercising with a full stomach can cause stomach pain and nausea. How much carbohydrate should be eaten? About 3–4 g/kg body weight should be consumed 3–4 hours prior to exercise.[4] For a 70 kg person, this is about 250 g of carbohydrate. Liquids can be consumed closer to beginning competition because they leave the stomach more quickly than solid food.

Fluids

Water is a critical nutrient for the athlete in training and competition. Working muscles produce heat, and water is lost during exercise as the body attempts to keep cool and dissipates heat through sweating. Ninety minutes of strenuous exercise in a 70-kg athlete will produce sweat water losses of 1.5–3.0 kg, depending on air temperature and humidity.[5]

Excessive loss of body water (dehydration) interferes with the ability of the body to circulate oxygen and nutrients and reduces performance. Muscular stamina and strength rapidly fall if only 1–2% of body water is lost – about a 1-kg sweat loss in a 70-kg person. Greater losses (5–7% of body weight) can cause muscular cramping, heat exhaustion, and collapse.[5] Thirst often lags behind water losses, so it is important to make a conscious effort to drink fluids before, during, and after activity.

Sweat contains trace amounts of electrolytes, particularly sodium and chloride. Although small amounts of these are lost in sweat, because the body loses much more water, concentrations of sodium actually rise in body fluids. Therefore, the need to replace water during and after exercise is much greater than the need to replace lost electrolytes. Because only very small amounts of electrolytes are lost, heavy sweating for periods of up to 2–3 hours has no significant effects on electrolyte concentrations in the body.[5] Although salt (sodium chloride) tablets are often promoted for athletes, only in ultra-long endurance events do electrolyte losses in sweat become significant. A single post-exercise meal replaces all the electrolytes lost in moderate exercise.

To estimate water needs, an athlete can weigh him/herself after a workout: if body weight drops more than 2% during exercise, fluid intake has probably been inadequate. In general, at least two large glasses of cool fluid should be consumed for every 0.5 kg of body weight lost. Fluids that are cool and diluted (containing less than 6% sugar) are absorbed more rapidly than concentrated fluids (more than 10% sugar).[5] Fruit juices, soft drinks, and many sports drinks have more than 10% sugar, and will be more rapidly absorbed if diluted with about two to three parts water. If exercise exceeds 60 minutes, a sports beverage containing sucrose, glucose, glucose polymers, or maltodextrin can be beneficial, providing energy for muscles and potentially increasing endurance.[3,5]

Protein for Bodybuilding

In bodybuilding increased muscle size is produced mainly by extensive weight training, not by eating large amounts of protein. However, weightlifters need about two and a half times the amount of protein of nonexercising individuals: about 1.8 g/kg/day, or about 120 g for a 70-kg person.[6] Increased protein requirements should be met by consuming high-quality protein foods, such as eggs, low-fat milk, lean meats, and fish. If the athlete is vegetarian, combining foods carefully (see pp. 19) will provide complete protein for new muscle synthesis. There is usually no need for protein or amino-acid supplements if ample high-quality protein is obtained from dietary sources.[6]

Vitamins and Minerals

Certain vitamins (such as thiamin, riboflavin, niacin, vitamin B6, and pantothenic acid) and minerals (iron, zinc, magnesium) play central roles in cellular energy production. Athletes have increased needs for these micronutrients during training. To cover these increased needs, diets need to be carefully selected and must include ample whole grains, lean meat, eggs, and fresh fruits and vegetables. However, the diets of many athletes in strenuous training do not provide adequate amounts of micronutrients. [7,8] Because even marginal deficiencies may adversely affect performance, a complete and balanced vitamin/mineral supplement may be beneficial.[7,9,10] Iron is a mineral of special concern in athletes. Low iron stores are common among athletes (especially runners) who exercise heavily: it is estimated that 50% of female runners have low iron stores and 10% of male athletes are iron deficient. Iron supplementation in athletes who are iron deficient can significantly improve performance.[11,12]

Strenuous exercise produces free radicals in muscle, and oxidative damage (see pp. 115) may contribute to slow recovery after exercise and early fatigue.[13] Foods rich in antioxidants such as the carotenoids, vitamins E and C, and selenium should be consumed daily. In addition, supplemental vitamin E, at doses above those found in usual diets, may help protect exercising muscle from free-radical damage.[14]

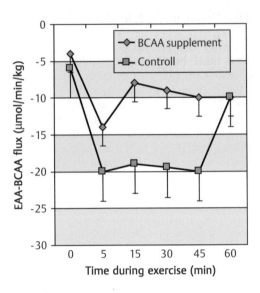

Fig. 5.**41**: **Branched-chain amino acids reduce protein breakdown during exercise.** 5 men were given an oral supplement of branched-chain amino acids (BCAAs) (77 mg/kg body weight) or placebo before exercising at 70% of maximal work capacity for 60 min. During exercise total release of essential amino acids (EAAs) minus BCAAs was lower for the BCAA trial than the control trial. This suggests that supplemental BCAAs during exercise suppress endogenous muscle protein breakdown.
(Adapted from MacLean DA, et al. Am J Physiol. 1994;267:E1010)

Micronutrients · Exercise

Nutrient	Suggested dialy dose	Comments
Multimineral supplement with iron	Balanced formula containing at least 10–20 mg zinc, 5–10 mg iron, and 200 µg chromium	Deficiencies of iron, zinc, or chromium are common among athletes and can impair performance[7,10,11]
Vitamin E plus selenium	50–100 mg vitamin E; 100 µg selenium	Helps protect muscles from free radical damage during exercise[13,14]
Vitamin B complex	Complete formula containing at least 25 mg thiamin, riboflavin, niacin, and vitamin B6, and pantothenic acid	In athletes whose diets are marginal, supplementation may enhance performance[7,9]

References

1. Coyle EF. Substrate utilization during exercise in active people. Am J Clin Nutr. 1995;61:968S.
2. Probart CK, et al. Diet and athletic performance. Med Clin North Am. 1993;77:757.
3. Hargreaves M. Carbohydrates and exercise performance. Nutr Rev. 1996;54:136S.
4. Coyle EF. Timing and method of increased carbohydrate intake to cope with heavy training, competition and recovery. In: Williams C, Devlin J, eds. Food, Nutrition and Sports Performance. London: E & FN Spon; 1992:35–61.
5. Maughan RJ. Fluid and electrolyte loss and replacement in exercise. In: Williams C, Devlin J, eds. Food, Nutrition and Sports Performance. London: E & FN Spon;1992:147–7.
6. Lemon PWR. Is increased dietary protein necessary or beneficial for individuals with a physically active lifestyle? Nutr Rev. 1996;54:S169.
7. Armstrong LA, Maresh CM: Vitamin and mineral supplements as nutritional aids to exercise performance and health. Nutr Rev. 1996;54:S149.
8. Telford RD, et al. The effect of 7 to 8 months of vitamin/mineral supplementation on the vitamin and mineral status of athletes. Int J Sport Nutr. 1992;2:123.
9. Suboticaneac K, et al. Effects of pyridoxine and riboflavin supplementation on physical fitness in young adolescents. Int J Vitam Nutr Res. 1990;60:81.
10. Clarkson PM. Minerals: Exercise performance and supplementation in athletes. J Sports Sci. 1991;9:91.
11. Hunding A, et al. Runners anemia and iron deficiency. Acta Med Scand. 1981;209:315.
12. Nickerson HJ, et al. Causes of iron deficiency in adolescent athletes. J Pediatr. 1989;114:657.
13. Kanter MM. Free radicals, exercise, and antioxidant supplementation. Int J Sport Nutr. 1994;4:205.
14. Rokitzki L, et al. Alpha-tocopherol supplementation in racing cyclists during extreme endurance training. Int J Sport Nutr. 1994;4:253.

Appendices

Appendix I

Drug-Micronutrient Interactions

Drug	Micronutrient	Interaction
Angiotension-converting enzyme inhibitors	Potassium	Increases blood potassium level
Adrenocorticotropic hormone	Potassium	Increases urinary potassium excretion
	Vitamin B6	Increases urinary vitamin B6 excretion
Adriamycin	Coenzyme Q10	Increases coenzyme Q10 requirements
Alcohol	B-complex and fat-soluble vitamins	Reduces vitamin absorption and impairs metabolism
	Magnesium	Increases urinary magnesium excretion
	Zinc	Reduces zinc absorption and increases urinary excretion
Allopurinol	Iron	Enhances storage of liver iron
Aminoglycosides	Potassium, magnesium, calcium, zinc	Increases urinary mineral excretion
	Vitamin K, biotin	Reduces endogenous vitamin production by colonic bacteria
Aminopterin	Folate	Impairs vitamin metabolism
Amitryptilline	Riboflavin	Impairs vitamin metabolism
Amphotericin B	Potassium, magnesium	Increases urinary mineral excretion
Androgens	Calcium	Reduces urinary calcium excretion, may produce hypercalcemia
Antacids	Vitamin-B complex, choline, vitamin A, vitamin C, calcium, phosphorus, iron, zinc, fluoride	Reduces vitamin and mineral absorption
Antibiotics (broad spectrum)	Vitamin K, biotin	Reduces endogenous vitamin production by colonic bacteria
Anticoagulants (warfarins)	Vitamin K	Antagonizes vitamin action
		High doses of vitamin K reduce activity of the coumarins
	Vitamin E, vitamin C	High doses of these vitamins may potentiate anticoagulant action
Atropine	Iron	Reduces iron absorption
Azathioprine	Vitamin B6	Increases urinary vitamin B6 excretion
	Folate	Impairs folate metabolism
Barbiturates	Biotin, vitamin B6, vitamin B12, riboflavin, folate	Impairs vitamin metabolism and decreases serum levels
	Calcium	Reduces calcium absorption
	Vitamin D, vitamin K	Increases vitamin breakdown and biliary excretion
	Vitamin C	Increases urinary vitamin C excretion
	Biotin	Decreases plasma biotin levels
	Potassium	Increases urinary potassium excretion
	Folate	High doses of folate may reverse the anticonvulsant effects
Beta-blockers	Niacin	High doses of niacin may enhance hypotensive action

Drug	Micronutrient	Interaction
Butyrophenone	Niacin, manganese	Impairs vitamin metabolism
Calcitonin	Vitamin C	Increases vitamin requirement
	Magnesium	Reduces urinary magnesium excretion
	Calcium	Decreases calcium release from bone
Carbamazine	Biotin, folate, vitamin B12	Increases vitamin requirements
Carbenoxolone	Potassium	Increases urinary potassium excretion
Carbutamide	Potassium	Increases urinary potassium excretion
Cephalosporins (e.g. moxalactam)	Vitamin K	Impairs vitamin metabolism
Chlorambucil	Vitamin B6	Increases urinary vitamin B6 excretion
Chloramphenicol	Vitamin B12	Reduces vitamin B12 absorption
	Folate	Increases folate requirements
	Vitamin K, biotin	Reduces endogenous vitamin production by colonic bacteria
	Vitamin B6	Increases urinary vitamin B6 excretion
Chlorpromazine	Riboflavin	Increases urinary riboflavin excretion and impairs metabolism
Cholesterol-lowering drugs:		
– Cholestyramine	Vitamin A, vitamin D, vitamin E , vitamin K, beta-carotene	Reduces vitamin and mineral absorption
	Calcium	Increases urinary calcium excretion
– Colestipol	Magnesium, folate, vitamin B12, iron, calcium,vitamin A, beta-carotene, vitamin D, vitamin E, vitamin K, calcium, magnesium	Reduces vitamin and mineral absorption, may lower plasma levels of vitamin A and vitamin E
– Clofibrate	Vitamin B12, beta-carotene, iron	Reduces vitamin and mineral absorption
– HMG-CoA reductase inhibitors	Coenzyme Q10	Impairs coenzyme Q10 metabolism
cis-Platin	Potassium, magnesium	Increases urinary mineral excretion
Colchicine	Vitamin A, vitamin D, vitamin E, vitamin K, vitamin B12, beta-carotene	Reduces vitamin absorption
	Magnesium	Increases urinary magnesium excretion
Corticosteroids	Vitamin C	Increases vitamin C turnover and urinary excretion
	Vitamin B6	Increases vitamin B6 urinary excretion
	Folate	Impairs folate metabolism
	Vitamin D	Increases vitamin D requirement
	Calcium, phosphorus	Reduces mineral absorption and increases urinary excretion
	Magnesium, potassium, zinc	Increases urinary mineral excretion
Cyclophosphamide	Vitamin B6	Increases urinary vitamin B6 excretion
Cycloserine	Folate, vitamin B12	Impairs vitamin metabolism
	Vitamin B6	Impairs vitamin B6 metabolism and increases urinary excretion
Digitalis	Potassium, magnesium	Increases urinary mineral excretion
Dimercaprol	Zinc, copper	Increases urinary mineral excretion
Dimethyl sulfoxide (DMSO)	Zinc, copper	Increases urinary mineral excretion
Doxorubicin	Vitamin E	Increases vitamin E oxidation
Ethosuximide	Vitamin D	Impairs vitamin metabolism

Drug	Micronutrient	Interaction
Fiber (e.g., psyllium, bran)	Beta-carotene, riboflavin, zinc, iron, copper, manganese	Reduces vitamin and mineral absorption
5-fluorouracil	Thiamin	Reduces thiamin absorption
Glutethimide	Vitamin D	Increases vitamin D requirement
Guanethidine	Niacin	Niacin enhances hypotensive action
Guanidine	Vitamin B12	Reduces vitamin B12 absorption
H₂-blockers	Vitamin B12, iron	Reduces vitamin and mineral absorption
Hydralazine	Folate	Impairs folate metabolism
	Vitamin B6	Increases urinary vitamin B6 excretion
Indomethacin	Vitamin C	Decreases plasma and leukocyte vitamin levels
Insulin	Chromium	Chromium enhances hypoglycemic action
Isoniazid	Vitamin D	Impairs vitamin D metabolism
	Vitamin B6	Impairs vitamin B6 metabolism and increases urinary excretion
	Folate	Increases folate requirement
	Niacin	Reduces conversion of tryptophan to niacin
	Zinc	Increases urinary zinc excretion
Potassium chloride	Vitamin B12	Reduces vitamin B12 absorption
Kaolin	Riboflavin	Reduces riboflavin absorption
Ketoconazole	Magnesium	Magnesium may reduce absorption
Oral contraceptives		
High-dose estrogen	Vitamin C	Increases vitamin C oxidation and decreases levels in plasma and leukocytes
	Vitamin B6, riboflavin, folate	Impairs vitamin metabolism
High-dose and low-dose estrogen	Calcium	Increases calcium absorption
	Manganese, zinc	Reduces blood mineral levels
	Carotenoids	Increases conversion to vitamin A
	Tryptophan	Increases conversion to niacin
	Vitamin A, iron, copper	Elevated vitamin and mineral levels in blood
Laxatives	Most vitamins and minerals	Reduces vitamin and mineral absorption due to accelerated transit time
Lithium	Magnesium, potassium	Increases blood mineral levels
	Iodine	Impairs iodine metabolism
L-dopa	Vitamin B6	Decreases L-dopa activity
Loop diuretics	Potassium, magnesium	Increases urinary mineral excretion
Mecamylamine	Magnesium	Reduces urinary excretion of mecamylamine
	Niacin	Niacin potentiates hypotensive effects
Mercaptopurine	Pantothenic acid	Impairs pantothenic acid metabolism
	Zinc	Increases zinc requirement
Metformin	Vitamin B12	Reduces vitamin absorption
	Folate	Decreases serum folate level
Methotrexate	Folate, riboflavin	Impairs vitamin metabolism
	Vitamin B12, folate, EFAs	Reduces vitamin and fatty acid absorption
	Zinc	Increases zinc requirement
Mineral oil (laxative)	Vitamin A, vitamin D, vitamin E, vitamin K, beta-carotene	Reduces vitamin absorption
Muscle relaxants	Thiamin	May enhance relaxant effect
Nitrofurantoin	Folate	Reduces folate absorption
Nitrous oxide	Vitamin B12	Increases vitamin B12 breakdown

Drug	Micronutrient	Interaction
Neomycin	Vitamin A, vitamin D, vitamin E, vitamin K, beta-carotene, vitamin B12, potassium, calcium, iron	Reduces vitamin and mineral absorption
	Vitamin K, biotin	Reduces endogenous vitamin production by colonic bacteria
	Magnesium	Increases urinary magnesium excretion
Neuroleptics	Thiamin	Reduces thiamin absorption and increases excretion
Estrogen replacement therapy	Vitamin D	Increases synthesis of 1,25 OH$_2$vitamin D
	Calcium	Increases calcium absorption and decreases urinary excretion
	Vitamin B6	Impairs vitamin B6 metabolism
p-Aminosalicylic acid	Vitamin B12, folate, iron	Reduces vitamin and mineral absorption
	Potassium	Increases urinary potassium excretion
Pargyline	Niacin	Niacin enhances hypotensive action
Penicillamine	Vitamin B6	Impairs B6 metabolism and increases urinary excretion
	Copper, zinc	Increases urinary mineral excretion
Penicillin	Potassium	Increases urinary potassium excretion
Pentamidine	Folate	Impairs folate metabolism
Phenothiazine	Manganese	Increases excretion of manganese
	Riboflavin	Impairs riboflavin metabolism and increases urinary excretion
Phenylbutazone	Potassium	Increases urinary potassium excretion
	Folate	Impairs folate utilization
Phenytoin	Folate	Reduces absorption and impairs metabolism, high doses of folate antagonize anticonvulsive effects
	Vitamin B12	Decreases serum and brain levels
	Magnesium	Decreases serum magnesium levels
	Vitamin D, vitamin K	Increases vitamin turnover
	Vitamin B6	High doses of B6 increase catabolism
	Calcium	Reduces calcium absorption
	Zinc	Increases zinc requirement
	Copper	Increases serum copper level
Potassium-sparing diuretics (spironolactone, triamterene)	Folate	Impairs metabolism
	Potassium, magnesium	Reduces urinary mineral excretion
Primidone	Folate	Impairs metabolism and reduces absorption, high doses of folate antagonize effects
	Vitamin B6, vitamin B12	Decreases serum vitamin levels
	Vitamin D, vitamin K	Increases vitamin breakdown and excretion
	Calcium	Reduces calcium absorption
Probenecid	Riboflavin	Reduces riboflavin absorption
	Calcium, magnesium, potassium	Increases urinary mineral excretion
Pyrimethamine	Folate, vitamin B12	Impairs vitamin metabolism, folate antagonizes activity
Quinidine	Vitamin K	Impairs vitamin K status
Quinine	Folate	Impairs folate status

Drug	Micronutrient	Interaction
Rifampicin	Vitamin D	Increases vitamin D turnover
	Calcium	Reduces calcium absorption due to decreased activity of vitamin D
Salicylates	Vitamin A, vitamin B6	Reduces vitamin clearance
	Vitamin C	Reduces vitamin C absorption, decreases uptake into leukocytes and levels in plasma and platelets; increases urinary excretion
	Vitamin K	Impairs vitamin metabolism
	Iron	Increases iron losses from the digestive tract
	Folate	Reduces serum folate levels
Sulfasalazine	Folate	Reduces folate absorption and impairs metabolism
Sodium nitroprusside	Vitamin B12	Increases urinary vitamin B12 excretion
Sulfonamide	Folate	Impairs folate metabolism
Sulfonylureas	Niacin	High doses of niacin may reduce effectiveness of certain oral hypoglycemic drugs
Tetracycline	Vitamin C	Impairs vitamin C metabolism and increases urinary excretion
	Magnesium, zinc, calcium, iron	Reduces both mineral and tetracycline absorption
	Zinc	Increases urinary excretion
	Vitamin K, biotin	Reduces endogenous vitamin production by colonic bacteria
	Riboflavin, vitamin C	Increases urinary vitamin excretion
Thiazides	Vitamin-B complex, vitamin C, potassium, magnesium, zinc	Increases urinary vitamin and mineral excretion
	Calcium	Decreases urinary calcium excretion
Theophylline	Vitamin B6	Impairs vitamin metabolism
Thyroxine	Riboflavin	Reduces riboflavin absorption
	Vitamin E	Impairs vitamin metabolism
Trimethoprim	Folate	Impairs folate metabolism and reduces absorption
Valproic acid	Copper, zinc, selenium	Reduces serum mineral levels

References

Handbook on Drug and Nutrient Interactions. Chicago: American Dietetic Association; 1994.

Knapp H. Nutrient-drug interactions. In: Ziegler EE, Filer LJ, eds. Present Knowledge in Nutrition. Washington, DC: ILSI Press; 1996.

Roe DA. Diet, nutrition and drug reactions. In: Shils ME, Olson JA, Shike M, eds. Modern Nutrition in Health and Disease. Philadelphia: Lea & Febiger; 1994.

Thomas JA. Drug-nutrient interactions. Nutr Rev. 1995;53:271.

Appendix II

Nutrient-Nutrient Interactions

Nutrient	Nutrient	Interaction
Calcium	Magnesium	High doses reduce calcium absorption, deficiency produces hypocalcemia
	Phosphorus	High intakes (> 2 g/d) increase urinary calcium excretion
	Protein	High intakes increase urinary calcium excretion
	Sodium	Increases urinary calcium excretion
	Vitamin D	Promotes calcium absorption, reduces urinary calcium excretion
	Zinc	High intakes (> 140 mg/d) reduce calcium absorption
Carnitine	Vitamin C	Deficiency increases carnitine requirements
Chromium	Calcium	High doses of calcium carbonate reduce chromium absorption
	Iron	Iron deficiency enhances chromium absorption. Saturating blood transferrin with iron reduces blood chromium transport and retention
Copper	Cadmium	Impairs copper absorption and utilization
	Iron	Large doses reduce copper absorption
	Molybdenum	Increases urinary copper excretion
	Vitamin B6	Deficiency reduces copper absorption
	Vitamin C	High levels reduce copper absorption and levels of ceruloplasmin, may stimulate copper utilization
	Zinc	High doses (> 80 mg/d) reduce copper absorption
Fluoride	Calcium	Reduces fluoride absorption
Folic acid	Vitamin B12	Deficiency impairs folate utilization and metabolism
	Niacin	Deficiency reduces activation of folate
	Vitamin C	Maintains body stores of folate and reduces urinary folate excretion
Iron	Calcium	Reduces absorption of both heme and nonheme iron
	Copper	High doses reduce iron absorption; deficiency impairs utilization of body iron
	Manganese	Reduces iron absorption
	Riboflavin	Deficiency may reduce iron absorption, impair iron metabolism, and increase risk of anemia
	Vitamin A	Deficiency impairs mobilization and utilization of body iron; plasma iron levels fall
	Vitamin B6	Deficiency impairs iron metabolism
	Vitamin E	May reduce hematologic response to iron in treatment of iron-deficiency anemia
	Vitamin C	Sharply increases absorption of iron and overcomes inhibition of iron absorption by phenols and phytates; enhances iron utilization by tissues
	Zinc	Reduces iron absorption
Magnesium	Calcium	High doses reduce magnesium absorption. Hypercalcemia increases and hypocalcemia reduces urinary magnesium excretion
	Iron	Reduces magnesium absorption
	Manganese	Reduces magnesium absorption

Nutrient	Nutrient	Interaction
	Phosphorus	Reduces magnesium absorption. Deficiency increases urinary magnesium excretion
	Potassium	Increases urinary magnesium excretion
	Sodium	Increases urinary magnesium excretion
	Vitamin B6	Increases intracellular magnesium levels and utilization
	Vitamin E	Deficiency reduces tissue levels of magnesium
	Vitamin D	Enhances bioavailability of magnesium
Manganese	Calcium	Reduces manganese absorption
	Copper	Reduces manganese absorption
	Phosphate	Reduces manganese absorption
	Iron	Reduces manganese absorption and impairs utilization
	Vitamin C	May increase manganese bioavailability
Molybdenum	Copper	High doses interfere with molybdenum metabolism
Niacin	Tryptophan	Precursor in niacin synthesis
	Riboflavin	Essential cofactor in synthesis of niacin from trytophan. Deficiency impairs synthesis of niacin
	Vitamin B6	Essential cofactor in synthesis of niacin from trytophan. Deficiency impairs synthesis of niacin
Omega-6 fatty acids (evening primrose oil, GLA)	Omega-3 fatty acids	Increased intake reduces utilization of omega-6 fatty acids
	Vitamin E	Reduces peroxidation of EFAs
Omega-3 fatty acids (fish oils, EPA, DHA)	Omega-6 fatty acids	Increased intake reduces utilization of omega-3 fatty acids
	Vitamin E	Reduces peroxidation of EFAs
Potassium	Magnesium	Deficiency increases urinary excretion
Riboflavin	Niacin	Important in activation of riboflavin
Selenium	Vitamin C	Deficiency impairs selenium utilization. High doses reduce absorption of inorganic forms of selenium (e.g., sodium selenite)
	Vitamin E	Deficiency increases selenium requirement
Thiamine	Magnesium	Deficiency impairs activation of thiamin to thiamin pyrophosphate
	Vitamin C	Protects thiamin from inactivation in gastrointestinal tract by polyphenols
	Folic acid	Deficiency reduces absorption of thiamin
Tryptophan	Protein	Reduces brain tryptophan levels when consumed with tryptophan supplements because dietary amino acids compete with tryptophan for transport into the brain and reduce brain uptake of tryptophan
	Carbohydrate	Increases brain tryptophan levels when consumed with tryptophan supplements because insulin secretion in response to carbohydrate promotes transport of competing amino acids out of bloodstream, increasing tryptophan uptake into the brain
	Vitamin B6	High doses increase brain tryptophan levels
Vitamin A	Vitamin C	May reduce toxicity from vitamin A
	Vitamin E	Enhances absorption, storage, and utilization of vitamin A, reduces toxicity of high doses of vitamin A
	Zinc	Deficiency impairs vitamin A metabolism and utilization
Vitamin B6	Niacin	Important in activation of vitamin B6

Nutrient	Nutrient	Interaction
	Riboflavin	Participates in conversion of vitamin B6 to active forms
	Zinc	Important in conversion of vitamin B6 to active forms
	Vitamin C	Deficiency may increase urinary vitamin B6 excretion
Vitamin B12	Potassium	Extended release potassium-chloride tablets reduce vitamin B12 absorption
	Folic acid	Large doses may mask hematologic signs of vitamin B12 deficiency
Vitamin C	Iron	Large doses reduce blood vitamin C levels through oxidation
	Vitamin A	Chronic high doses may reduce tissue levels of vitamin C and increase urinary excretion
	Vitamin B6	Deficiency may increase risk of vitamin C deficiency
Vitamin D	Vitamin E	Deficiency impairs vitamin D metabolism
	Magnesium	Deficiency impairs vitamin D activity
	Calcium	Hypocalcemia stimulates vitamin D conversion to active forms; hypercalcemia inhibits vitamin D activation
	Phosphorus	Hypophosphatemia stimulates vitamin D conversion to active forms; hyperphosphatemia inhibits vitamin D activation
Vitamin E	Iron	Large doses increase vitamin E requirements
	Copper	Large doses increase vitamin E requirements
	Zinc	Deficiency reduces vitamin E blood levels
	Selenium	Poor status increases vitamin E requirements
	Vitamin C	Reduces oxidized tocopherol back to active tocopherol, thereby conserving vitamin E stores
	EFAs	Increases vitamin E requirements
Vitamin K	Calcium	High doses of calcium, or a dietary calcium : phosphorus ratio > 2:1 may impair vitamin K status
	Vitamin E	Large doses (> 1200 mg/d) may reduce absorption and activity of vitamin K
	Vitamin A	High doses reduce absorption of vitamin K, and hypothrombinemia may occur
Zinc	Calcium	High doses reduce zinc absorption
	Copper	Reduces zinc absorption
	Folic acid	Reduces zinc absorption
	Iron	A dietary iron : zinc ratio > 2:1 reduces absorption of zinc
	Cysteine	Enhances zinc absorption
	Histidine	Enhances zinc absorption
	Vitamin A	Enhances zinc absorption
	Vitamin B6	Enhances zinc absorption, vitamin B6 deficiency reduces plasma zinc levels
	Vitamin E	Deficiency reduces plasma zinc levels and may exacerbate zinc deficiency

Appendix III

Laboratory Diagnosis of Micronutrient Status

Micronutrient	Values	Comments
Vitamins:		
Vitamin A and the carotenoids		
Plasma retinol	Levels < 1.05 μmol/l indicate deficiency	Plasma retinol levels are maintained at the expense of liver vitamin A. Thus, plasma retinol levels begin to fall only when vitamin A deficiency is severe. Retinol-binding protein transports retinol in the blood. Even with adequate body stores of vitamin A, if retinol-binding protein levels fall (for example, if liver synthesis is inadequate) plasma retinol levels will be low
Measurement of vitamin A content of liver by biopsy	Levels < 0.07 μmol/g indicate deficiency	An accurate measure of body stores
Plasma beta-carotene	Normal levels are 0.3–0.6 μmol/l	
Serum total carotenoids	Levels < 50 μmol/l indicate deficiency	
Vitamin D		
Plasma 25-(OH) vitamin D	Levels < 25 μmol/l indicate deficiency	Reflects body reserves
Plasma 1–25-(OH)$_2$ vitamin D	Normal levels are 48–100 pmol/l	Measures current biologic activity of vitamin
Vitamin E		
Plasma total vitamin E	Levels < 11.6 μmol/l indicate deficiency	
Plasma alpha-tocopherol (μmol/l)/ plasma cholesterol (mmol/l)	Ratio < 2.2 indicates deficiency	Vitamin E level in the blood is directly correlated with the blood triglyceride level. Therefore, to accurately measure vitamin E status, ratio of vitamin E : total lipids is used
Plasma alpha-tocopherol	Levels < 10 μmol/l generally indicate deficiency	Normally, > 90% of total vitamin E is alpha-tocopherol
Vitamin K		
Plasma vitamin K	Normal levels are 0.4–5.0 nmol/l	
Prothrombin time and/or clotting factors (X, IX, VII, and protein C)	Normal prothrombin time is 11–14 sec. Normal values for clotting factors are 100% or 1.0 unit/ml	Because of the central role of vitamin K in blood coagulation, status is measured by indexes of blood clotting. Deficiency results in prolongation of the prothrombin time and reduced function of vitamin K-dependent clotting factors
Vitamin C		
Plasma ascorbate	Levels < 23 μmol/l indicate deficiency	
Leukocyte ascorbate	Levels < 114 nmol/ 10^8 cells (buffy coat) indicate deficiency	

Micronutrient	Values	Comments
Urinary ascorbate	Excretion of <10 mg/d indicates severe deficiency	Insensitive index of status except in severe deficiency
Ascorbate loading test	Urinary ascorbate is measured after an oral dose of 0.5–2.0 g over 4 days; excretion of < 60% of dose indicates tissue ascorbate depletion.	
Thiamin (vitamin B1) Whole blood thiamin	Levels < 70 nmol/l indicate deficiency	
Measurement of the activity of red blood transketolase (ETKA) and its stimulation after addition of thiamin pyrophosphatase (TTP)	Deficiency is indicated by low ETKA(< 5 U/mmol hemoglobin) and > 16% increase after addition of TTP	
Riboflavin (vitamin B2) Erythrocyte riboflavin	Levels below 15 µg/dl cells indicate deficiency	Not a sensitive index
Urinary riboflavin	Excretion <100 µg/d indicates deficiency	
Erythrocyte glutathione reductase (a riboflavin-dependent enzyme) and its stimulation by addition of flavin adenine dinucleotide (FAD)	Expressed as an activity ratio: > 1.2 indicates deficiency	A reliable indicator of status
Niacin (vitamin B3) Urinary 1-N-methyl-nicotinamide (NMN) and 2-N-pyridone (2-N-P)	Deficiency is indicated by excretion of < 0.8 mg NMN/d and/or < 1.0 mg 2-N-P/d	Excretion of these major niacin metabolites are good indexes of niacin status
Erythrocyte nicotinamide adenine nucleotide (NAD)	A ratio of NAD to nicotinamide nucleotide phosphate (NADP) < 1.0 may indicate deficiency	Sensitive indicator of status
Vitamin B6 Plasma pyridoxal-5-phosphate (PLP)	Levels <30 nmol/l indicate deficiency	Active form of vitamin B6
Plasma total vitamin B6	Levels < 40 nmol/l indicate deficiency	
Urinary excretion of 4-pyridoxic acid	Levels < 3.0 µmol/d indicate deficiency	Major urinary metabolite
Erythrocyte alanine transaminase index	Ratio > 1.25 indicates deficiency	Activity of this PLP-dependent enzyme is measured before and after addition of PLP
Tryptophan load test	Urinary xanthenuric acid (XA) excretion > 65 µmol/l indicates deficiency	Because tryptophan catabolism is PLP dependent, a 2-g oral tryptophan load is given and XA measured
Folic acid Serum folate	Normal levels are 4.5–30 nmol/l	Reflects recent dietary intake

Micronutrient	Values	Comments
Red blood cell folate	Levels < 312 nmol/l indicate deficiency	Reflects body folate stores
Hypersegmentation index of the nuclei of neutrophils	Ratio of neutrophils with ≥ 5 lobes to those with ≤ 4 lobes; values > 30% indicate deficiency	Can also result from vitamin B12 deficiency and is not reliable during pregnancy
Vitamin B12 Serum vitamin B12	Levels < 150 pmol/l indicate clear deficiency	Levels may remain normal even when anemia or neurologic symptoms due to vitamin B12 deficiency are present
Urinary methylmalonic acid	Levels > 5 µg/mg creatinine indicate deficiency	Sensitive index of status
Hypersegmentation index of the nuclei of neutrophils	Ratio of neutrophils with ≥ 5 lobes to those with ≤ 4 lobes; values > 30% indicate deficiency	Can also result from vitamin B12 deficiency and is not reliable during pregnancy
Pantothenic acid Whole blood pantothenic acid	Levels < 1.6 µmol/l indicate deficiency	
Urinary pantothenic acid	Reliable indicator; excretion of < 1 mg/d indicates deficiency	
Biotin Plasma biotin	Levels < 1.02 nmol/l indicate deficiency	Literature values are variable and inconsistent
Urinary biotin	Normal levels are 35 ± 14 nmol/d	
Minerals and trace elements: *Calcium* Serum calcium	Normal levels are 2.2–2.6 mmol/l	Poor indicator of status, as < 1% of body calcium is in serum and serum level is under tight physiologic control
Ionized (unbound) serum calcium	Normal levels are 1.17–1.29 mmol/l	Low levels may indicate negative calcium balance
Urinary calcium	Normal levels are approximately 200–300 mg/d for men, 150–250 mg/d for women	
Magnesium Serum magnesium	Normal levels are 0.75–1.05 mmol/l	Insensitive index of body stores, as levels fall only if deficiency is advanced
Serum ionized magnesium	Normal levels are 0.5–0.66 mmol/l	Superior to serum levels because the portion of blood magnesium that is ionized is not affected by conditions that alter serum proteins
Leukocyte magnesium	Normal levels are 3.0–4.0 ± 0.09 fmol/cell	Levels may reflect tissue levels
Urinary magnesium	Excretion of <1 mmol/d indicates deficiency	A sensitive measure of status
Sodium Serum sodium	Normal levels are 135–145 mEq/l	

Micronutrient	Values	Comments
Urinary sodium	Normal levels are 130–260 mEq/d	Level varies with dietary intake
Potassium		
Serum potassium	Normal levels are 3.5–5.1 mmol/l	
Erythrocyte potassium level	Normal levels are approximately 100 mmol/l red blood cells	An index of tissue potassium stores
Urinary potassium	Normal levels are 26–123 mmol/d	Level varies with dietary intake
Zinc		
Serum zinc	Levels < 10.7 µmol/l indicate deficiency; levels 10.7–13.0 µmol/l indicate marginal status	Levels are decreased in moderate to severe deficiency. Infection and/or stress may shift zinc from plasma to liver and decrease plasma levels without affecting body stores
Zinc tolerance test	A 2–3 fold increase in plasma zinc indicates zinc deficiency	After a baseline plasma zinc measurement, an oral load of 50 mg elemental zinc is given. 120 min later plasma zinc is remeasured
Copper		
Erythrocyte Cu/Zn superoxide dismutase	Normal values are 0.47 ± 0.067 mg/g Hb	Levels are a good index of copper status
Serum copper	Levels < 12 µmol/l indicate deficiency	Can be used to detect copper deficiency, but serum copper levels are elevated by a variety of conditions and can vary independent of body copper
Plasma ceruloplasmin	Normal levels are 0.1–0.5 g/l	> 90 % of blood copper is bound to ceruloplasmin. Although ceruloplasmin levels can be used to detect copper deficiency, ceruloplasmin is an acute-phase protein. Therefore, ceruloplasmin is elevated by a variety of conditions and can vary independent of body copper
Urinary copper	Normal levels are 0.47–0.94 µmol/d	
Iron		
Serum iron	Normal levels are 9–29 µmol/l	Serum levels are an insensitive indicator of status, falling only after iron stores are completely exhausted
Serum ferritin	Normal levels are 12–200 µg/l	Good indicator of body stores
Iron saturation of transferrin	Saturation of < 16 % of available binding sites indicates iron deficiency	
Serum transferrin receptor	> 8 mg/l indicates deficiency	Indicates body stores independent of inflammation or infection
Measurement of iron in bone marrow by biopsy	Absence of stainable iron indicates severe deficiency	Accurately measures body stores
Manganese		
Whole blood manganese	Normal levels are 72–255 nmol/l	
Urinary manganese	Normal levels are 10.6 ± 1.9 nmol/d; > 180 nmol/l indicates toxicity	

Micronutrient	Values	Comments
Molybdenum Serum molybdenum	Normal values are 6.0–8.3 ± 2.1 nmol/l	
Chromium Serum chromium	Levels < 2.0 nmol/l may indicate deficiency	A relatively insensitive indicator of tissue stores
Whole blood chromium	Normal range is 14–185 nmol/l	
Urinary chromium	Normal range is approximately 3–4 nmol/l; > 38 nmol indicates toxicity	Of limited value in assessing chromium status due to the very low concentrations and the fact that they often do not respond to chromium supplementation. However, they can be used to measure overexposure to chromium
Iodine Urinary iodine	Excretion <0.78 µmol/d indicates deficiency	Reliable indicator of status
Serum total thyroxine (T$_4$)	Normal range 68–182 nmol/l	Severe iodine deficiency may cause hypothyroidism
Serum thyroid-stimulating hormone (TSH)	Values > 4.0 mU/l may indicate iodine deficiency or another cause of thyroid impairment	Iodine deficiency will increase serum TSH level
Selenium Blood glutathione peroxidase	Activity < 30 E/g hemoglobin indicates deficiency	Sensitive index of status
Serum selenium	Normal range is 0.9–1.9 µmol/l	Index of short-term dietary intake
Flouride Whole blood fluoride	Normal levels are 0.1–0.25 mg/l	
Plasma fluoride	Normal levels are 4–14 µg/l	
Urinary fluoride	Normal levels are 0.3–1.5 mg/d	
Toxic metals: *Aluminum* Hair aluminum	Normal levels are 3–40 µg/g	Hair analysis is a reliable measure of tissue levels
Cadmium Hair cadmium levels	Levels > 1.6 µg/g hair may indicate elevated tissue levels	Hair analysis is a reliable measure of tissue levels and is superior to blood levels as an index of long-term exposure
Lead Blood lead	Levels > 200 µg/l indicate elevated tissue levels and toxicity	Blood levels are a relatively insensitive index of chronic exposure because most body lead is deposited in the skeleton
Hair lead	Levels > 15 µg/g may indicate elevated tissue levels	Hair analysis is a reliable measure of tissue levels

Micronutrient	Values	Comments
Erythrocyte zinc protoporphyrin	Levels > 40 µmol/mol heme may indicate elevated tissue levels	Lead interferes with normal synthesis of hemoglobin. Elevated levels may also be caused by iron deficiency.
Mercury Urinary mercury	Levels > 1.5 µg/d indicate elevated tissue levels	Urinary excretion is a good index of total body burden
Hair mercury	Levels > 3.0 µg/g may indicate elevated tissue levels	Hair analysis is a reliable measure of tissue levels
Essential fatty acids: *Polyunsaturated fatty acids of the n-6 series* Triene (20:3 n-9) to tetraene (20:4 n-6) ratio in blood	Ratio > 0.4 indicates deficiency	Sensitive indicator of deficiency
Polyunsaturated fatty acids of the n-3 series Measurement of n-3 fatty acids in erythrocyte membranes	Low levels (reference ranges vary between laboratories) indicate deficiency	Sensitive indicator of deficiency

References

Brody T. Nutritional Biochemistry. San Diego: Academic Press; 1994.

Fidanza F, ed. Nutritional Status Assessment. London: Chapman & Hall; 1991.

Ziegler EE, Filer LJ, eds. Present Knowledge in Nutrition. Washington, DC: ILSI Press; 1996.

Friedrich W. Vitamins. Berlin: de Gruyter; 1988.

Shils ME, Olson JA, Shike M, eds. Modern Nutrition in Health and Disease. Philadelphia: Lea & Febiger; 1994.

Mertz W. Chromium in human nutrition: A review. J Nutr. 1993;123:626.

Werbach MR. Foundations of Nutritional Medicine. Tarzana, CA: Third Line Press; 1997.

World Health Organization. Trace Elements in Human Nutrition and Health. Geneva: WHO; 1996.

Mertz W, et al. (eds.) Risk Assessment of Essential Trace Elements. Washington DC: ILSI Press; 1994.

Index

Page numbers in **bold type** denote major references